Mixed and Augmented Reality in Medicine

T0253444

Series in Medical Physics and Biomedical Engineering

Series Editors: John G. Webster, E. Russell Ritenour, Slavik Tabakov, and Kwan Hoong Ng

For more information about this series, please visit: https://www.crcpress.com/Series-in-Medical-Physics-and-Biomedical-Engineering/book-series/CHMEPHBIOENG

Mixed and Augmented Reality in Medicine

Edited by

Terry M. Peters
Robarts Research Institute, Western University, Canada

Cristian A. Linte
Department of Biomedical Engineering and
Chester F Carlson Center for Imaging Science
Rochester Institute of Technology, USA

Ziv Yaniv
Office of High Performance Computing and
Communications, National Library of Medicine
National Institutes of Health, and TAJ Technologies Inc, USA

Jacqueline Williams
Robarts Research Institute, Western University, Canada

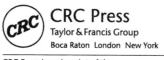

CRC Press
Taylor & Francis Group
Boca Raton London New York

CRC Press is an imprint of the
Taylor & Francis Group, an **informa** business

CRC Press
Taylor & Francis Group
6000 Broken Sound Parkway NW, Suite 300
Boca Raton, FL 33487-2742

First issued in paperback 2020

© 2019 by Taylor & Francis Group, LLC
CRC Press is an imprint of Taylor & Francis Group, an Informa business

No claim to original U.S. Government works

ISBN 13: 978-0-367-57076-7 (pbk)
ISBN 13: 978-1-138-06863-6 (hbk)

Visit the Taylor & Francis Web site at
http://www.taylorandfrancis.com

and the CRC Press Web site at
http://www.crcpress.com

About the Series

The Series in Medical Physics and Biomedical Engineering describes the applications of physical sciences, engineering, and mathematics in medicine and clinical research.

The series seeks (but is not restricted to) publications in the following topics:

- Artificial organs
- Assistive technology
- Bioinformatics
- Bioinstrumentation
- Biomaterials
- Biomechanics
- Biomedical engineering
- Clinical engineering
- Imaging
- Implants
- Medical computing and mathematics
- Medical/surgical devices
- Patient monitoring
- Physiological measurement
- Prosthetics
- Radiation protection, health physics, and dosimetry
- Regulatory issues
- Rehabilitation engineering
- Sports medicine
- Systems physiology
- Telemedicine
- Tissue engineering
- Treatment

The Series in Medical Physics and Biomedical Engineering is an international series that meets the need for up-to-date texts in this rapidly developing field. Books in the series range in level from introductory graduate textbooks and practical handbooks to more advanced expositions of current research. The Series in Medical Physics and Biomedical Engineering is the official book series of the International Organization for Medical Physics.

THE INTERNATIONAL ORGANIZATION FOR MEDICAL PHYSICS

The International Organization for Medical Physics (IOMP) represents over 18,000 medical physicists worldwide and has a membership of 80 national and 6 regional organizations, together with a number of corporate members. Individual medical physicists of all national member organisations are also automatically members.

The mission of IOMP is to advance medical physics practice worldwide by disseminating scientific and technical information, fostering the educational and professional development of medical physics, and promoting the highest quality medical physics services for patients.

A World Congress on Medical Physics and Biomedical Engineering is held every three years in cooperation with International Federation for Medical and Biological Engineering (IFMBE) and International Union for Physics and Engineering Sciences in Medicine (IUPESM). A regionally based international conference, the International Congress of Medical Physics (ICMP) is held between world congresses. IOMP also sponsors international conferences, workshops, and courses.

The IOMP has several programmes to assist medical physicists in developing countries. The joint IOMP Library Programme supports 75 active libraries in 43 developing countries, and the Used Equipment Programme coordinates equipment donations. The Travel Assistance Programme provides a limited number of grants to enable physicists to attend the world congresses.

IOMP co-sponsors the *Journal of Applied Clinical Medical Physics*. The IOMP publishes, twice a year, an electronic bulletin, *Medical Physics World*. IOMP also publishes e-Zine, an electronic news letter about six times a year. IOMP has an agreement with Taylor & Francis for the publication of the Medical Physics and Biomedical Engineering series of textbooks. IOMP members receive a discount.

IOMP collaborates with international organizations, such as the World Health Organizations (WHO), the International Atomic Energy Agency (IAEA), and other international professional bodies such as the International Radiation Protection Association (IRPA) and the International Commission on Radiological Protection (ICRP), to promote the development of medical physics and the safe use of radiation and medical devices.

Guidance on education, training, and professional development of medical physicists is issued by IOMP, which is collaborating with other professional organizations in development of a professional certification system for medical physicists that can be implemented on a global basis.

The IOMP website (www.iomp.org) contains information on all the activities of the IOMP, policy statements 1 and 2, and the 'IOMP: Review and Way Forward,' which outlines all the activities of IOMP and plans for the future.

Contents

Preface

The origins of this book date back to the MICCAI Workshop on Augmented Environments for Computer-assisted Interventions (AE-CAI) held October 2015 in Munich, Germany. The AE-CAI workshop, which this year (2018) celebrates its 12th edition, continues to serve as a leading platform for dissemination of cutting-edge work in augmented, virtual, and mixed reality visualization for image-guided interventions, simulation, and training.

After being approached by Taylor & Francis to consider editing a book on the topic of the workshop, we discussed the idea and agreed that such a collection would fit an under-represented sector in the literature. It also would serve as a timely, ten-year update and augmentation of the 2008 publication, *Image-guided Interventions: Technology and Applications*, edited by Peters and Cleary. However, to do a new book justice, it would need to be focused more specifically on mixed reality in the context of interventions, simulation, and training. During the 2015 edition of AE-CAI in Munich, we received overwhelming enthusiasm from authors, presenters, and attendees to contribute to this book.

Jacqueline Williams generously agreed to take on the role of Executive Editor, and during the past 18 months, we received contributions from the authors represented in the 18 chapters in this book. The title, *Mixed and Augmented Reality in Medicine* was selected to represent the widest range of visualization environments across the reality-virtuality continuum, ranging from purely real to purely virtual. Although all such environments fall under mixed reality, depending on the extent of their real to virtual content, augmented reality has evolved as the widely agreed upon terminology to describe even mixed realities.

This book overviews a variety of mixed reality environments and their application in medicine. It begins with a historical overview chapter on medical augmented realities. Subsequent chapters focus on the fundamental technologies for building augmented reality environments, including surgical tracking, registration, display technologies, and haptics. Additional chapters focus on applications in education and training, visualization for medical education and rehabilitation, cost-effective simulations, augmented reality visualization for an ultrasound and ultrasound-enhanced laparoscopic applications, X-ray guided procedures, minimally invasive cardiac diagnosis and therapy, surgical navigation and intervention, as well as augmented haptic perception in surgery. Finally, the collection would be incomplete without discussing perceptual capacities and constraints, interaction paradigms and cognitive-oriented design, and assessment of medical augmented realities. These topics are covered in three chapters dedicated to perception and cognition in augmented reality.

We sincerely thank our colleagues for joining us in this endeavor to make this book happen and for their patience and continued support and commitment despite incessant demands during this long process.

Terry M. Peters
London, ON, Canada

Cristian A. Linte
Rochester, NY, USA

Ziv Yaniv
Bethesda, MD, USA

Jacqueline Williams
London, ON, Canada

Editors

Terry M. Peters is a scientist in the Imaging Research Laboratories at the Robarts Research Institute (RRI), and Professor in the Departments of Medical Imaging and Medical Biophysics at Western University London, Canada. He is also the Director of the Biomedical Imaging Research Centre at Western, and Associate Director (Graduate Studies) of the School of Biomedical Engineering.

Cristian A. Linte is a faculty member in the Department of Biomedical Engineering and Chester F. Carlson Center for Imaging Science at Rochester Institute of Technology. His research has focused on intelligent solutions for computer-assisted diagnosis, therapy planning, and guidance for which augmented and mixed reality environments have been a key component for effective display and interaction with multimodality imaging data.

Ziv Yaniv is a senior computer scientist in the Office of High Performance Computing and Communications at the National Library of Medicine, U.S. National Institutes of Health, and at TAJ Technologies, Inc. His main areas of research are image-guided interventions, biomedical image analysis, and software engineering. He believes in the curative power of open research, and this past decade has been involved in the development of free open source software for image-guided interventions and biomedical image analysis.

Jacqueline Williams is the Executive Director of the Biomedical Imaging Research Centre at Western University, and previously was the Manager of the CIHR Vascular Training Program at Western. An experienced scientific editor, she also has been involved in writing and managing large imaging grants, and, for the past 15 years, she has served as Recording Secretary for the MICCAI Board.

Contributors

Seyed Farokh Atashzar
Canadian Surgical Technologies and
    Advanced Robotics (CSTAR)
and
Department of Electrical and Computer
    Engineering
Western University
London, Ontario, Canada

Elvis C. S. Chen
Robarts Research Institute
Western University
London, Ontario, Canada

D. L. Collins
McConnell Brain Imaging Centre
Montreal Neurological Institute
McGill University
Montreal, Quebec, Canada

Håvard Dalen
Department of Circulation and Medical
    Imaging
Norwegian University of Science and
    Technology
Trondheim, Norway

Simon Drouin
McConnell Brain Imaging Centre
Montreal Neurological Institute
McGill University
Montreal, Quebec, Canada

Roy Eagleson
Department of Electrical and Computer
    Engineering
Western University
London, Ontario, Canada

Ulrich Eck
Lehrstuhl fuer Informatikanwendungen
    in der Medizin
Technische Universität München
Munich, Germany

Pascal Fallavollita
Interdisciplinary School of Health
    Sciences
Faculty of Health Science
University of Ottawa
Ottawa, Ontario, Canada

Zhencheng Fan
Department of Biomedical Engineering
School of Medicine
Tsinghua University
Beijing, China

Ren Hui Gong
School of Computing
Queen's University
Kingston, Ontario, Canada

Özgür Güler
eKare Inc.
Fairfax, Virginia

Bjørn Olav Haugen
Department of Circulation and Medical
    Imaging
Norwegian University of Science and
    Technology
Trondheim, Norway

Pierre Jannin
MediCIS Group
Faculty of Medicine
University of Rennes 1
Rennes, France

Uditha L. Jayarathne
Northern Digital Inc.
Waterloo, Ontario, Canada

M. Kersten-Oertel
McConnell Brain Imaging Centre
Montreal Neurological Institute
McGill University
Montreal, Quebec, Canada

Gabriel Hanssen Kiss
Operating Room of the Future
St. Olavs University Hospital
and
Department of Circulation and Medical
    Imaging
Norwegian University of Science and
    Technology
Trondheim, Norway

Roberta L. Klatzky
Department of Psychology
Carnegie Mellon University
Pittsburgh, Pennsylvania

Randy Lee
Department of Bioengineering
University of Pittsburgh
Pittsburgh, Pennsylvania

Hongen Liao
Department of Biomedical Engineering
School of Medicine
Tsinghua University
Beijing, China

Cristian A. Linte
Biomedical Engineering and Center for
    Imaging Science
Rochester Institute of Technology
Rochester, New York

Wen Pei Liu
Intuitive Surgical
Sunnyvale, California

Xinyang Liu
Sheikh Zayed Institute
Children's National Health System
Washington, DC

Burton Ma
Department of Electrical Engineering
    and Computer Science
York University
Toronto, Ontario, Canada

Cong Ma
Department of Biomedical
    Engineering
School of Medicine
Tsinghua University
Beijing, China

Lena Maier-Hein
Division of Computer Assisted Medical
    Interventions (CAMI)
German Cancer Research Center
    (DKFZ)
Heidelberg, Germany

Ole Christian Mjølstad
Department of Circulation and Medical
    Imaging
Norwegian University of Science and
    Technology
Trondheim, Norway

Thierry Morineau
Centre de Recherches en
    Psychologie, Cognition,
    Communication
Universit e de Bretagne-Sud
Vannes, France

Michael Naish
Canadian Surgical Technologies and
    Advanced Robotics (CSTAR)
and
Department of Mechanical and
    Materials Engineering
Western University
London, Ontario, Canada

Nassir Navab
Computer Aided Medical Procedures
Fakultät für Informatik
Technische Universität München
Munich, Germany
and
Computer Aided Medical Procedures
Department of Computer Science
Johns Hopkins University
Baltimore, Maryland

Nicolas Padoy
Research Group CAMMA
University of Strasbourg
Strasbourg, France

Cameron Lowell Palmer
Department of Circulation and Medical
    Imaging
Norwegian University of Science and
    Technology
Trondheim, Norway

Rajni V. Patel
Canadian Surgical Technologies and
    Advanced Robotics (CSTAR)
Department of Electrical and Computer
    Engineering
Department of Surgery
Western University
London, Ontario, Canada

Terry M. Peters
Robarts Research Institute and School
    of Biomedical Engineering
Western University
London, Ontario, Canada

Sandrine de Ribaupierre
Clinical Neurological Sciences
Western University
London, Ontario, Canada

Nicolas Loy Rodas
ICube Laboratory
Centre National de la Recherche
    Scientifique
IHU Strasbourg
University of Strasbourg
Strasbourg, France

Michael S. Sacks
Institute for Cardiovascular Engineering
    and Sciences
University of Texas
Austin, Texas

Raj Shekhar
George Washington School of Medicine
    & Health Sciences
Children's National Health System
Washington, District of Columbia

Tobias Sielhorst
Lehrstuhl fuer Informatikanwendungen
    in der Medizin
Technische Universität München
Munich, Germany

Stefanie Speidel
Division of Translational Surgical
    Oncology (TSO)
National Center for Tumor Diseases
    (NCT)
Dresden, Germany

Esther Stenau
Division of Computer Assisted Medical
    Interventions (CAMI)
German Cancer Research Center
    (DKFZ)
Heidelberg, Germany

George D. Stetten
Department of Bioengineering
University of Pittsburgh
and
Robotics Institute
Carnegie Mellon University
Pittsburgh, Pennsylvania

Russell H. Taylor
Department of Computer Science
Johns Hopkins University
Baltimore, Maryland

Hans Torp
Department of Circulation and Medical
    Imaging
Norwegian University of Science and
    Technology
Trondheim, Norway

Ziv Yaniv
Office of High Performance Computing
    and Communications
National Library of Medicine
U.S. National Institutes of Health
Bethesda, Maryland
and
TAJ Technologies, Inc.
Bethesda Maryland

Xinran Zhang
Department of Biomedical Engineering
School of Medicine
Tsinghua University
Beijing, China

1 Overview of Mixed and Augmented Reality in Medicine

Terry M. Peters

CONTENTS

1.1 DEFINITIONS

From the outset, let us define what we mean by "augmented and mixed reality" (as well as "virtual reality," for that matter). The most concise definition, and one that has endured for several decades, is contained in the taxonomy introduced by Milgram and Kishino (1994), through which they established a "reality-virtuality continuum" between the real and virtual worlds (Figure 1.1). Milgram described an "augmented reality" (AR) as virtual images fused with the real world and "augmented virtuality" (AV) as a largely virtual (computer-generated) world augmented by additional components that represent the "real" world. Together, AR and AV form the "reality-virtuality continuum," which is spanned by "mixed reality" (MR). In practice, however, we encounter examples at multiple points on this spectrum, and common usage has gravitated towards (perhaps somewhat loosely) using the term "augmented reality" to describe any technique that combines artificially generated information with information from the physical world, be it visual, tactile, or auditory, while the term "virtual reality" refers to an entirely "virtual" environment with no "real" components. In accordance with common usage, the term "augmented reality" is employed in this book sometimes according to Milgram's strict definition and sometimes to encompass the more general term of "mixed reality."

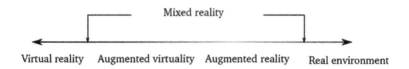

FIGURE 1.1   The reality-virtuality continuum. (Adapted from Milgram, P. and Kishino F., *IEICE Trans Inform Sys.*, 77, 1321–1329, 1994.)

1.2   WHY USE AR?

The use of AR in medicine clearly has been driven by the ever-increasing power of computational resources that have made it possible to not only fuse images in real time but also to perform computational simulations for increasingly complex models. Its use has manifested in two distinct domains: simulation and intervention. AR is employed to add information to a visualized scene, most commonly to integrate images from some medical image modality with the patient—much like the science fiction concept of "x-ray vision"—to see organs and surgical targets inside the human body. Registering a simple x-ray projection with the patient, while helpful, is not optimal, and today's imaging modalities allow so much more functionality, as cross-sectional, three-dimensional (3D), and dynamic imaging modalities are available. Within this context, we also consider the fusion of two to three imaging modalities, such as ultrasound (US) and video, US and CT, or even US, CT, and video as examples of AR. In this example, the "real" scene may not exist but is represented by a surrogate image (video, for example) that represents the real world. AR may also be used to provide expert annotation on images, in much the same manner that consumer AR applications can label buildings or items of interest in a digital image of a scene.

1.3   BEGINNINGS

The examples given below are far from exhaustive but represent the author's view of the significant events that influenced his own research in the area. One of the earliest demonstrations of the value of AR in a surgical procedure was that outlined by Bajura et al. (1992), who demonstrated the methodology for fusing a US image with a patient using a head-mounted display (HMD). Shortly thereafter, the same researchers demonstrated the use of AR visualization during laparoscopic surgery, as reported in their MICCAI paper (Fuchs et al. 1998), which demonstrated that accurate calibration and tracking could achieve robust registration of the virtual scene (the surgical target) with the real-world environment. They explored the use of a custom-built video pass through an HMD device, which was a structured light projector combined with a laparoscope that enabled the capture of both depth and color data, and a "keyhole" display method that unambiguously placed the virtual image in the appropriate context of the real world. Their HMD preceded similar devices that have rapidly become commodity items in the gaming world in the past 30 years. Around the same time, Pisano et al. (1998), also affiliated with Fuchs's laboratory, demonstrated the use of AR applied to US-guided breast cyst aspiration, wherein the operator also employed an HMD that displayed a US image *in situ* using the same keyhole approach described above to visualize the breast lesion (Figure 1.2).

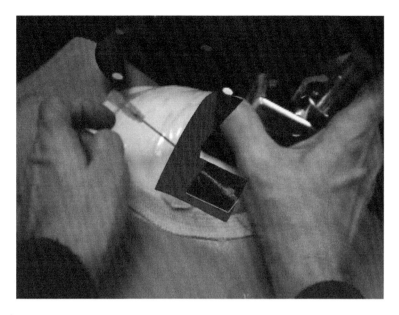

FIGURE 1.2   Pisano and Fuchs's pioneer demonstration of an AR application integrating a US image with the real world for a breast biopsy. (Courtesy of UNC Chapel Hill Department of Computer Science, Chapel Hill, NC.)

Shortly after this, Rosenthal et al. (2002) employed a similar US/AR setup and reported the results of a randomized, controlled trial that compared the accuracy of standard US-guided needle biopsies to that obtained using a 3D AR guidance system. Fifty core biopsies of breast phantoms were randomly assigned to one of the methods, the raw ultrasound data from each biopsy was recorded, and the distance of the biopsy from the ideal position was measured. These results demonstrated that the HMD used to provide an AR display led to a statistically significant smaller mean deviation from the desired target than did the standard display method. This was one of the first studies to suggest that AR systems can offer improved accuracy over traditional biopsy guidance methods.

An adaptation of this approach was developed by Stetten et al. (2001, 2002). In their system, the US image was viewed directly *in situ* without the need for additional visual aids. Rather, the image was viewed simply by reflecting the image, which was displayed on a small screen attached to the US probe, via a half-silvered mirror, so that the image appeared to be located in the same space as the actual US image. Ever since, this "Sonic Flashlight" approach has been the topic of multiple publications (Stetten et al. 2005; Shelton et al. 2007).

The concept of using a half-silvered mirror was also exploited by Fichtinger et al. (2005) and Baum et al. (2016, 2017) (Figure 1.3) to overlay, in the correct plane, a CT image with the direct view of the patient in a CT scanner to guide a needle to a target in the spine. In both the Stetten and Fichtinger cases, there are 2D images displayed on a monitor, whose reflections via a half-silvered mirror are arranged to coincide with the anatomical plane being imaged. Thus, the virtual (reflected) images are locked in

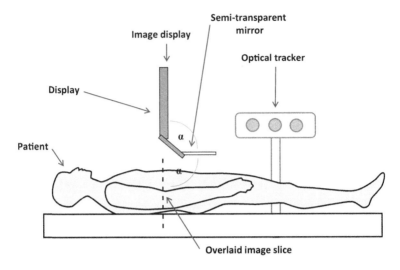

FIGURE 1.3 Schematic of the reflection technique used in both the "Sonic Flashlight" of Stetten and the CT-based AR system of Fichtinger. In both cases, an image generated by a tomographic imaging modality is displayed on the monitor and reflected to the appropriate plane within the patient via the half-silvered mirror. Liao's "Integral Videography" (IV) approach employs a similar configuration, except that the 2D image is replaced by an IV display that consists of an array of hemispherical lenses matched to a high-resolution screen. This combination is able to produce a true 3D virtual image that is reflected onto the appropriate region of the patient. (Courtesy of Dr. G. Fichtinger, Queen's University, Kingston, Canada.)

space relative to the coordinate systems of the US probe or the CT scanner and can be observed by multiple viewers via the half-silvered mirrors, without the need for special eye ware. In Stetten's US device, the imaged planes are shifted in 3D space by moving the US transducer. In the CT-based approach employed by Fichtinger, the imaged planes are shifted by moving the mirror-monitor frame while simultaneously updating the displayed image slice. Several researchers have since evaluated this approach in multiple scenarios (e.g., Fritz et al. 2012; Marker et al. 2017).

An elegant system that was tested in a neurosurgical operating room (OR) was presented by Edwards et al. (1999). They demonstrated a system that allowed surgeons to view objects extracted from preoperative radiological images by accurately registering and overlaying 3D stereoscopic images in the optical path of a surgical microscope. The objective of this system was to provide the surgeon with a view of structures, in the correct 3D positions, beneath the brain surface, which would normally be viewed through a microscope (Figure 1.4). In this case, patient registration to preoperative images was achieved using bone-implanted markers, and a dental splint equipped with optical tracking markers was used for patient tracking. The microscope also was tracked optically. An added feature (and complication) of their system was that the focus and zoom of the microscope optics had to be modeled. The accuracy of their system was in the order of 1 mm. However, there are several psychophysical issues with the system; for example, just because the virtual image is in

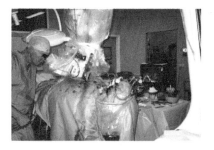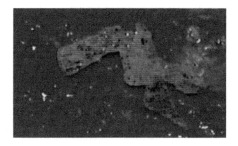

FIGURE 1.4 Edwards's implementation of AR in a neurosurgery microscope as embodied in the "microscope-assisted guided interventions" (MAGI) system. Left: Surgeon using MAGI-equipped OR microscope; Right: Fused image of neuroma as seen through the microscope. (Courtesy of Dr. P. J. "Eddie" Edwards.)

the correct place geometrically, this does not guarantee that the human visual system perceives it to be in this position (see Section 1.4 Psychophysical Issues).

Motivated by Edwards's earlier work, Cheung et al. (2010) evaluated the role of AR for the resection of kidney tumors under US and laparoscopic guidance. To overcome the cognitive workload difficulties associated with the lack of cohesion between the endoscopic and US images that were displayed on separate screens, the researchers fused the US and laparoscopic images such that the latter was positioned spatially in its correct position and orientation. The goal of this work was to allow the surgeon to more accurately locate the tumor, establish safety margins, and, because speed is essential for patient safety during the procedure, resect the tumor more rapidly. Their intuitive visualization platform, which required the surgeon to observe a single fused image, was used to assess surgeon performance using both the standard of care approach as well as the AR system. Using a phantom study that mimicked the tumor resection of a partial nephrectomy, they achieved a registration error of around 2.5 mm. While faster planning time for the resection was achieved using their fusion visualization system, benefits in terms of the overall speed of the speed of the procedure were not obvious in this limited study. However, a real benefit was the more accurate specification of tumor resection margins.

One research group that has arguably had more impact than any other on AR in medicine, particularly with respect to image-guided interventions, has been that of Nassir Navab at the Technical University of Munich. Beginning in 2006, this group published multiple seminal papers discussing perceptual issues in AR (Sielhorst et al. 2006); the development of AR-based platforms for orthopedic surgery (Traub et al. 2006); the fusion of ultrasound and gamma/beta images for cancer detection, (Wendler et al. 2006, 2007); the development of a "Virtual Mirror" (Bichlmeier et al. 2009) to provide a more intuitive user interface than direct image fusion; and an AR x-ray C-Arm (Navab et al. 2010; Fallavollita et al. 2016) that permits real-time fusion of x-ray and optical images. These applications represent just a sample of the many contributions of this group. A compelling example of their work is shown in Figure 1.5, which demonstrates the effective fusion of a CT image of an ankle with a direct view of the limb.

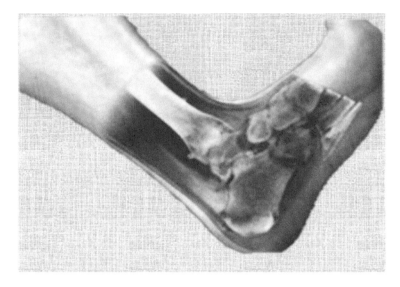

FIGURE 1.5   One of the many examples of compelling AR that has come from the Navab laboratory at the Technical University of Munich. A CT representation of an ankle fused with a real image in a manner that preserves realism. (Courtesy of Dr. Nassir Navab, Technical University of Munich, Munich, Germany.)

In the neurosurgery domain, Wang et al. (2011) developed an AR approach to combine a real environment with virtual models to plan epilepsy surgery. During such procedures, it is important for the surgeon to correlate preoperative cortical morphology (from preoperative images) with the actual surgical field. This team developed an alternate approach to providing enhanced visualization by fusing a direct (photographic) view of the surgical field with the 3D patient model during image-guided epilepsy surgery. To achieve this goal, they correlated the preoperative plan with the intraoperative surgical scene, first by a manual landmark-based registration and then by an intensity-based perspective 3D-2D registration for camera pose estimation. The 2D photographic image was then texture-mapped onto the standard 3D preoperative model created by an image-guidance platform using the calculated camera pose. This approach was validated clinically as part of a neuronavigation system, and the efficacy of this alternative to sophisticated AR environments for assisting in epilepsy surgery was demonstrated. Requiring no specialized display equipment, the approach also requires minimal changes to existing systems and workflow, thus making it well suited to the OR environment.

An additional example was presented by Abhari et al. (2015), who exploited AR systems during neurosurgical planning. Planning surgical interventions is a complex task that demands a high degree of perceptual, cognitive, and sensorimotor skills to reduce intra- and postoperative complications. It also requires a great deal of spatial reasoning to coordinate between the preoperatively acquired medical images and patient reference frames. In the case of neurosurgical interventions, traditional approaches to planning tend to focus on ways to visualize preoperative images but rarely support transformation between different spatial reference frames.

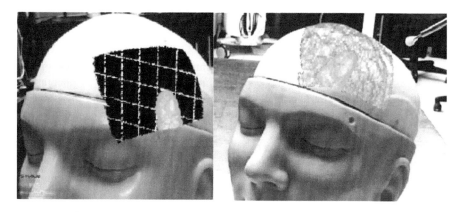

FIGURE 1.6 AR view of a tumor inside the brain, as visualized via a head-mounted video pass-through headset (VusixIinc Rochester NY). Left: Tumor fused on image of cortex. Right: Tumor viewed via a keyhole with gridlines to provide context. (Courtesy of Kamyar Abhari, Robarts Research Institute, London, Canada.)

Consequently, surgeons usually rely on their previous experience and intuition to perform mental transformations. In the case of surgical trainees, this may lead to longer operation times or increased chances of error as a result of additional cognitive demands. To help this situation, Abhari et al. introduced an augmented/virtual (mixed) reality system (Figure 1.6) to facilitate the training of brain tumor resection. Their system was designed and evaluated with human factors explicitly in mind, with the goal of reducing the degree of cognitive overload.

Compared to conventional planning environments, their proposed system greatly improved the novice's performance, independent of the sensorimotor tasks that were undertaken. Furthermore, when clinicians used the system it resulted in a significant reduction in time to perform clinically relevant tasks. This demonstrated that AR and MR systems could assist residents to develop the necessary spatial reasoning skills needed for planning neurosurgical procedures to improve patient outcomes.

Similar work was reported by Kersten-Oertel et al. (2015), who, similar to Wang, developed an AR system that employed an external camera to capture a live view of a patient on an OR table and merged this view with volume-rendered versions of vascularity acquired preoperatively. They demonstrate AR to be useful for tailoring craniotomies, localizing vessels of interest, and planning resection corridors and find that AR is a promising technology for neurovascular surgery planning and guidance. This research group expands on their earlier work in Chapter 7 by focusing on observer interaction with AR environments.

Laparoscopic imaging is a modality for which AR is a natural contender. Given the narrow field of view of the typical endoscope or laparoscope, it makes perfect sense to augment the video image with a model of the organ being examined. This can include an extended surface representation of the organ (to add context to the video image) or a depiction of internal organ structures that are blocked from view in the standard laparoscopic image.

This topic has been addressed extensively by the ICube group at the University of Strasbourg, who have written a number of comprehensive reviews and papers on this topic (Nicolau et al. 2011; Bernhardt et al. 2016). They have addressed many of the technical aspects related to the accurate registration and visualization of preoperative imagery with the laparoscopic view, including image registration, segmentation, calibration, visualization, tracking, and intraoperative imaging, including MRI, CT, and US. Bernhardt et al. (2017) is a particularly valuable document that provides not only the basics of the building blocks of AR in laparoscopy, but also a comprehensive view of the current state of the art.

Often, when hidden critical structures must be observed in the context of the surface laparoscopic image, laparoscopic US is employed using a US probe designed to be introduced into the body cavity and manipulated by either a rigid laparoscopic instrument or a robot. These probes are usually cylindrical in shape and have a linear or a curvilinear array of transducing elements that create a 2D tomographic image. While numerous attempts to provide real-time volumetric imaging using 2D laparoscopic transducer arrays can be found in the literature (Light et al. 2005), very little has appeared since this 2005 publication, and this technology has not made its way to clinical practice. Recent developments by Jayarathne et al. (2017) are now showing promise. For example, by optically tracking the US probe, 3D US images may be reconstructed and displayed unambiguously within the context of the surface images delivered by the laparoscope. Further elaboration of this approach is provided in Chapter 12 of this book.

In 2004, Liao et al. (2004) described an autostereoscopic image overlay technique that could be integrated into a surgical navigation system to superimpose a real, 3D image onto the patient. This approach employed "integral videography" (IV), which is a dynamic extension of integral photography that records multiple views of a scene within a single image placed behind a microconvex lens array. IV can display geometrically accurate 3D autostereoscopic images and reproduce motion parallax without the need for special devices. The researchers used a half-silvered mirror to make the 3D image appear to be inside the patient's body, in a manner similar to that illustrated in Figure 1.3. In this early publication, Liao's team demonstrated that using this dynamic IV rendering technique, virtual and real images can be registered accurately to approximately 1 mm, and initial targeting tasks showed that the system could guide a needle toward a target with an average error of 2.6 mm. Recent developments related to this technology are discussed in Chapter 17.

The value of AR is truly appreciated during interventions in which the surgeon cannot directly visualize the targets to be treated, such as during cardiac procedures performed on the beating heart. Linte et al. (2010a, 2010b) recognized that the displayed virtual environments must accurately represent the real surgical field and require the seamless integration of preoperative and intraoperative imaging, surgical tracking, and visualization technology in a common framework centered on the patient. Their review begins with an overview of minimally invasive cardiac interventions; describes the architecture of a typical surgical guidance platform, including imaging, tracking, registration and visualization; highlights both clinical and engineering accuracy limitations in cardiac image guidance; and discusses the translation of the work from the laboratory into the OR together with typically encountered challenges. This work was subsequently followed up by a description of a system that employed a simple AR platform to facilitate the navigation of an instrument from the apex of the heart to the mitral valve annulus during a procedure to repair the mitral valve itself. Not only did this approach provide a much more intuitive means of performing the procedure, but it also could be executed four times faster than using standard-of-care echo-cardiographic imaging and reduced the potential for intracardiac injury by 95% (Moore et al. 2013).

Luo et al. (2013) described a navigation system for transcatheter aortic valve implantation that employed a magnetic tracking system (MTS) together with a dynamic aortic model and intraoperative US images. This work was motivated by the desire to minimize or eliminate the use of radiation in the interventional suite or OR. The dynamic 3D aortic model was constructed from a preoperative 4D-computed tomography data set whose motion was synchronized with the patient's ECG, and preoperative planning was performed to determine the target position of the aortic valve prosthesis. The contours of the aortic root were extracted automatically in real time from short-axis US images to register the 2D, intraoperative US image to the dynamic, preoperative aortic model. This platform guided the interventionist during the positioning and delivery of the aortic valve prosthesis to the target in a porcine model and demonstrated acceptable deployment error and computation time to render this approach as a viable alternative to the use of fluoroscopy during the procedure. A similar approach, which involved guiding the aortic valve to the target via the apex rather than the femoral vein, was recently described by McLeod et al. (2016).

Minimally invasive valvular intervention commonly requires intraprocedural navigation to provide spatial and temporal information of relevant cardiac structures and device components. Recently, intraprocedural transesophageal echocardiography (TEE) has been exploited for this purpose due to its accessibility, low cost, ease of use, and real-time imaging capability. However, the position and orientation of tissue targets relative to surgical tools can be challenging to perceive, particularly when using 2D imaging planes. Li et al. (2015) proposed the use of CT images to generate a high-quality 3D context to enhance US images using image registration and provide an augmented guidance system with minimal impact on standard clinical workflow. They also described the generation of synthetic 4D CT images via deformable registration to the TEE US image to avoid the excessive radiation required for dynamic CT. Their results show that synthetically generated dynamic CT images are a suitable surrogate for real, dynamic CT images with respect to providing context for the US image. Chapter 16 of this book elaborates on these approaches in more depth.

1.4 PSYCHOPHYSICAL ISSUES

The difficulties experienced when visualizing 3D scenes beneath a solid surface, as highlighted by Edwards et al., were further investigated by Johnson et al. (2003), who critically examined the use of stereoscopic displays to present surgeons with an accurate perception of surgical targets in 3D space. While the researchers noted that stereopsis is a powerful binocular cue that can supplement any monocular information in the scene, they also highlighted several difficulties. They showed that when employing a simple optical AR system that superimposes stereoscopic images onto a physical scene, an accurate sense of depth cannot be easily achieved from the stereoscopic images when the visualized target lies beneath a physical surface. In their AR system, they used stereo images of anatomical structures overlaid on the patient in a simulated surgical guidance scenario. The objective was to position the target stereoscopic image at a location beneath the patient surface to enable accurate localization in 3D space. However, when the stereo images were presented behind the transparent physical surface, they demonstrated that the perception of the depth of the images can become unstable and ambiguous despite appropriate system calibration, registration, and tracking.

Sielhorst et al. (2006) also tackled this problem and observed that even if the virtual data were presented at the appropriate location in space, the observer often would misperceive the spatial position of the visualization because of virtual/real overlay. Their work evaluated novel visualization techniques designed to overcome misleading depth perception of virtual images when combined with a real view. The researchers concluded that techniques that render the surface transparent, or simulate a "keyhole" for viewing the virtual subcutaneous image, outperformed methods that simply fused the images or replaced the original surface with a triangular mesh.

This topic was further elaborated by Lerotic et al. (2007) in the context of integrating AR with minimally invasive robotic surgery. In an attempt to overcome the problems elaborated by Johnston, the researchers presented a new AR method that could be implemented in systems using video pass-through displays (through which the "real" scene is captured by video and merged with the virtual environment). They employed a novel "pq-space"-based, nonphotorealistic rendering technique to provide a see-through vision of the embedded virtual object whilst maintaining salient anatomical details of the exposed anatomical surface. Here "p" and "q" relate to the slope of the surface along the x- and y-axes of the surface, and following application of a "pq filter," surface components normal to the viewing direction are suppressed, while sloping areas are emphasized. The same visual effect can also be achieved by applying a simple, radial 3D high-pass filter to the image of the surface. The key message is that the human visual system responds to the resulting high-frequency components on the surface, thus building a sparse representation of the surface in 3D. The buried virtual object no longer appears to overlay a solid-looking surface, and the correct relative depth perception of the buried object is restored. Experimental results with both phantom and *in vivo* data demonstrated that the visual realism achieved is appropriate for high-fidelity AR depth perception. The take-home message of this work is that one must take extreme care when designing the user interface of AR systems in medicine. The moment the image ceases to be believable or becomes ambiguous, an otherwise robust system may become useless. This topic is further elaborated by Drouin and colleagues in Chapter 7 of this book.

A different potential psychophysical effect of AR in surgery is that of "inattentional blindness," which refers to when the enhanced display technology to render a navigation procedure more accurate produces a corollary impact in the form of distraction from image details. Dixon et al. (2013) demonstrated this phenomenon during a simulated laparoscopic procedure, during which the video image was augmented by fused anatomic contours. Using two groups of subjects (surgeons and trainees) assigned to perform a task under normal and augmented laparoscopic guidance, they found that while AR improved the accuracy and speed of task completion, the AR group was less likely to identify significant, unexpected findings that were clearly within view. This study is one of the first to identify one of the downsides of using AR in a surgical context and provides a valuable warning that the display must be designed to mitigate such inattentional blindness.

1.5 CONCLUSION

This chapter sets the stage for the topics in the remainder of the book. There is clearly an increasing interest in the use of mixed, augmented, and virtual reality approaches to facilitate many areas of medical imaging, from therapy to simulation and training. While much has already been accomplished, there remain numerous challenges to address, including cost, usability, intrusiveness, workflow integration, validation, and comfort. I hope that the remaining chapters shed some light on these issues.

REFERENCES

Abhari, K., J. S. Baxter, E. C. Chen, A. R. Khan, T. M. Peters, S. de Ribaupierre, and R. Eagleson. 2015. Training for planning tumour resection: Augmented reality and human factors. *IEEE Trans Biomed Eng* 62(6):1466–1477. doi:10.1109/TBME.2014.2385874.

Bajura, M., H. Fuchs, and R. Ohbuchi. 1992. Merging virtual objects with the real-world—Seeing ultrasound imagery within the patient. *Siggraph 92: Conference Proceedings* 26:203–210.

Baum, Z., A. Lasso, T. Ungi, and G. Fichtinger. 2016. Real-time self-calibration of a tracked augmented reality display. *Medical Imaging 2016: Image-Guided Procedures, Robotic Interventions, and Modeling* 9786. doi:10.1117/12.2217270.

Baum, Z., T. Ungi, A. Lasso, and G. Fichtinger. 2017. Usability of a real-time tracked augmented reality display system in musculoskeletal injections. *Medical Imaging 2017: Image-Guided Procedures, Robotic Interventions, and Modeling* 10135. doi:10.1117/12.2255897.

Bernhardt, S., S. A. Nicolau, V. Agnus, L. Soler, C. Doignon, and J. Marescaux. 2016. Automatic localization of endoscope in intraoperative CT image: A simple approach to augmented reality guidance in laparoscopic surgery. *Med Image Anal* 30:130–143. doi:10.1016/j.media.2016.01.008.

Bernhardt, S., S. A. Nicolau, L. Soler, and C. Doignon. 2017. The status of augmented reality in laparoscopic surgery as of 2016. *Med Image Anal* 37:66–90. doi:10.1016/j.media.2017.01.007.

Bichlmeier, C., S. M. Heining, M. Feuerstein, and N. Navab. 2009. The virtual mirror: A new interaction paradigm for augmented reality environments. *IEEE Trans Med Imaging* 28(9):1498–1510. doi:10.1109/TMI.2009.2018622.

Cheung, C. L., C. Wedlake, J. Moore, S. E. Pautler, and T. M. Peters. 2010. Fused video and ultrasound images for minimally invasive partial nephrectomy: A phantom study. *Med Image Comput Comput Assist Interv* 13(Pt 3):408–415.

Dixon, B. J., M. J. Daly, H. Chan, A. D. Vescan, I. J. Witterick, and J. C. Irish. 2013. Surgeons blinded by enhanced navigation: The effect of augmented reality on attention. *Surg Endosc* 27(2):454–461. doi:10.1007/s00464-012-2457-3.

Edwards, P. J., A. P. King, D. J. Hawkes, O. Fleig, C. R. Maurer, Jr., D. L. Hill, M. R. Fenlon et al. 1999. Stereo augmented reality in the surgical microscope. *Stud Health Technol Inform* 62:102–128.

Fallavollita, P., A. Brand, L. Wang, E. Euler, P. Thaller, N. Navab, and S. Weidert. 2016. An augmented reality C-arm for intraoperative assessment of the mechanical axis: A preclinical study. *Int J Comput Assist Radiol Surg* 11(11):2111–2117. doi:10.1007/s11548-016-1426-z.

Fichtinger, G., A. Deguet, K. Masamune, E. Balogh, G. S. Fischer, H. Mathieu, R. H. Taylor, S. J. Zinreich, and L. M. Fayad. 2005. Image overlay guidance for needle insertion in CT scanner. *IEEE Trans Biomed Eng* 52(8):1415–1424. doi:10.1109/TBME.2005.851493.

Fritz, J., P. U-Thainual, T. Ungi, A. J. Flammang, N. B. Cho, G. Fichtinger, Iordachita, II, and J. A. Carrino. 2012. Augmented reality visualization with image overlay for MRI-guided intervention: Accuracy for lumbar spinal procedures with a 1.5-T MRI system. *AJR Am J Roentgenol* 198(3):W266–W273. doi:10.2214/AJR.11.6918.

Fuchs, H., M. Livingston, R. Raskar, D. Colluci, K. Ketter, A. State, J. Crawford, P. Rademacher, S. Drake, and A. Meyer. 1998. *Augmented Reality Visualization for Laparoscopic Surgery*. Medical Image Computing and Computer-Assisted Interventions, New York.

Jayarathne, U. L., J. Moore, E. C. S. Chen, S. E. Pautler, T. M. Peters. 2017. *Real-Time 3D Ultrasound Reconstruction and Visualization in the Context of Laparoscopy*. MICCAI, Quebec City, Canada.

Johnson, L. G., P. Edwards, and D. Hawkes. 2003. Surface transparency makes stereo overlays unpredictable: The implications for augmented reality. *Stud Health Technol Inform* 94:131–136.

Kersten-Oertel, M., I. Gerard, S. Drouin, K. Mok, D. Sirhan, D. S. Sinclair, and D. L. Collins. 2015. Augmented reality in neurovascular surgery: Feasibility and first uses in the operating room. *Int J Comput Assist Radiol Surg* 10(11):1823–1836. doi:10.1007/s11548-015-1163-8.

Lerotic, M., A. J. Chung, G. Mylonas, and G. Z. Yang. 2007. Pq-space based non-photorealistic rendering for augmented reality. *Med Image Comput Comput Assist Interv* 10(Pt 2):102–109.

Li, Feng P., M. Rajchl, J. A. White, A. Goela, and T. M. Peters. 2015. Ultrasound guidance for beating heart mitral valve repair augmented by synthetic dynamic CT. *IEEE Trans Med Imaging* 34(10):2025–2035. doi:10.1109/TMI.2015.2412465.

Liao, H., N. Hata, S. Nakajima, M. Iwahara, I. Sakuma, and T. Dohi. 2004. Surgical navigation by autostereoscopic image overlay of integral videography. *IEEE Trans Inf Technol Biomed* 8(2):114–121.

Light, E. D., E. G. Dixon-Tulloch, P. D. Wolf, S. W. Smith, and S. F. Idriss. 2005. Real-time 3D ultrasound laparoscopy. *2005 IEEE Ultrasonics Symposium* 1–4:796–799.

Linte, C. A., J. Moore, C. Wedlake, and T. M. Peters. 2010a. Evaluation of model-enhanced ultrasound-assisted interventional guidance in a cardiac phantom. *IEEE Trans Biomed Eng* 57(9):2209–2218.

Linte, C. A., J. White, R. Eagleson, G. M. Guiraudon, and T. M. Peters. 2010b. Virtual and augmented medical imaging environments: Enabling technology for minimally invasive cardiac interventional guidance. *IEEE Rev Biomed Eng* 3:25–47. doi:10.1109/RBME.2010.2082522.

Luo, Z., J. Cai, T. M. Peters, and L. Gu. 2013. Intra-operative 2-D ultrasound and dynamic 3-D aortic model registration for magnetic navigation of transcatheter aortic valve implantation. *IEEE Trans Med Imaging* 32(11):2152–2165. doi:10.1109/TMI.2013.2275233.

Marker, D. R., P. U-Thainual, T. Ungi, A. J. Flammang, G. Fichtinger, Iordachita, II, J. A. Carrino, and J. Fritz. 2017. 1.5 T augmented reality navigated interventional MRI: Paravertebral sympathetic plexus injections. *Diagn Interv Radiol* 23(3):227–232. doi:10.5152/dir.2017.16323.

McLeod, A. J., M. E. Currie, J. T. Moore, D. Bainbridge, B. B. Kiaii, M. W. A. Chu, and T. M. Peters. 2016. Phantom study of an ultrasound guidance system for transcatheter aortic valve implantation. *Comput Med Imag Grap* 50:24–30. doi:10.1016/j.compmedimag.2014.12.001.

Milgram, P., and F. Kishino. 1994. A taxonomy of mixed reality visual displays. *IEICE Trans Inform Sys* 77(12):1321–1329.

Moore, J. T., M. W. Chu, B. Kiaii, D. Bainbridge, G. Guiraudon, C. Wedlake, M. Currie, M. Rajchl, R. V. Patel, and T. M. Peters. 2013. A navigation platform for guidance of beating heart transapical mitral valve repair. *IEEE Trans Biomed Eng* 60(4):1034–1040. doi:10.1109/TBME.2012.2222405.

Navab, N., S. M. Heining, and J. Traub. 2010. Camera augmented mobile C-arm (CAMC): Calibration, accuracy study, and clinical applications. *IEEE Trans Med Imaging* 29(7):1412–1423. doi:10.1109/TMI.2009.2021947.

Nicolau, S., L. Soler, D. Mutter, and J. Marescaux. 2011. Augmented reality in laparoscopic surgical oncology. *Surg Oncol-Oxford* 20(3):189–201. doi:10.1016/j.suronc.2011.07.002.

Pisano, E. D., H. Fuchs, A. State, M. A. Livingston, G. Hirota, W. F. Garrett, and M. C. Whitton. 1998. Augmented reality applied to ultrasound-guided breast cyst aspiration. *Breast Dis* 10(3–4):221–230.

Rosenthal, M., A. State, J. Lee, G. Hirota, J. Ackerman, K. Keller, E. Pisano, M. Jiroutek, K. Muller, and H. Fuchs. 2002. Augmented reality guidance for needle biopsies: An initial randomized, controlled trial in phantoms. *Med Image Anal* 6(3):313–320.

Shelton, D., B. Wu, R. Klatzky, and G. Stetten. 2007. Design and calibration of a virtual tomographic reflection system. *2007 4th IEEE International Symposium on Biomedical Imaging: Macro to Nano* 1–3:956–959. doi:10.1109/Isbi.2007.357012.

Sielhorst, T., C. Bichlmeier, S. M. Heining, and N. Navab. 2006. Depth perception—A major issue in medical AR: Evaluation study by twenty surgeons. *Med Image Comput Comput Assist Interv* 9(Pt 1):364–372.

Stetten, G., A. Cois, W. Chang, D. Shelton, R. Tamburo, J. Castellucci, and O. von Ramm. 2005. C-mode real-time tomographic reflection for a matrix array ultrasound sonic flashlight. *Acad Radiol* 12(5):535–543. doi:10.1016/j.acra.2004.06.011.

Stetten, G., V. Chib, D. Hildebrand, and J. Bursee. 2001. Real time tomographic reflection: Phantoms for calibration and biopsy. *IEEE and ACM International Symposium on Augmented Reality, Proceedings*, pp. 11–19. doi:10.1109/Isar.2001.970511.

Stetten, G., D. Shelton, W. Chang, V. Chib, R. Tamburo, D. Hildebrand, L. Lobes, and J. Sumkin. 2002. Towards a clinically useful sonic flashlight. *2002 IEEE International Symposium on Biomedical Imaging, Proceedings*, Washington, DC, pp. 417–420.

Traub, J., P. Stefan, S. M. Heining, T. Sielhorst, C. Riquarts, E. Euler, and N. Navab. 2006. Hybrid navigation interface for orthopedic and trauma surgery. *Med Image Comput Comput Assist Interv* 9(Pt 1):373–80.

Wang, A., S. M. Mirsattari, A. G. Parrent, and T. M. Peters. 2011. Fusion and visualization of intraoperative cortical images with preoperative models for epilepsy surgical planning and guidance. *Comp Aid Surg* 16(4):149–160. doi:10.3109/10929088.2011.585805.

Wendler, T., M. Feuerstein, J. Traub, T. Lasser, J. Vogel, F. Daghighian, S. I. Ziegler, and N. Navab. 2007. Real-time fusion of ultrasound and gamma probe for navigated localization of liver metastases. *Med Image Comput Comput Assist Interv* 10(Pt 2):252–260.

Wendler, T., J. Traub, S. I. Ziegler, and N. Navab. 2006. Navigated three dimensional beta probe for optimal cancer resection. *Med Image Comput Comput Assist Interv* 9(Pt 1):561–569.

2 Tracking and Calibration

Elvis C. S. Chen and Burton Ma

CONTENTS

2.1 INTRODUCTION

The spatial measuring device, i.e. tracking system, is an integral component of an image-guided intervention workflow. The primary utilization of these devices is to determine the pose (orientation and position) of surgical instruments intraoperatively in real time. Patient registration (Chapter 3) is typically facilitated using a tracked and calibrated surgical instrument. Because the tracking system can only track its dynamic reference frame (DRF) directly, the pose of the tool with respect to its DRF must be determined through a calibration process. This chapter provides a short overview on the principles of tracking technology and error propagation and the specifics of surgical tool calibration.

2.2 SPATIAL MEASUREMENT DEVICES

Spatial measurement is the enabling technology for surgical navigation. Perhaps the first spatial measurement used for computer-assisted surgery was the stereotactic frame introduced by Horsley and Clarke [1], and stereotactic frames are still the dominant approach for many types of neuronavigation. Many other types of tracking system have been applied to surgery, including mechanical linkage, optical, magnetic, and vision-based systems. Each type of system differs with respect to the physics and mathematical principles from which the tracking information is inferred. In general, an optical tracking system operates on the principal of triangulation: it offers submillimeter accuracy but suffers from line-of-sight issues. Magnetic-based tracking[1] employs the principle of sensing the strength and orientation of an artificially generated magnetic field. It too offers submillimeter accuracy, but this may be compromised by the presence of ferromagnetic metals inside the surgical field. A comprehensive review and brief history of these types of tracking system can be found in this chapter [2], and the principle of vision-based tracking is described in detail in Chapter 3.

Optical tracking systems are either videometric or infrared (IR)-based. In a videometric tracking system, the poses of marker patterns are determined on video image sequences using one or more cameras. Using only a monoscopic camera, the pose of a planar marker can be determined through homography. A dictionary of unique markers can be built, such as those freely available in ArUco [3], allowing robust tracking of multiple patterns simultaneously. The size of these planar patterns must be optimized with respect to the size of the viewing frustum to ensure visibility and tracking accuracy.

The principle of pose tracking for all IR-based and videometric systems with multiple cameras is based on triangulation and registration. A set of fiducial markers is rigidly arranged in a known configuration and defines a DRF. During tracking, the location of each fiducial marker is determined via triangulation, and the pose of the DRF is determined by registering fiducial locations to the known configuration. Both the number and spatial distribution of the fiducial marker influences the tracking accuracy of the DRF [4]. At least three fiducial markers must be arranged in a noncollinear configuration to resolve the pose of the DRF in six degrees-of-freedom. Passive tracking systems, such as MicronTracker (ClaroNav, Toronto, Ontario Canada) and Polaris (Northern Digital Inc., Waterloo, Ontario Canada), are wireless. In active tracking systems, power supplied to the infrared emitting diode (IRED) emitter can be wired (as in Certus (Northern Digital Inc., Waterloo, Ontario, Canada)) or wireless and battery-powered (as in FusionTrack (Atracsys, Switzerland)). Hybrid systems are capable of tracking both passive and active fiducial markers.

The design of an optical DRF must follow vendor-specific criteria, both with respect to the intra- (i.e. location of individual fiducial marks of a DRF) and inter-compatibility of multiple DRFs. Intra-DRB criteria assures that each fiducial marker can be localized accurately, whereas inter-DRF criteria assures that each DRF can be identified uniquely. The integration of optical DRF into surgical instruments is limited by the finite DRF size and its inability to track flexible surgical tools.

Magnetic tracking systems represent another type of spatial measuring technology commonly used in computer-assisted intervention. The physical principle of magnetic tracking is the generation of an artificial magnetic field in which the strength and the orientation of the magnetic field can be detected using either a search coil (for an

---

[1] We refer throughout this chapter to "Magnetic Tracking System" (MTS), as these systems respond to magnetic, rather than electromagnetic, fields. Nonetheless, it is not uncommon for these systems to be referred to as Electromagnetic (EM) Tracking Systems. The two terms are synonymous.

alternating current driven field) or a fluxgate coil (for a direct current driven field) [5]. Magnetic tracking systems are sensitive to the presence of ferromagnetic objects. Due to the small size of these coils, a magnetic tracking system is particularly suitable in a scenario in which optical DRF is too large to be integrated into the surgical instrument or within flexible instruments such as transesophageal echocardiography ultrasounds.

2.3   TARGET REGISTRATION ERROR ESTIMATION MODELS

The solution to the rigid point-based registration problem is the rotation, $\mathbf{R}$, and translation, $\mathbf{t}$, that best aligns a set of points, $\{\mathbf{x}_i\}$, to a set of corresponding points, $\{\mathbf{y}_i\}$. The distance between a measured point, $\mathbf{x}_i$, and the unknown true location of the point before the registration transformation is computed is called the fiducial localization error (FLE). If the FLE is not zero, then the $\{\mathbf{x}_i\}$ will not coincide exactly with the $\{\mathbf{y}_i\}$ after the registration transformation is applied to $\{\mathbf{x}_i\}$; the root-mean-squared (rms) distance between $\{\mathbf{x}_i\}$ and $\{\mathbf{y}_i\}$ after registration is called the fiducial registration error (FRE). For N points, FRE is given by

$$\mathbf{FRE}^2 = \frac{1}{N} \sum_{1}^{N} \left\| \mathbf{R}\mathbf{x}_i + \mathbf{t} - \mathbf{y}_i \right\|^2, \tag{2.1}$$

where the vector $\mathbf{FRE}_i = \mathbf{R}\mathbf{x}_i + \mathbf{t} - \mathbf{y}_i$ is the residual displacement error between the registered point, $\mathbf{x}_i$, and its corresponding point, $\mathbf{y}_i$.

In most surgical applications, the target of interest does not coincide with a fiducial marker. When the registration is applied to some point $\mathbf{r}$ not used in computing the registration, then the distance between $\mathbf{r}$ and its corresponding point $\mathbf{r}$ is called the target registration error (TRE).

The expected value of the squared magnitude of TRE as a function of zero-mean, independent, identical, isotropic, normally distributed FLE is given by [6]

$$\left\langle \mathrm{TRE}^2(\mathbf{r}) \right\rangle = \frac{1}{N} \left(1 + \frac{1}{3} \sum_{k=1}^{3} \frac{d_k^2}{f_k^2} \right) \left\langle \mathrm{FLE}^2 \right\rangle, \tag{2.2}$$

where N is the number of markers, d_k is the distance of $\mathbf{r}$ from the principal axis, k, of the noise-free fiducial markers defined in $\{Y\}$, f_k^2 is the mean of the squared distances of the markers from axis k, and FLE^2 is the expected value of the squared magnitude of FLE. Equation 2.2 concisely describes the behavior of the magnitude of TRE: TRE magnitude is proportional to the standard deviation of FLE, inversely proportional to the square root of the number of markers, and minimized at the centroid of the markers, and the isocontours of TRE are ellipsoidal.

Many other results are known regarding the behavior of TRE for point-point registration (see Section 3.2), but less work has been performed regarding the behavior of TRE when measured points are registered to lines or surfaces. In the following section, we describe the spatial stiffness approach to modelling TRE for point-point, point-line, and point-surface registration.

2.3.1 SPATIAL STIFFNESS MODEL OF TRE

The spatial stiffness model approach for predicting the magnitude of TRE models the registration problem as the elastic displacement of a passive mechanical system; it has been used for point-point [7], point-line [8], and point-surface registration [9]. To construct the mechanical system corresponding to a registration problem, the spatial stiffness model approach assumes that FLE causes the computed registration transformation to differ from the true registration transformation by a small rigid displacement. Noisy registration point measurements, $\mathbf{z}_i$, are modelled by displacing the noise-free points, $\mathbf{y}_i = [x_i \ y_i \ z_i]^T$, by a small rotation: $\boldsymbol{\Omega} = \mathbf{R}_z(\omega_z)\mathbf{R}_y(\omega_y)\mathbf{R}_x(\omega_x)$, where $\mathbf{R}_x(\omega_x)$, $\mathbf{R}_y(\omega_y)$, and $\mathbf{R}_z(\omega_z)$ are the 3×3 rotation matrices representing rotations about the x, y, and z axes by the small amounts of ω_x, ω_y, and ω_z, respectively, and a translation vector of $\boldsymbol{\delta} = [\delta_x \ \delta_y \ \delta_z]^T$. The locations, $\mathbf{z}_i$, of the displaced registration points are given by $\mathbf{z}_i = \boldsymbol{\Omega}\mathbf{y}_i + \boldsymbol{\delta}$. For each displaced point $\mathbf{z}_i$ the point $\bar{\mathbf{y}}_i$ on the shape that is nearest to $\mathbf{z}_i$ is computed; if FLE is not isotropic, then $\bar{\mathbf{y}}_i$ is the shape point that is nearest in terms of the Mahalanobis distance. The squared Mahalanobis distance between $\mathbf{z}_i$ and $\bar{\mathbf{y}}_i$.

$$d_{M,i}^2 = \left(\mathbf{z}_i - \bar{\mathbf{y}}_i\right)^T \Sigma_i \left(\mathbf{z}_i - \bar{\mathbf{y}}_i\right) \tag{2.3}$$

where Σ_i is the FLE covariance matrix for point $\mathbf{z}_i$.

The spatial-stiffness model assumes that there is a linear spring associated with each registration point that stores an amount of potential energy: $U_i = 1/2 \, d_{M,i}^2$. The matrix of second-order partial derivatives of U_i taken with respect to the translation and rotation parameters and evaluated at $\omega_x = \omega_y = \omega_z = \delta_x = \delta_y = \delta_z$ yields the Hessian matrix $\mathbf{H}_i$. The stiffness matrix is then given by

$$\mathbf{K} = \sum_{i=1}^{N} \mathbf{H}_i = \begin{bmatrix} \mathbf{A} & \mathbf{B} \\ \mathbf{B}^T & \mathbf{D} \end{bmatrix}, \tag{2.4}$$

where $\mathbf{A}$, $\mathbf{B}$, and $\mathbf{D}$ are 3×3 block matrices. The stiffness matrix $\mathbf{K}$ is symmetric positive-definite for stable springs and small displacements from equilibrium. The eigenvalues of $\mathbf{K}$ are not immediately useful because they are not frame invariant; however, it can be shown that the eigenvalues of

$$\mathbf{K}_V = \mathbf{D} - \mathbf{B}^T \mathbf{A}^{-1} \mathbf{B} \tag{2.5}$$

$$\mathbf{C}_W = \mathbf{A}^{-1} \tag{2.6}$$

are frame invariant [7]. The eigenvalues, μ_1, μ_2, and μ_3, of $\mathbf{K}_V$ are the principal rotational stiffnesses, and the eigenvalues, σ_1, σ_2, and σ_3, of $\mathbf{C}_W^{-1}$ are the principal translational stiffnesses. Given the principal stiffnesses, the expected squared RMS value of TRE can be computed as follows:

$$\left\langle \mathrm{TRE}^2(\mathbf{r}) \right\rangle = \frac{1}{\sigma_1} + \frac{1}{\sigma_2} + \frac{1}{\sigma_3} + \frac{1}{\mu_{eq,1}} + \frac{1}{\mu_{eq,2}} + \frac{1}{\mu_{eq,3}}, \tag{2.7}$$

where the $\mu_{eq,i}$ are called the equivalent rotational stiffnesses and depend on the principal rotational stiffnesses, μ_i, the target location, $\mathbf{r}$, and the eigenvectors of $\mathbf{K}_V$; please see [7] for full details.

2.3.1.1 Point-Point Registration

For point-point registration, the Hessian matrix is given by [7]:

$$\mathbf{H}_i^P = \begin{bmatrix} \Sigma_i & \Sigma_i [\mathbf{y}_i]_\times^T \\ [\mathbf{y}_i]_\times^T \Sigma_i & [\mathbf{y}_i]_\times^T \Sigma_i [\mathbf{y}_i]_\times^T \end{bmatrix} \text{where} [\mathbf{y}_i]_\times^T = \begin{bmatrix} 0 & -\mathbf{z}_i & \mathbf{y}_i \\ \mathbf{z}_i & 0 & -\mathbf{x}_i \\ -\mathbf{y}_i & \mathbf{x}_i & 0 \end{bmatrix} \quad (2.8)$$

2.3.1.2 Point-Surface Registration

For point-surface registration, the Hessian matrix is given by [9]:

$$\mathbf{H}_i^S = \frac{1}{\mathbf{n}_i^T \Sigma_i \mathbf{n}_i} \begin{bmatrix} \mathbf{n}_i \\ \mathbf{y}_i \times \mathbf{n}_i \end{bmatrix} \begin{bmatrix} \mathbf{n}_i \\ \mathbf{y}_i \times \mathbf{n}_i \end{bmatrix}^T, \quad (2.9)$$

where the noise-free registration point, $\mathbf{y}_i$, is assumed to lie on a plane with unit surface normal $\mathbf{n}_i$.

2.3.1.3 Point-Line Registration

For point-line registration, the Hessian matrix is given by [8]:

$$\mathbf{H}_i^L = \mathbf{H}_i^P - \frac{1}{\mathbf{n}_i^T \Sigma_i \mathbf{n}_i} \begin{bmatrix} \Sigma_i \mathbf{n}_i \\ \mathbf{y}_i \times \Sigma_i \mathbf{n}_i \end{bmatrix} \begin{bmatrix} \Sigma_i \mathbf{n}_i \\ \mathbf{y}_i \times \Sigma_i \mathbf{n}_i \end{bmatrix}^T, \quad (2.10)$$

where the noise-free registration point, $\mathbf{y}_i$, is assumed to lie on a line with the unit direction of $\mathbf{n}_i$, and $\mathbf{H}_i^P$ is the Hessian matrix for point-point registration.

2.3.2 TRE MODELS IN TRACKING AND CALIBRATION

West and Maurer described the use of a TRE model to design targets for optically tracked surgical instruments [4]. They primarily studied planar target configurations although they briefly discussed some of the expected effects of using nonplanar targets.

Wiles and Peters [10] studied the problem of predicting TRE of an optically tracked target when a reference target was used, while Wiles and Peters [11] described a method to estimate the FLE of a tracked optical target in real time. A TRE model incorporating the estimated FLE was used to predict the TRE of a tracked optical tool. Seginer [12] described a method to predict the TRE directly from the vector fiducial registration errors. Sielhorst [13] described a covariance propagation technique to predict the covariance of the TRE for an optically tracked target.

The point-line spatial stiffness model of TRE has been used to optimize the collection of calibration data for B-mode ultrasound calibration [8] and hand-eye calibration of a surgical camera [14,15].

2.4   NUMERICAL SOLUTIONS

The problem of registration of homologous point-sets is more appropriately known as the Orthogonal Procrustes Problem [16]. It is normally formulated as a minimization of the FRE between two datasets through a similarity transform, consisting of scaling (or weighting) factors, followed by rotation and then translation. If $\mathbf{X}$ denotes a mobile measurement point-set with $\mathbf{n}$ points, and $\mathbf{Y}$ denotes the homologous stationary model points, then the FRE is defined as follows:

$$\mathrm{FRE}^2 = \frac{1}{N} \sum_{1}^{N} \left\| \mathbf{R}\,\mathbf{S}\,x_i + \mathbf{t} - y_i \right\|^2, \qquad (2.11)$$

where $\mathbf{R}$ is the orthonormal rotation, and $\mathbf{t}$ is the translation. Equation 2.11 is a generalization of Equation 2.1 with the addition of the matrix $\mathbf{S}$.

The matrix $\mathbf{S}$ serves dual purposes and is often underutilized in the field of image-guided interventions. It can serve as an *a priori* weighting factor for each pair of homologous $(\mathbf{X}_i, \mathbf{Y}_i)$. When $\mathbf{S}_i$ are isotropic, closed-form solutions exist [17,18]. These solutions are, in fact, optimal if the FLE is isotropic and identically distributed (i.i.d.). When $\mathbf{S}_i$ is anisotropic, Balachandran and Fitzpatrick presented an iterative solution [19]. When $\mathbf{S}_i$ is a full covariance matrix, Matei and Meer presented an optimal solution [20] but at the expense of computational complexity. The matrix $\mathbf{S}$ can also serve as an *a posteriori*, unknown scaling factor. For example, ultrasound probe calibration can be formulated using Equation 2.11, where the matrix $\mathbf{S}$ represents the pixel size of an ultrasound image [8]. Closed-form solutions can be used to solve Equation 2.11 with isotropic $\mathbf{S}$. Chen et al. [21] presented a solution to solve anisotropic scaling factors, $\mathbf{S}$, that is guaranteed to converge to a local minimum.

Equation 2.1 can be further generalized, where the dataset y_i represents geometrical primitives, such as a line or a plane. Assuming zero-mean, isotropic, and i.i.d. FLE, an optimal solution for homologous point-point, point-line, and point-plane can be achieved [22]. No optimal solution exists in the current literature when the FLE is anisotropic or heteroscedastic for Equation 2.1 when y_i is a line or a plane.

2.5   TOOL CALIBRATION

Because the spatial measuring device can only determine the pose of the DRFs directly, the geometrical relationship between a tracked instrument to its DRF must be determined through a calibration process. The outcome of the calibration process can be a rigid (rotation plus translation) or affine (scaling followed by rotation and translation) transformation. The DRF is assumed to be rigidly attached to the surgical instrument, which allows the calibration to be performed prior to the surgical interventions. For clinical deployment, it is beneficial to have an "on-line" (intraoperative) calibration and validation workflow, with the assurance that the calibration transformation is accurate immediately prior to its clinical usage. However, such an on-line calibration workflow requires the calibration process to be accurate, robust, and computationally efficient.

2.5.1 STYLUS TIP CALIBRATION

The surgical stylus is a ubiquitous component for any surgical navigational system and is used to digitize (localize) the spatial location of a fiducial. It is a pen-shaped instrument, and the objective of the calibration is to determine the location of the tip relative to its tracking DRF. If an optical tracking system is used, then the spatial configuration of the tracking fiducial and its geometrical relationship to the tip dictates how accurate the digitization process can be. West and Maurer [4] investigated this issue in detail although their findings were mainly focused on planar DRF.

Stylus tip calibration is typically performed by pivoting the tip about a stationary point: the motion of the DRF falls onto a sphere where the stylus tip is located at the center. The shape of the stylus tip to the pivoting surface dictates the quality of the pivoting data. In a clinical scenario, the shape of the stylus tip is often blunt to avoid accidental tissue injury during the digitization process: calibration of a blunt-tip stylus should be performed against a conforming surface to promote spherical motion of the DRF. In this manner, the calibrated tip location is a mathematical construct that resides within the physical construct of the tip. Consequently, it introduces the FLE during the digitization process (Figure 2.1).

In a typical clinical scenario in which pivoting data are noisy, Yaniv [23] demonstrated that algebraic formulation of pivot calibration, which utilizes both the position and the orientation of the DRF and thus provides a more accurate tip calibration

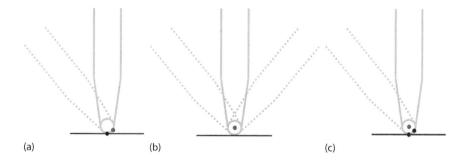

(a)   (b)   (c)

FIGURE 2.1 A surgical stylus is often equipped with a dull tip to avoid accidental tissue damage during digitization. (a) Pivoting a dull tip against a flat surface does not guarantee pivoting about a stationary point, (b) pivoting about a confirming surface produces a calibrated tip that is located inside the physical construct of the dull tip, and (c) in both cases, digitizing a fiducial on a non-conforming surface results in digitizing FLE.

than the sphere-fitting formation [23]. When the pivot data are good, Ma et al. [24] suggested that the sphere-fitting formulation provides a more accurate tip calibration result compared to the algebraic formulation.

For an optically tracked stylus, after calibration Equation 2.2 can be used following calibration on the digitizing accuracy. In this scenario, the target $\mathbf{r}$ denotes the calibrated tip location. Because d^2_k is proportional to the distance between the tip location to DRF, the longer the stylus the worse the digitizing accuracy will be.

2.5.2   ULTRASOUND PROBE CALIBRATION

Probe calibration of freehand ultrasound has long been an active research area [25]. The objective of ultrasound calibration is to determine the geometrical relationship between the coordinate system of the US 2D image/3D volume and its DRF. This process is often facilitated by using a calibration phantom, in which the geometry and the physical property of the phantom is known by construction (Figure 2.2).

The majority of the calibration methods can be categorized into three categories: single-point or line, 2D alignment, and freehand methods. Lindseth et al. [26] concluded the freehand methods achieved the best calibration accuracy. The common calibration phantom used in freehand calibration includes a tracked pointer stylus [27], a single-wall [28,29], single-line [8,30], and lines arranged in a Z-configuration [31]. Categorically, methods using a tracked stylus or Z-fiducial can be formulated as point-point registration, where Procrustean solutions [17] apply.

Chen et al. [8] introduced the concept of guided calibration, by which sequential placement of fiducials is facilitated by the use of the TRE prediction model. The calibration used in this framework is a single tracked line fiducial, and the ultrasound calibration is formulated as a homologous point-line registration (Section 2.4). After bootstrapping an initial calibration transformation using n measurements, the scalar TRE for every pixel on the ultrasound image is estimated using a point-line TRE model (Section 2.3.1.3). The TRE estimation model is used to exhaustively search for

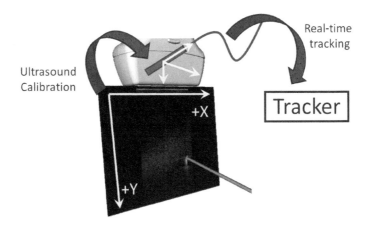

FIGURE 2.2   In tracked ultrasound, probe calibration refers to the geometrical relationship (scaling, rotation, and translation) between the ultrasound image coordinate to its DRF.

the next fiducial placement (coinciding pixel location and line orientation) such that the predicted TRE for a given target would be reduced maximally. In general, TRE using guided calibration decreases monotonically, reaching a submillimeter TRE when 12 to 15 measurements are collected [8].

In the context of computer-assisted orthopedic surgery, a tracked A-mode ultrasound is used as a variable-length stylus to digitize the surface of bony structures [32,33]. The calibration of A-mode ultrasound is typically formulated as a variation of pivot calibration (Section 2.5.1). Alternatively, it can also be formulated as line-to-lines registration [34], where the distance to the object is not needed.

2.5.3 SURGICAL CAMERA HAND-EYE CALIBRATION

A surgical camera such as endoscopic video is another real-time imaging modality commonly employed in image-guided interventions. Hand-eye calibration refers to the process of determining the geometrical relationship between the optical axis of the camera lens and its tracking sensor. Hand-eye calibration in a surgical environment is non-trivial [35], as issues such as sterilization, DRF attachment, and real-time computation requirement remain challenging.

Most camera hand-eye calibration used in image-guided intervention borrows techniques from the robotic literature [36–38]. Similar to ultrasound calibration using a stationary point, these hand-eye calibration techniques often acquire images of a stationary feature (fiducial) and solve the calibration algebraically as the $AX = BX$ problem [36,37]. Alternatively, calibration using a stationary feature can also be solved using dual quaternion [39] or in a branch-and-bound optimization framework [40]. The quality of this hand-eye calibration approach is highly dependent upon the data used for computing the unknown transformation. Schmidt and Neimann [41] examined the issue of data selection for this type of hand-eye calibration.

A surgical robot such as the da Vinci system has a built-in camera. Hand-eye calibration of the da Vinci camera can be achieved using the $AX = BX$ solution [42]. An interesting approach is to use the end-effector of the da Vinci robot as a calibration phantom [43]. In this manner, the requirement of a custom sterile object for intraoperative calibration is removed.

Using a spatial measuring device, an additional tracked phantom may be used to aid the process of hand-eye calibration. Perhaps the simplest method is the Procrustean approach, where the hand-eye calibration is reduced to homologous point-point registration (Section 2.3.1.1). Both Voruganti and Bartz [44] and Chen et al. [45] used a calibrated, tracked planar chessboard pattern for hand-eye calibration, in which the 3D positions of the chessboard corners are determined both in the tracker's coordinate system (via tracking) and the camera's optical axis (by solving some forms of Perspective-n-Point problem).

Using a tracked ball-tip stylus, surgical hand-eye calibration can also be formulated as homologous point-line registration [14,15]: the point is the 3D location of the calibrated stylus tip, and the line is the line-of-sight ray emanating from the camera origin. In this formulation, a TRE estimation model can be used to guide the placement of the calibration fiducial [15]. Submillimeter accuracy can be achieved using as little as 12 to 15 tracked images [14].

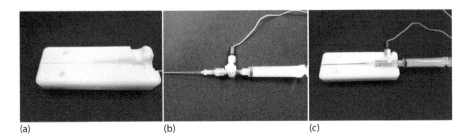

(a)   (b)   (c)

FIGURE 2.3 Example of a template-based calibration: (a) a calibration template with the exact negative imprint of the surgical instrument; (b) a sharp, tracked surgical needle; and (c) calibration is performed by mating the tracked surgical instrument to the template.

2.5.4 TEMPLATE-BASED TOOL CALIBRATION

The calibration of other surgical instruments such as a sharp needle or surgical drill can be facilitated using a tracked template. A template is a tracked object with the exact negative imprint of the surgical instrument, and the geometry of this negative imprint is known to its DRF by manufacturing (or via another calibration process).

When the surgical instrument is placed onto its negative imprint, the spatial relationship between the two tracked DRF provides the calibration transformation (Figure 2.3). Template-based calibration is particularly useful when the geometry of the surgical instrument is complex. Using 3D scanner and 3D printing technology, such a template can be manufactured precisely and inexpensively.

2.6 CONCLUSION

The tracking of calibrated instruments is a fundamental requirement in many mixed and augmented reality surgical applications. The use of error analysis techniques and numerical methods developed for registration purposes has many applications in tracking and calibration. In tracking, registration techniques have been used to optimize the design of tracked targets, estimate tracking error, and optimize tracking accuracy. In calibration, registration techniques have been used for effective calibration of a tracked B-mode ultrasound probe and hand-eye calibration of a tracked surgical camera. There is great potential for the increased use of registration techniques in calibration given the ubiquitous use of calibrated instruments in augmented reality surgical application.

REFERENCES

1. V. Horsley and R. H. Clarke. The structure and functions of the cerebellum examined by a new method. *Brain*, 31(1):45–124, 1908.
2. W. Birkfellner, J. Hummel, E. Wilson, and K. Cleary. Tracking devices. In T. M. Peters and K. Cleary (Eds.), *Image-Guided Interventions: Technology and Applications*, Chapter 2, pp. 23–44. Springer, New York, 2008.
3. S. Garrido-Jurado, R. Munoz Salinas, F. J. Madrid-Cuevas, and M. J. Marn-Jimenez. Automatic generation and detection of highly reliable fiducial markers under occlusion. *Pattern Recognition*, 47(6):2280–2292, 2014.

4. J. B. West and C. R. Maurer, Jr. Designing optically tracked instruments for image-guided surgery. *IEEE Transactions on Medical Imaging*, 23(5):533–545, 2004.
5. A. M. Franz, T. Haidegger, W. Birkfellner, K. Cleary, T. M. Peters, and L. Maier-Hein. Electromagnetic tracking in medicine – A review of technology, validation, and applications. *IEEE Transactions on Medical Imaging*, 33(8):1702–1725, 2014.
6. J. M. Fitzpatrick, J. B. West, and C. R. Maurer. Predicting error in rigid-body point-based registration. *IEEE Transactions on Medical Imaging*, 17(5):694–702, 1998.
7. B. Ma, M. H. Moghari, R. E. Ellis, and P. Abolmaesumi. Estimation of optimal fiducial target registration error in the presence of heteroscedastic noise. *IEEE Transactions on Medical Imaging*, 29(3):708–723, 2010.
8. E. C. S. Chen, T. M. Peters, and B. Ma. Guided ultrasound calibration: Where, how, and how many calibration fiducials. *International Journal of Computer Assisted Radiology and Surgery*, 11(6):889–898, 2016.
9. B. Ma, J. Choi, and H. M. Huai. Target registration error for rigid shape-based registration with heteroscedastic noise. In *Proceedings of the SPIE*, vol. 9036, 2014.
10. A. D. Wiles and T. M. Peters. Improved statistical tre model when using a reference frame. In N. Ayache, S. Ourselin, and A. Maeder (Eds.), *Medical Image Computing and Computer-Assisted Intervention – MICCAI 2007: 10th International Conference*, Brisbane, Australia, October 29–November 2, 2007, *Proceedings, Part I*, pp. 442–449. Springer, Berlin, Germany, 2007.
11. A. D. Wiles and T. M. Peters. Real-time estimation of fle statistics for 3-d tracking with point-based registration. *IEEE Transactions on Medical Imaging*, 28(9):1384–1398, 2009.
12. A. Seginer. Rigid-body point-based registration: The distribution of the target registration error when the fiducial registration errors are given. *Medical Image Analysis*, 15(4):397–413, 2011.
13. T. Sielhorst, M. Bauer, O. Wenisch, G. Klinker, and N. Navab. Online estimation of the target registration error for n-ocular optical tracking systems. In *Medical Image Computing and Computer-Assisted Intervention (MICCAI 2007)*, pp. 652–659, Brisbane, Australia. Springer-Verlag, Berlin, Germany, 2007.
14. I. Morgan, U. Jayarathne, A. Rankin, T. M. Peters, and E. C. S. Chen. Hand-eye calibration for surgical cameras: A procrustean perspective-n-point solution. *International Journal of Computer Assisted Radiology and Surgery*, 12(7):1141–1149, 2017.
15. E. C. S. Chen, I. Morgan, U. Jayarathne, B. Ma, and T. M. Peters. Hand-eye calibration using a target registration error model. *Healthcare Technology Letters*, 4(5):157–162, 2017.
16. J. C. Gower and G. B. Dijksterhuis. *Procrustes Problems*. Oxford University Press, Oxford, UK, 2004.
17. B. K. P. Horn. Closed-form solution of absolute orientation using unit quaternions. *Journal of the Optical Society of America*, 4:629–642, 1987.
18. K. S. Arun, T. S. Huang, and S. D. Blostein. Least-squares fitting of two 3-D point sets. *IEEE Transactions on Pattern Analysis and Machine Intelligence*, 9(5):698–700, 1987.
19. R. Balachandran and J. M. Fitzpatrick. Iterative solution for rigid-body point-based registration with anisotropic weighting. In *Proceedings of the SPIE*, vol. 7261, 2009.
20. B. Matei and P. Meer. Optimal rigid motion estimation and performance evaluation with bootstrap. In *Computer Vision and Pattern Recognition, 1999. IEEE Computer Society Conference on*, vol. 1, pp. 339–345, 1999.
21. E. C. S. Chen, A. J. McLeod, U. L. Jayarathne, and T. M. Peters. Solving for free-hand and real-time 3D ultrasound calibration with anisotropic orthogonal procrustes analysis. In *Proceedings of the SPIE*, vol. 9036, p. 90361Z, 2014.
22. C. Olsson, F. Kahl, and M. Oskarsson. Branch-and-bound methods for euclidean registration problems. *IEEE Transactions on Pattern Analysis and Machine Intelligence*, 31(5):783–794, 2009.

23. Z. Yaniv. Which pivot calibration? In *Proceedings of the SPIE*, vol. 9415, 2015.

24. B. Ma, N. Banihaveb, J. Choi, E. C. S. Chen, and A. L. Simpson. Is pose-based pivot calibration superior to sphere fitting? In *Proceedings of the SPIE*, vol. 10135, 2017.

25. L. Mercier, T. Lang, F. Lindseth, and L. D. Collins. A review of calibration techniques for freehand 3-D ultrasound systems. *Ultrasound in Medicine & Biology*, 31(4):449–471, 2005.

26. F. Lindseth, G. A. Tangen, T. Lang, and J. Bang. Probe calibration for freehand 3-D ultrasound. *Ultrasound in Medicine & Biology*, 29(11):1607–1623, 2003.

27. D. M. Muratore and R. L. Galloway, Jr. Beam calibration without a phantom for creating a 3-D freehand ultrasound system. *Ultrasound in Medicine & Biology*, 27(11):1557–1566, 2001.

28. R. W. Prager, R. N. Rohling, A. H. Gee, and L. H. Berman. Rapid calibration for 3-D freehand ultrasound. *Ultrasound in Medicine & Biology*, 24(6):855–869, 1998.

29. F. Rousseau, P. Hellier, and C. Barillot. Confhusius: A robust and fully automatic calibration method for 3D freehand ultrasound. *Medical Image Analysis*, 9(1):25–38, 2005.

30. A. Khamene and F. Sauer. A novel phantom-less spatial and temporal ultrasound calibration method. In J. S. Duncan and G. Gerig (Eds.), *Medical Image Computing and Computer-Assisted Intervention – MICCAI 2005: 8th International Conference*, Palm Springs, CA, October 26–29, *Proceedings, Part II*, pp. 65–72. Springer, Berlin, Germany, 2005.

31. R. M. Comeau, A. Fenster, and T. M. Peters. Integrated MR and ultrasound imaging for improved image guidance in neurosurgery. In *Proceedings of the SPIE*, vol. 3338, pp. 747–754, 1998.

32. C. R. Maurer, R. P. Gaston, D. L. G. Hill, M. J. Gleeson, M. G. Taylor, M. R. Fenlon, P. J. Edwards, and D. J. Hawkes. Acoustick: A tracked a-mode ultrasonography system for registration in image-guided surgery. In C. Taylor and A. Colchester (Eds.), *Medical Image Computing and Computer-Assisted Intervention – MICCAI'99: Second International Conference*, Cambridge, UK, September 19–22. *Proceedings*, pp. 953–962. Springer, Berlin, Germany, 1999.

33. D. De Lorenzo, E. De Momi, E. Beretta, P. Cerveri, F. Perona, and G. Ferrigno. Experimental validation of A-mode ultrasound acquisition system for computer assisted orthopaedic surgery. In *Proceedings of the SPIE*, vol. 726502, 2009.

34. E. C. S. Chen, B. Ma, and T. M. Peters. Contact-less stylus for surgical navigation: Registration without digitization. *International Journal of Computer Assisted Radiology and Surgery*, 12(7):1231–1241, 2017.

35. S. Thompson, D. Stoyanov, C. Schneider, K. Gurusamy, S. Ourselin, B. Davidson, D. Hawkes, and M. J. Clarkson. Hand–eye calibration for rigid laparoscopes using an invariant point. *International Journal of Computer Assisted Radiology and Surgery*, 11(6):1071–1080, 2016.

36. Y. C. Shiu and S. Ahmad. Calibration of wristmounted robotic sensors by solving homogeneous transform equations of the form ax=xb. *IEEE Transactions on Robotics and Automation*, 5(1):16–29, 1989.

37. R. Y. Tsai and R. K. Lenz. A new technique for fully autonomous and efficient 3D robotics hand/eye calibration. *IEEE Transactions on Robotics and Automation*, 5(3):345–358, 1989.

38. F. Dornaika and R. Horaud. Simultaneous robot-world and hand-eye calibration. *IEEE Transactions on Robotics and Automation*, 14(4):617–622, 1998.

39. K. Daniilidis. Hand-eye calibration using dual quaternions. *The International Journal of Robotics Research*, 18(3):286–298, 1999.

40. J. Heller, M. Havlena, and T. Pajdla. Globally optimal hand-eye calibration using branch-and-bound. *IEEE Transactions on Pattern Analysis and Machine Intelligence*, 38(5):1027–1033, 2016.

41. J. Schmidt and H. Niemann. Data selection for handeye calibration: A vector quantization approach. *The International Journal of Robotics Research*, 27(9):1027–1053, 2008.

42. Z. Zhang, L. Zhang, and G. Z. Yang. A computationally efficient method for hand–eye calibration. *International Journal of Computer Assisted Radiology and Surgery*, 12(10):1775–1787, 2017.

43. K. Pachtrachai, M. Allan, V. Pawar, S. Hailes, and D. Stoyanov. Hand-eye calibration for robotic assisted minimally invasive surgery without a calibration object. In *2016 IEEE/RSJ International Conference on Intelligent Robots and Systems (IROS)*, pp. 2485–2491, 2016.

44. A. K. R. Voruganti and D. Bartz. Alternative online extrinsic calibration techniques for minimally invasive surgery. In *Proceedings of the 2008 ACM Symposium on Virtual Reality Software and Technology*, VRST'08, pp. 291–292. ACM, 2008.

45. E. C. S. Chen, K. Sarkar, J. S. H. Baxter, J. Moore, C. Wedlake, and T. M. Peters. An augmented reality platform for planning of minimally invasive cardiac surgeries. In *Proceedings of the SPIE*, vol. 8316, 2012.

3 Registration

Lena Maier-Hein, Stefanie Speidel, Esther Stenau,
Elvis C. S. Chen, and Burton Ma

CONTENTS

3.1 INTRODUCTION

In computer assisted surgery (CAS), the term registration typically refers to aligning pre-operative patient-specific models with intraoperatively acquired data. It can be used to augment the surgeon's view by visualizing of structures below the tissue surface. This chapter provides a short overview of the principles behind intra-operative registration reviews the related literature on error estimation and presents representative registration methods developed in the context of minimally invasive surgery (MIS).

3.2 PRINCIPLES OF INTRAOPERATIVE REGISTRATION

Methods for intraoperative registration can roughly be divided into the following categories:

Manual registration: In manual registration the actual data fusion is performed by a human. This is typically done by shifting, rotating, and scaling preoperative data until a good match with intraoperative data is obtained.

Point-based registration: In point-based registration a set of corresponding natural or artificial landmarks are located in the planning image (typically preoperatively) as well as on the patient (typically intraoperatively), and a point-based registration is applied to register the data (see Figure 3.1). Line fiducials are used in a variant of this approach.

Shape-based registration: In surface-based registration (or *shape-based* registration) intraoperative data—typically a surface mesh or a point cloud—is registered to the planning image based on geometrical shape information, as illustrated in Figure 3.2.

Volume-based registration: In volume-based registration subsurface information, such as three-dimensional (3D) geometric information (e.g., the vessel geometry obtained from a computed tomography [CT] scan) is acquired during surgery and mapped to corresponding information from a 3D planning image.

Calibration-based registration: In calibration-based registration multiple intraoperative imaging modalities (e.g., an endoscope and ultrasound [US] device) are calibrated to each other to fuse imaging information (see Figure 3.3). Most frequently, it is implemented by a tracking system being used to establish a spatial relationship between the two image coordinate systems.

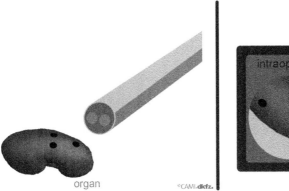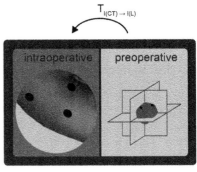

FIGURE 3.1 Example of point-based registration in MIS. Fiducials are attached to the organ's surface and their 3D configuration is determined from a preoperative 3D image (e.g., C-arm CT image, transrectal US image). During surgery, the fiducials are continuously tracked in the 2D laparoscopic image, and a 2D-3D registration algorithm is applied to compute the pose of the laparoscope relative to the 3D image (transformation $T_{I(CT)\to I(L)}$ from the image coordinate system of the CT $I(CT)$ to the image coordinate system of the laparoscope $I(L)$).

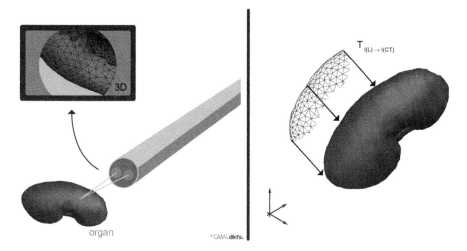

FIGURE 3.2 Example of surface-based registration in MIS. Parts of the surface of an organ are reconstructed with a stereo laparoscope and then matched to the preoperatively recorded shape of the same organ. A transformation $T_{I(CT)\to I(L)}$ is thus established from the image coordinate system of the CT to the image coordinate system of the laparoscope.

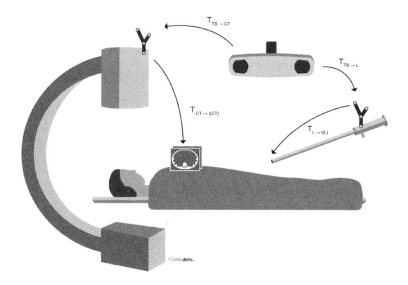

FIGURE 3.3 Example of calibration-based registration. Optical markers are attached to both an intraoperative 3D imaging modality (here: C-arm) and a laparoscope. Preoperatively, both devices are calibrated with respect to the tracking system so that extrinsic camera parameters are known. Given that both devices are tracked during surgery, all image information can be transformed to the same coordinate system.

Some representative methods and systems developed in the context of the MIS are shown in Section 3.3.

3.3 ERROR ESTIMATION IN INTRAOPERATIVE REGISTRATION

Error estimation is important for two reasons: it can be used as a stop criterion during an iterative registration process, and it provides feedback on the quality of the registration to the surgeons. The following sections introduce approaches to error methods in point-based registration and other registration types.

3.3.1 ERROR ESTIMATION IN POINT-BASED REGISTRATION

Error estimation for point-based registration depends on three quantities: the fiducial localization error (FLE), the fiducial registration error (FRE), and the target registration error (TRE). FLE is the error that occurs in localizing a registration fiducial. FRE is the distance between the physical fiducial and its corresponding point in the preoperative image after the fiducial has been registered to the image. TRE is the distance between a point of interest (the target) on the patient and its corresponding point on the preoperative image after the registration has been performed.

FRE, while easy to compute, is not a useful metric for registration error because FRE and TRE are uncorrelated [1]. Several models for predicting TRE in point-based registration have been described that account for zero-mean heteroscedastic FLE [1,2]. Methods for predicting the distribution of TRE have also been proposed [1–4]. An alternative error metric to TRE is the metric based on registration circuits [5]. TRE modeling of point-based registration has been incorporated into robotic bone milling [6] and surgical navigation systems [3].

One issue with using a TRE model is specifying the FLE magnitude or covariance matrix. Wiles and Peters [7] described an algorithm for real-time estimation of FLE for tracked optical targets. A different approach completely avoids estimating FLE by using the FRE vectors to estimate TRE for a single registration instance [4].

3.3.2 ERROR ESTIMATION IN OTHER REGISTRATION CATEGORIES

Literature on error estimation for other registration categories is sparse. Modeling TRE for point-line registration and applying a TRE model to calibration problems is discussed in Chapter 2. Registration error prediction has been used to optimize registration point selection in point-surface registration for computer-assisted surgery [8,9].

3.4 INTRAOPERATIVE REGISTRATION IN LAPAROSCOPY

While computer-assisted *open* surgery generally requires the application of additional imaging modalities to acquire intraoperative anatomical information, the advantage of MIS is that the endoscope itself can be used for this purpose. Although numerous methods have been proposed for multimodal image registration in general, the literature on registration in computer-assisted *laparoscopic* interventions is relatively sparse. Registration in laparoscopic interventions is particularly challenging due to the continuously changing morphology of the organ. While several authors have proposed the manual alignment of preoperatively and intraoperatively acquired images, current research also focuses on semiautomatic and fully automatic registration methods that are simultaneously robust and reduce the amount of required user interaction. Once an initial registration has been established across modalities, it is typically sufficient to register all subsequent movements of the endoscopic camera to the first registration. The next section provides a brief review of initial registration methods, and Section 3.3.2 gives an overview of continuous multimodal registration in laparoscopy.

3.4.1 Initial Multimodal Registration

Following the categorization of registration methods proposed in Section 3.1, the approaches to initially registering the endoscopic image data with pre- or intraoperatively acquired 3D anatomical data can roughly be divided into the following categories: *manual* methods, *point-based* methods, *surface-based* methods, *volume-based* registrations, and *calibration-based* registrations. The following sections give an overview of sample applications and their advantages or disadvantages in laparoscopic surgery for all categories.

3.4.1.1 Manual

One of the first intraoperative laparoscopic registrations in humans was proposed by Maresceaux et al. [10] in 2004. An assistant manually rotated and shifted a preoperative CT scan until the view of the preoperative data matched the laparoscopic image. Manual registration can also be facilitated or complemented by algorithmic components [11,12]. Those that are based on manual localization of landmarks as initialization are detailed in the next section. Manual approaches are robust and easy to implement. Furthermore, approval and certification for clinical usage is comparatively easy to achieve [13]. On the other hand, the method is not well-suited for non-rigid registration, is extremely time-consuming, and the quality of the registration depends heavily on the caregiver's experience.

3.4.1.2 Point-Based

In point-based registration, a set of corresponding points (natural or artificial landmarks) are identified in the planning image and in the laparoscopic image or on the intraoperatively constructed surface, and a point-based registration is applied to register the data (Figure 3.1). However, because laparoscopic images and 3D planning images, such as CT images or magnetic resonance images (MRI), share few common landmarks, the automatic identification of corresponding landmarks is extremely challenging given the limited field of view (FoV) of the endoscope. Hence, the majority of approaches proposed so far require manual interaction for the registration. If tracking systems are used for the point localization, point-based approaches are very similar to calibration-based approaches. For example, an optically and/or magnetically tracked pointer can be used to locate landmarks intraoperatively that have previously been identified in the planning image. The landmarks may be artificial, anatomical, or both and can be located on the target organ [14] or on the skin surface [15]. In robotic-assisted surgery, the robot tool tip can be used as a pointing device. Alternatively, laparoscopic instruments can be tracked, and the position of incisions can be recorded and matched to the preoperatively planned cutting position [16]. Anatomical landmarks can also be selected manually in the laparoscopic image to avoid tracking systems.

The main drawback of manually locating the points is that the registration becomes invalid as soon as the tissue and/or the camera moves. To address this issue, Simpfendörfer et al. [17] proposed attaching radio-opaque, needle-shaped markers that can be tracked in real time to the target organ. An intraoperative 3D US or C-arm CT image yields the 3D configuration of these fiducials in relation to the patient anatomy. This in turn allows continuous computation of the poses of the endoscope from their known positions in the 2D endoscopic images. While this approach is generally very robust in the presence of rigid organ motion, attaching fiducials to internal organs is not ideally suited to the current surgical workflow. Also, the detection of the fiducials is challenging in the presence of smoke, blood, or tissue in the FoV of the laparoscope. The usage of near-infrared fluorescent markers solves these detection issues [18], but the approval of such markers for usage in humans has not yet been addressed. Furthermore, the extension of both approaches to nonrigid registration is not straightforward, but first attempts have been made that combine fluorescent markers with a biomechanical model for nonrigid registration [19].

In summary, point-based registration is a popular practical method for fast, accurate, and robust compensation of rigid organ motion. The remaining challenges involve workflow integration and deformable registration.

3.4.1.3   Surface-Based

In the most common implementation of surface-based registration, the surface is either reconstructed from the image itself using stereo information (see e.g., [20]) or recorded with tracked instruments that are used as a stylus [21]. Alternatively, other reconstruction methods such as structured light or time-of-flight cameras can potentially be used (see [22]).

The registration problem is usually posed as an optimization problem, where the metric to be optimized represents the goodness of fit. It should be mentioned that the majority of literature on shape matching is not related to medical applications, but comprehensive reviews have been published by the computer vision community. Regardless of the application, shape matching methods can be classified into two categories: *fine* registration methods that assume a rough alignment of the input data and *global* matching methods that establish correspondences between the input shapes without any prior knowledge of their poses relative to each other. The latter are often used to compute an initial alignment for the fine registration algorithm (as detailed in Section 3.3.2). Despite many influential publications on surface matching in general, the methods that are typically proposed do not adequately address all of the challenges related to intraoperative surface registration, namely the need for *partial* and *nonrigid* registration of surfaces that typically *lack salient features* but are subject to *systematic errors* and *noise* (cf. [23]).

A promising approach to nonrigid surface registration is to incorporate a priori knowledge of the mechanical properties of the tissue via biomechanical modeling. Using elasticity theory, the approach can be described as a boundary value problem with displacement boundary conditions generated from the intraoperative surface.

In general, the finite element method is used to solve the resulting set of partial differential equations. This has been successfully applied, for example in neurosurgery to compensate the brain shift (cf. e.g., [24]) or in open liver surgery (cf. e.g., [25]), and is becoming increasingly popular in laparoscopic settings (cf. e.g., [26,27]).

It is not necessary to intraoperatively reconstruct the surface in 3D to incorporate shape information. In a variant of the surface-based registration approach, a reconstructed pre-operative surface obtained by segmenting the preoperative data for the target organ is deformed according to visual cues extracted in a single or multiple intraoperative laparoscopy images. A very important visual cue in this approach is the organ silhouette. It was used in conjunction with a small number of point-landmarks for the uterus in multiple extrinsically calibrated images [28] and in conjunction with curve-landmarks for the liver in a single image [29].

A major advantage of surface-based registration in general is that it requires no additional hardware (at least in some implementations), as the surface information can be directly computed from the endoscopic images. In addition, the method may often be carried out in real-time, as typically no manual interaction is required. However, accurate and robust registration based on partial surface data is extremely challenging, especially in the presence of deformations.

3.4.1.4   Volume-Based

In contrast to surface-based methods, volume-based approaches include subsurface information for the registration process. These approaches are relatively new and are based on very different concepts. Until now there have only been a few attempts at volume-based registration in laparoscopic surgery, such as using pre- and intraoperative CT images [30–32] or tracked US as an intraoperative device [33]. In general, volume-based registration methods need some kind of intraoperative volume data, which can be supplied by a 3D US, a tracked US, an open MRI scanner, or by intraoperative CT scans.

If the intraoperative modality is tracked, then the positional information is usually only used as a first rough positioning step, and the final registration is based on the information in the volumes themselves and can thus incorporate and compensate the soft-tissue deformation of the organ. When comparing volumetric data, a common strategy is to deform the preoperative image data so as to maximize its similarity to the intraoperative image. This is often done using an optimization algorithm that incorporates a similarity measure, such as the sum of squared distances, mutual information, or cross-correlation between the images. Furthermore, a biomechanical model can be used for registration [31,32]. A comprehensive overview and comparison of slice-to-volume registration in medical image registration can be found in [34].

An interesting variant works without any additional hardware, and registration can be achieved by estimating the vessel structure using pulse motion detected in the laparoscopic image [35].

The key advantage of volume-based registration is that it is potentially the most accurate method. On the other hand, reliable deformable registration can still be regarded as an unsolved challenge, especially if topological changes resulting from cutting, for example, are taken into account.

3.4.1.5 Calibration-Based

This type of registration method is based on directly calibrating two image modalities with each other. In the most common implementation, both the laparoscope and a second intraoperative imaging modality are equipped with fiducials in order to enable localization by a tracking system (see Figure 3.3). Transforming all image data to one common coordinate system (e.g., the tracking coordinate system) then enables for AR visualization of subsurface anatomical structures in the endoscopic video data. Commonly used tracking systems for laparoscopic registration are either based on purely optical marker detection, electromagnetic markers, or optical and electromagnetic (magneto-optic) measurements. Hybrid approaches may take magnetic distortion correction into account. In robotic-assisted interventions, the kinematic parameters can also be used to determine the pose of a device [36].

The transformation between the different modalities and the reference world coordinate system is calculated via a calibration routine, typically performed once before the intervention. US transducers, which provide either 2D or 3D images, are usually used as intraoperative imaging devices to augment the laparoscopic images [37,38]. Rendered views of intraoperative CT [39], C-arm data [40], or single photon emission computed tomography images [41] are also used for registration with the laparoscope. Furthermore, virtual views from preoperative CTs can be rendered, which correspond with the tracked laparoscope pose [42].

An alternative method for calibration-based registration does not require an additional tracking system and relies on detecting or tracking one modality in a calibration image of the second modality. For example, if an intraoperative CT is recorded, then the shape of the laparoscope detected in the CT data can be registered to a model of the laparoscope to determine the position and orientation of it relative to the imaging device. This pose information can be used to view the recorded CT data from the angle of the laparoscope [43]. As the laparoscope is symmetric with respect to the viewing axis, the missing degree of freedom for the laparoscope pose needs to be determined, either by sensors or image processing methods. In general, the problem of detecting the second device in an image can be facilitated using a calibration pattern, such as by attaching it to a laparoscopic US probe in order to determine the pose of the US probe in relation to the laparoscope [44].

Calibration-based methods have the advantage that they are typically real-time capable and that the clinical workflow is not severely interrupted during the actual procedure. On the other hand, they are generally only suitable for rigid registration. Furthermore, the specific drawbacks of using tracking systems in the operation theater (e.g., robustness problems due to electromagnetic distortions or line-of-sight requirements) must be taken into account [45].

3.4.2 CONTINUOUS MULTIMODAL REGISTRATION

While interventions on sufficiently rigid structures, such as bones, may only require an initial registration at the beginning of the operation, soft-tissue interventions rely on fast, nonrigid registration methods in order to account for the continuously changing morphology of the organs. To avoid the computational demands of repeating the registration process over time with one of the previously described methods, an alternative registration approach can be used that involves continuously updating a registration that is performed at the beginning. This can be carried out using tracking devices, via tissue tracking or surface reconstruction using the endoscopic image information acquired during surgery, or via volume-based approaches. As the advantages and disadvantages of the different methods are similar to those mentioned in the previous section, they are not explicitly discussed.

3.4.2.1 Tracking-Based

For organs that only have minor organ deformations and organ movement (e.g., kidney), a continuous update of the laparoscope pose relative to the initial registration may be sufficient. This can be done using tracking devices and sensors or markers attached to the laparoscope (as described in the previous section).

3.4.2.2 Image-Based

Alternatively, information extracted from the endoscopic image can be used to enable continuous registration. Feature detection and correspondence search are challenging tasks given the homogeneous nature of tissue, specular reflections, and the presence of blood and smoke in the FoV. A correspondence search of the endoscopic images is often performed using salient features detected on the basis of pixel intensities, high-dimensional image descriptors, or artificial landmarks.

Feature tracking methods fall within either iterative strategies or those which use matching between feature descriptors. Iterative strategies such as optical flow [46] rely on knowledge of the location of a feature in the previous frame to limit a search for the corresponding feature in the next frame, assuming a small degree of motion and intensity coherence. They have been used extensively in laparoscopic images with varying degrees of success. Given that these assumptions are often violated under the imaging conditions of laparoscopy, these methods have been combined with predictive models of feature localization based on prior knowledge of anatomical periodicity, machine learning approaches, and predictive filtering (e.g., [47–49]. Matching techniques using feature descriptors involve comparing descriptors from one image to another and assuming specific criteria to establish correspondence between feature vectors. Recent advances use deep learning for tracking and matching [50], which poses new challenges regarding training data, especially in the context of laparoscopic surgery.

Generally speaking, feature tracking methods can either be used to update a manual initial registration [51]; to compensate breathing and pulsation [20]; to correct for changing camera parameters like zooming, changing distortion, or focus parameters [52]; or to calculate constraints for biomechanical models [53].

3.4.2.3 Surface-Based

In the medical domain, the proposed surface matching methods concentrate on fine registration, using a manually defined rough alignment of the data. In rigid surface registration, the most popular fine registration algorithm is the well-known iterative closest point (ICP) algorithm [54,55]. Given two roughly aligned shapes represented by two point sets, the algorithm iteratively (1) establishes point correspondences when given the current alignment of the data and (2) computes a rigid transformation accordingly. As both steps in the algorithm reduce the (Euclidean) distance between corresponding points, the algorithm converges to an at least local minimum with respect to a mean-square distance metric. Several generalizations of the algorithm have been proposed that enable partially overlapping surface registration [56] or allow integration of a priori knowledge [57] without altering the favorable convergence properties. Most surface-based intraoperative registration methods presented for laparoscopic interventions rely on the ICP algorithm or one of its many variants [58]. Hence, the initial alignment required in order for the ICP to converge to the global optimum is typically obtained by manual initialization [58]. Furthermore, biomechanical models can also be used to continuously update the registration using surface reconstructions and corresponding projections as displacement constraints [59,60].

The patient's skin (as opposed to the reconstructed organ's surface) may also be used for surface-based intraoperative registration [61]. In this case, however, problems may arise because exterior landmarks on the surface of the body do not rigidly correspond to target structures inside the body, especially in the presence of a pneumoperitoneum. As discussed in Section 3.4.2.2, silhouette-based or contour-based methods can also be used to perform a continuous registration based on shape information.

3.4.2.4 Volume-Based

Volume-based methods for continuous registration are effectively applied for neurosurgical applications and are often based on preoperative tomographic images and intra-operative US [34]. An example of this approach [62] generates pseudo-US images from a tracked US probe and preoperative MRI images. The deformation is estimated by comparing the actual and simulated US image, followed by an optimization algorithm applied to the MRI data. Until now, there have only been a few approaches available in laparoscopic surgery. All the attempts rely on an intraoperative, tracked US probe that is continuously registered to preoperative CT data [63,64]. After the initial alignment of the data according to the tracking information, the approaches differ in how they modify the data to account for deformation. An early approach applies a modified phase-correlation approach to find the displacement between an US image and a CT volume without considering deformation [63]. Recent approaches segment the intraoperative US images to find the center points of vessels on each image, which are then used to compute the corresponding 3D point by using the tracking information of the US probe [64]. The 3D vessel centers are then matched to vessel center points of the preoperative, segmented CT data using an ICP approach. A similar method is described by [65]. In addition, a breathing model is proposed to compensate for breathing motion.

3.5 DISCUSSION

This chapter described basic concepts for intraoperative registration along with methods proposed for error estimation and specific implementations presented in the context of MIS. It is worth mentioning that the categorization provided is only one of multiple ways to distinguish the different methods. Also, there is a lot of overlap between the categories. Many practical implementations of calibration-based registration, for example, implicitly rely on principles of point-based registration if they apply an optical tracking system. Similarly, surface-based and volume-based registration are closely related—for example, both information on the vessel topology and surface data may be used for intraoperative registration with biomechanical models.

While rigid point-based and surface-based registration are already commercially applied by a number of companies, such as Brainlab (Munich, Germany), Medtronic (Fridley, MN), Stryker (Kalamazoo, MI), and CAScination (Bern, Switzerland), over a broad range of clinical applications from brain surgery, spine, and knee surgery to open liver surgery, deformable registration is far from being solved. In the previous section, we reviewed state-of-the-art registration approaches in the specific context of MIS. While the advances in the field are promising, few methods have been applied in humans to date, as shown in Table 3.1. For a successful transfer from bench to bedside, deformable registration methods will need to fulfill several requirements. Most importantly, the methods should be very robust for a number of factors, such as occlusion, changing conditions like camera zooming or movement, and deformations or topological changes in the organ. Furthermore, the approaches should work quickly, preferably in real time, and should not require a long preparation time (e.g., for calibration steps or hardware setup). In general, the approaches should be easy to integrate into the existing clinical workflow and not be reliant on complex additional hardware.

TABLE 3.1

Overview of Laparoscopic Registration Methods That Have Already Been Used in Humans

Author	Year		Number of Treated Patients	Method	Update
Marescaux et al.	2004	[10]	1	Manual	–
Su et al.	2009	[12]	2	Manual	Surface
Nakamura et al.	2010	[66]	2	Manual	–
Pratt et al.	2012	[11]	3	Manual	–
Marzano et al.	2013	[67]	1	Manual	–
Haouchine et al.	2014	[68]	1	Manual	Surface
Pessaux et al.	2015	[69]	3	Manual	–
Vemuri et al.	2012	[70]	12	Manual	–
Ukimura et al.	2008	[71]	1	Calibration	n.n.
Brouwer et al.	2012	[41]	1	Calibration	n.n.
Pratt et al.	2015	[44]	1	Calibration	n.n.
Hayashi et al.	2016	[42]	23	Calibration	Tracking
Konishi et al.	2005	[72]	20	Point (nat.)	[b]
Suzuki et al.	2008	[73]	1	Point (nat.)	Tracking
Buchs et al.	2013	[74]	2	Point (nat.)	Tracking
Conrad et al.	2016	[75]	1	Point (nat.)	Tracking
Hayashi et al.	2016	[16]	20	Point (nat.)	n.n.
Teber et al.	2009	[76]	10	Point (art.)	n.n.

(Continued)

TABLE 3.1 (*Continued*)
Overview of Laparoscopic Registration Methods That Have Already Been Used in Humans

Author	Year		Number of Treated Patients	Method	Update
Simpfendörfer et al.	2011	[17]	1	Point (art.)	n.n.
Ieiri et al.	2012	[15]	6	Point (art.)[a]	Tracking
Tsutsumi et al.	2013	[77]	5	Point (art.)	Tracking
Souzaki et al.	2013	[78]	6	Point (art.)	Tracking
Tinguely et al.	2017	[14]	51	Point (nat.)	–
Marques et al.	2015	[20]	?	Surface	Image
Kleemann et al.	2012	[33]	1	Volume	–
Kenngott et al.	2014	[30]	1	Volume	–

Source: Adapted with major modifications from Bernhardt, S. et al., *Med. Image Anal.*, 2017.
Note: The last column refers to the method used for updating the registration, as introduced in Section 3.1. ?: no information given, n.n.: update not necessary because the initial registration can be done in real time, –: no update of the initial registration.
[a] Additional surface registration.
[b] Additional calibration-based registration for US probe.

In conclusion, there has been tremendous progress in the field of intraoperative registration in the past two decades, leading to widely applied commercial solutions for a number of different clinical applications involving sufficiently rigid structures, such as bones or the brain. The key technical challenge is how to ensure robust registration of multimodal data in the presence of motion, deformation, and topological changes.

ACKNOWLEDGMENTS

The authors would like to thank Carolin Feldmann (CAMI, DKFZ) for providing the figures and Micha Pfeiffer (TSO, NCT) for assisting in reviewing the literature.

REFERENCES

1. Danilchenko, A.; Fitzpatrick, J. M.: General approach to first-order error prediction in rigid point registration. *IEEE Transactions on Medical Imaging* 30(3) (2011), 679–693.
2. Moghari, M. H.; Abolmaesumi, P.: Distribution of fiducial registration error in rigid-body point-based registration. *IEEE Transactions on Medical Imaging* 28(11) (2009), 1791–1801.
3. Sielhorst, T.; Bauer, M.; Wenisch, O.; Klinker, G.; Navab, N.: Online estimation of the target registration error for n-ocular optical tracking systems. In: *International Conference on Medical Image Computing and Computer-Assisted Intervention (MICCAI)*, Ayache, N., Ourselin, S., Maeder, A. (Eds.), Vol. 4792 (2007), pp. 652–659.
4. Seginer, A.: Rigid-body point-based registration: The distribution of the target registration error when the fiducial registration errors are given. *Medical Image Analysis* 15(4) (2011), 397–413.

5. Datteri, R. D.; Dawant, B. M.: Estimation and reduction of target registration error. Ayache, N. (Hrsg.); Delingette, H. (Hrsg.); Golland, P. (Hrsg.); Mori, K. (Hrsg.): *International Conference on Medical Image Computing and Computer-Assisted Intervention (MICCAI)*, Springer, Berlin, Germany, 2012, pp. 139–146.

6. Siebold, M. A.; Dillon, N. P.; Fichera, L.; Labadie, R. F.; Webster, R. J.; Fitzpatrick, J. M.: Safety margins in robotic bone milling: From registration uncertainty to statistically safe surgeries. *The International Journal of Medical Robotics and Computer Assisted Surgery* 13(3) (2017), e1773.

7. Wiles, A. D.; Peters, T. M.: Real-time estimation of FLE statistics for 3-D tracking with point-based registration. *IEEE Transactions on Medical Imaging* 28(9) (2009), 1384–1398.

8. Simon, D. A.; Hebert, M.; Kanade, T.: Techniques for fast and accurate intrasurgical registration. *Journal of Image Guided Surgery* 1(1) (1995), 17–29.

9. Ma, B.; Ellis, R. E.: A point-selection algorithm based on spatial-stiffness analysis of rigid registration. *Computer Aided Surgery* 10(4) (2005), 209–223.

10. Marescaux, J.; Rubino, F.; Arenas, M.; Mutter, D.; Soler, L.: Augmented-reality-assisted laparoscopic adrenalectomy. *Journal of the American Medical Association* 292(18) (2004), 2214–2215. doi:10.1001/jama.292.18.2214-c.

11. Pratt, P.; Mayer, E.; Vale, J.; Cohen, D.; Edwards, E.; Darzi, A.; Yang, G.-Z.: An effective visualisation and registration system for image-guided robotic partial nephrectomy. *Journal of Robotic Surgery* 6(1) (2012). doi:10.1007/s11701-011-0334-z.

12. Su, L.-M.; Vagvolgyi, B. P.; Agarwal, R.; Reiley, C. E.; Taylor, R. H.; Hager, G. D.: Augmented reality during robotassisted laparoscopic partial nephrectomy: Toward real-time 3D-CT to stereoscopic video registration. *Urology* 73(4) (2009). doi:10.1016/j.urology.2008.11.

13. Bernhardt, S.; Nicolau, S. A.; Soler, L.; Doignon, C.: The status of augmented reality in laparoscopic surgery as of 2016. *Medical Image Analysis* (2017). doi:10.1016/j.media.2017.01.007.

14. Tinguely, P.; Fusaglia, M.; Freedman, J.; Banz, V.; Weber, S.; Candinas, D.; Nilsson, H.: Laparoscopic image-based navigation for microwave ablation of liver tumors—A multi-center study. *Surgical Endoscopy* 31(10) (2017), 4315–4324.

15. Ieiri, S.; Uemura, M.; Konishi, K.; Souzaki, R.; Nagao, Y.; Tsutsumi, N.; Akahoshi, T. et al.: Augmented reality navigation system for laparoscopic splenectomy in children based on preoperative CT image using optical tracking device. *Pediatric Surgery International* 28(4) (2012). doi:10.1007/s00383-011-3034-x.

16. Hayashi, Y.; Misawa, K.; Hawkes, D. J.; Mori, K.: Progressive internal landmark registration for surgical navigation in laparoscopic gastrectomy for gastric cancer. *International Journal of Computer Assisted Radiology and Surgery* 11(5), 837–845. doi:10.1007/s11548-015-1346-3.

17. Simpfendörfer, T.; Baumhauer, M.; Müller, M.; Gutt, C. N.; Meinzer, H.-P.; Rassweiler, J. J.; Guven, S.; Teber, D.: Augmented reality visualization during laparoscopic radical prostatectomy. *Journal of Endourology* 25(12) (2011). doi:10.1089/end.2010.0724.

18. Wild, E.; Teber, D.; Schmid, D.; Simpfendörfer, T.; Müller, M.; Baranski, A.-C.; Kenngott, H.; Kopka, K.; Maier-Hein, L.: Robust augmented reality guidance with fluorescent markers in laparoscopic surgery. In: *International Journal of Computer Assisted Radiology and Surgery* (2016). doi:10.1007/s11548-016-1385-4.

19. Kong, S.-H.; Haouchine, N.; Soares, R.; Klymchenko, A.; Andreiuk, B.; Marques, B.; Shabat, G. et al.: Robust augmented reality registration method for localization of solid organs' tumors using CT-derived virtual biomechanical model and fluorescent fiducials. *Surgical Endoscopy* 31(7) (2017), 2863–2871.

20. Marques, B.; Plantefève, R.; Roy, F.; Haouchine, N.; Jeanvoine, E.; Peterlik, I.; Cotin, S.: Framework for augmented reality in minimally invasive laparoscopic surgery. In: *E-health Networking, Application & Services (HealthCom), 2015 17th International Conference on* IEEE, 2015, pp. 22–27.

21. Altamar, H. O.; Ong, R. E.; Glisson, C. L.; Viprakasit, D. P.; Miga, M. I.; Herrell, S. D.; Galloway, R. L.: Kidney deformation and intraprocedural registration: A study of elements of image-guided kidney surgery. *Journal of Endourology* 25(3) (2011), 511–517. doi:10.1089/end.2010.0249.

22. Maier-Hein, L.; Mountney, P.; Bartoli, A.; Elhawary, H.; Elson, D.; Groch, A.; Kolb, A. et al.: Optical techniques for 3D surface reconstruction in computer-assisted laparoscopic surgery. *Medical Image Analysis* 17(8) (2013). doi:10.1016/j.media.2013.04.003.

23. Santos, T. R. D.: *Muti-Modal Partial Surface Matching For Intraoperative Registration*, Dissertation, Ruprecht-Karls-Universität Heidelberg, 2012.

24. Clatz, O.; Delingette, H.; Talos, I.-F.; Golby, A. J.; Kikinis, R.; Jolesz, F. A.; Ayache, N.; Warfield, S. K.: Robust nonrigid registration to capture brain shift from intraoperative MRI. *IEEE Transactions on Medical Imaging* 24(11) (2005), 1417–1427.

25. Rucker, D. C.; Wu, Y.; Clements, L. W.; Ondrake, J. E.; Pheiffer, T. S.; Simpson, A. L.; Jarnagin, W. R.; Miga, M. I.: A mechanics-based nonrigid registration method for liver surgery using sparse intraoperative data. *IEEE Transactions on Medical Imaging* 33(1) (2014), 147–158.

26. Suwelack, S.; Röhl, S.; Bodenstedt, S.; Reichard, D.; Dillmann, R.; Santos, T. D.; Maier-Hein, L. et al.: Physics-based shape matching for intraoperative image guidance. *Medical Physics* 41(11) (2014). doi:10.1118/1.4896021.

27. Peterlík, I.; Courtecuisse, H.; Rohling, R.; Abolmaesumi, P.; Nguan, C.; Cotin, S.; Salcudean, S.: Fast elastic registration of soft tissues under large deformations. *Medical Image Analysis* 45 (2017), 24–40.

28. Collins, T.; Pizarro, D.; Bartoli, A.; Bourdel, N.; Canis, M.: Computer-aided laparoscopic myomectomy by augmenting the uterus with Pre-operative MRI data. *International Symposium on Mixed and Augmented Reality*, Munich, Germany, 2014.

29. Koo, B.; Özgür, E.; Roy, B. L.; Buc, E.; Bartoli, A.: Deformable registration of a preoperative 3D liver volume to a laparoscopy image using contour and shading cues. In: *Medical Image Computing and Computer-Assisted Intervention*, Springer, Cham, Switzerland, 2017, pp. 326–334.

30. Kenngott, H. G.; Wagner, M.; Gondan, M.; Nickel, F.; Nolden, M.; Fetzer, A.; Weitz, J. et al.: Real-time image guidance in laparoscopic liver surgery: First clinical experience with a guidance system based on intraoperative CT imaging. *Surgical Endoscopy* 28(3) (2014), 933–940.

31. Oktay, O.; Zhang, L.; Mansi, T.; Mountney, P.; Mewes, P.; Nicolau, S.; Soler, L.; Chefd'hotel, C.: Biomechanically driven registration of pre-to intra-operative 3D images for laparoscopic surgery. In: *International Conference on Medical Image Computing and Computer-Assisted Intervention*, Springer, Berlin, Germany, 2013, 1–9.

32. Bano, J.; Nicolau, S. A.; Hostettler, A.; Doignon, C.; Marescaux, J.; Soler, L.: Registration of preoperative liver model for laparoscopic surgery from intraoperative 3d acquisition. In: Li Ao, H.; Linte, C.A.A.; M As Amune, K.; Peters, T.M.; Zheng, G. (Eds.) *Augmented Reality Environments for Medical Imaging and Computer-Assisted Interventions*, Springer, Berlin, Germany, 2013, pp. 201–210.

33. Kleemann, M.; Deichmann, S.; Esnaashari, H.; Besirevic, A.; Shahin, O.; Bruch, H.-P.; Laubert, T.: Laparoscopic navigated liver resection: Technical aspects and clinical practice in benign liver tumors. *Case Reports in Surgery* 2012 (2012), 1–8. doi:10.1155/2012/265918.

34. Ferrante, E.; Paragios, N.: Slice-to-volume medical image registration: A survey. *Medical Image Analysis* 39 (2017), 101–123.

35. Amir-Khalili, A.; Hamarneh, G.; Peyrat, J.-M.; Abinahed, J.; Al-Alao, O.; Al-Ansari, A.; Abugharbieh, R.: Automatic segmentation of occluded vasculature via pulsatile motion analysis in endoscopic robot-assisted partial nephrectomy video. *Medical Image Analysis* 25(1) (2015), 103–110.

36. Leven, J.; Burschka, D.; Kumar, R.; Zhang, G.; Blumenkranz, S.; Dai, X. D.; Awad, M. et al.: DaVinci canvas: A telerobotic surgical system with integrated, robot-assisted, laparoscopic ultrasound capability. In: *International Conference on Medical Image Computing and Computer-Assisted Intervention (MICCAI)*, Springer, Berlin, Germany, 2005, pp. 811–818.

37. Feuerstein, M.; Reichl, T.; Vogel, J.; Schneider, A.; Feussner, H.; Navab, N.: Magneto-optic tracking of a flexible laparoscopic ultrasound transducer for laparoscope augmentation. In: *International Conference on Medical Image Computing and Computer-Assisted Intervention*, Springer, Berlin, Germany, pp. 458–466.

38. Jayarathne, U. L.; Moore, J.; Chen, E. C.; Pautler, S. E.; Peters, T. M.: Real-Time 3D ultrasound reconstruction and visualization in the context of laparoscopy. In: *International Conference on Medical Image Computing and Computer-Assisted Intervention*, Springer, Berlin, Germany, 2017, pp. 602–609.

39. Shekhar, R.; Dandekar, O.; Bhat, V.; Philip, M.; Lei, P.; Godinez, C.; Sutton, E. et al.: Live augmented reality: A new visualization method for laparoscopic surgery using continuous volumetric computed tomography. *Surgical Endoscopy* 24 (2010), 1976–1985.

40. Feuerstein, M.; Mussack, T.; Heining, S.; Navab, N.: Intraoperative laparoscope augmentation for port placement and resection planning in minimally invasive liver resection. *IEEE Transactions on Medical Imaging* 27(3) (2008), 355–369. doi:10.1109/TMI.2007.907327.

41. Brouwer, O. R.; Buckle, T.; Bunschoten, A.; Kuil, J.; Vahrmeijer, A. L.; Wendler, T.; Valdés-Olmos, R. A.; Poel, H. G. D.; Leeuwen, F. W. B.: Image navigation as a means to expand the boundaries of fluorescence-guided surgery. *Physics in Medicine and Biology* 57(10) (2012). doi:10.1088/0031-9155/57/10/3123.

42. Hayashi, Y.; Misawa, K.; Oda, M.; Hawkes, D. J.; Mori, K.: Clinical application of a surgical navigation system based on virtual laparoscopy in laparoscopic gastrectomy for gastric cancer. *International Journal of Computer Assisted Radiology and Surgery* 11(5) (2016), 827–836.

43. Bernhardt, S.; Nicolau, S. A.; Agnus, V.; Soler, L.; Doignon, C.; Marescaux, J.: Automatic localization of endoscope in intraoperative CT image: A simple approach to augmented reality guidance in laparoscopic surgery. *Medical Image Analysis* 30 (2016). doi:10.1016/j.media.2016.01.008.

44. Pratt, P.; Jaeger, A.; Hughes-Hallett, A.; Mayer, E.; Vale, J.; Darzi, A.; Peters, T.; Yang, G.-Z.: Robust ultrasound probe tracking: Initial clinical experiences during robot-assisted partial nephrectomy. *International Journal of Computer Assisted Radiology and Surgery* 10(12) (2015), 1905–1913. doi:10.1007/s11548-015-1279-x.

45. Franz, A. M.; Haidegger, T.; Birkfellner, W.; Cleary, K.; Peters, T. M.; Maier-Hein, L.: Electromagnetic tracking in medicine—A review of technology, validation, and applications. *IEEE Transactions on Medical Imaging* 33(8) (2014), 1702–1725. doi:10.1109/TMI.2014.2321777.

46. Lucas, B. D.; Kanade, T.: An iterative image registration technique with an application to stereo vision. In: *International Joint Conference on Artificial Intelligence*, Vancouver, Canada, 1981, pp. 674–679.

47. Bogatyrenko, E.; Pompey, P.; Hanebeck, U. D.: Efficient physics-based tracking of heart surface motion for beating heart surgery robotic systems. *International Journal of Computer Assisted Radiology and Surgery* 6(3) (2011), 387–399.

48. Giannarou, S.; Visentini-Scarzanella, M.; Yang, G. Z.: Probabilistic tracking of affine-invariant anisotropic regions. *IEEE Transactions on Pattern Analysis and Machine Intelligence* 35(1) (2012), 130–143.

49. Mahadevan, V.; Vasconcelos, N.: Saliency-based discriminant tracking. In: *IEEE International Conference on Computer Vision and Pattern Recognition (CVPR)*, 2009, pp. 1007–1013.

50. Li, P.; Wang, D.; Wang, L.; Lu, H.: Deep visual tracking: Review and experimental comparison. *Pattern Recognition* 76 (2018), 323–338.

51. Nicolau, S.; Diana, M.; Agnus, V.; Soler, L.; Marescaux, J.: Semi-automated augmented reality for laparoscopic surgery: First in-vivo evaluation. *International Journal of Computer Assisted Radiology and Surgery* 8(1) (2013).

52. Lourenço, M.; Barreto, J. P.; Fonseca, F.; Ferreira, H.; Duarte, R. M.; Correia-Pinto, J.: Continuous zoom calibration by tracking salient points in endoscopic video. In: *International Conference on Medical Image Computing and Computer-Assisted Intervention*, Springer, Berlin, Germany, 2014, pp. 456–463.

53. Pratt, P.; Stoyanov, D.; Visentini-Scarzanella, M.; Yang, G.-Z.: Dynamic guidance for robotic surgery using image-constrained biomechanical models. In: *International Conference on Medical Image Computing and Computer-Assisted Intervention*, Springer, Berlin, Germany, 2010, pp. 77–85.

54. Besl, P. J.; McKay, N. D.: A method for registration of 3-D shapes. *IEEE Transactions of Pattern Analysis and Machine Intelligence* 14 (1992), 239–256.

55. Chen, Y.; Medioni, G.: Object modeling by registration of multiple range images. *Computer Vision and Image Understanding* 10 (1992), 145–155.

56. Chetverikov, D.; Stepanov, D.; Krsek, P.: Robust Euclidean alignment of 3D point sets: The trimmed iterative closest point algorithm. *Image and Vision Computing* 23 (2005), 299–309.

57. Maier-Hein, L.; Franz, A.; Santos, T. D.; Schmidt, M.; Fangerau, M.; Meinzer, H.-P.; Fitzpatrick, J. M.: Convergent iterative closest-point algorithm to accomodate anisotropic and inhomogenous localization error. *IEEE Transactions on Pattern of Analysis and Machine Intelligence* 34(8) (2012), 1520–1532.

58. Rauth, T. P.; Bao, P. Q.; Galloway, R. L.; Bieszczad, J.; Friets, E. M.; Knaus, D. A.; Kynor, D. B.; Herline, A. J.: Laparoscopic surface scanning and subsurface targeting: Implications for image-guided laparoscopic liver surgery. *Surgery* 142(2) (2007), 207–214. doi:10.1016/j.surg.2007.04.016.

59. Reichard, D.; Häntsch, D.; Bodenstedt, S.; Suwelack, S.; Wagner, M.; Kenngott, H.; Müller-Stich, B.; MaierHein, L.; Dillmann, R.; Speidel, S.: Projective biomechanical depth matching for soft tissue registration in laparoscopic surgery. *International Journal of Computer Assisted Radiology and Surgery* 12(7) (2017), 1101–1110.

60. Plantefeve, R.; Peterlik, I.; Haouchine, N.; Cotin, S.: Patient-specific biomechanical modeling for guidance during minimally-invasive hepatic surgery. *Annals of Biomedical Engineering* 44(1) (2016), 139–153.

61. Soler, L.; Nicolau, S.; Fasquel, J. B.; Agnus, V.; Charnoz, A.; Hostettler, A.; Moreau, J.; Forest, C.; Mutter, D.; Marescaux, J.: Virtual reality and augmented reality applied to laparoscopic and notes procedures. In: *IEEE International Symposium on Biomedical Imaging (ISBI): From Nano to Macro*, 2008, pp. 1399–1402.

62. Arbel, T.; Arbel, T.; Morandi, X.; Comeau, R. M.; Collins, D. L.: Automatic non-linear MRI-ultrasound registration for the correction of intra-operative brain deformations. *Computer Aided Surgery* 9(4) (2004), 123–136.

63. Estépar, R. S. J.; Westin, C.-F.; Vosburgh, K. G.: Towards real time 2D to 3D registration for ultrasound-guided endoscopic and laparoscopic procedures. *International Journal of Computer Assisted Radiology and Surgery* 4(6) (2009), 549.

64. Song, Y.; Totz, J.; Thompson, S.; Johnsen, S.; Barratt, D.; Schneider, C.; Gurusamy, K. et al.: Locally rigid, vessel-based registration for laparoscopic liver surgery. *International Journal of Computer Assisted Radiology and Surgery* 10(12) (2015), 1951–1961.

65. Ramalhinho, J.; Robu, M.; Thompson, S.; Edwards, P.; Schneider, C.; Gurusamy, K.; Hawkes, D.; Davidson, B.; Barratt, D.; Clarkson, M. J.: Breathing motion compensated registration of laparoscopic liver ultrasound to CT. In: *Medical Imaging 2017: Image-Guided Procedures, Robotic Interventions, and Modeling* Bd. 10135 International Society for Optics and Photonics, Orlando, FL, 2017, p. 101352V.

66. Nakamura, K.; Naya, Y.; Zenbutsu, S.; Araki, K.; Cho, S.; Ohta, S.; Nihei, N.; Suzuki, H.; Ichikawa, T.; Igarashi, T.: Surgical navigation using three-dimensional computed tomography images fused intraoperatively with live video. *Journal of Endourology* 24(4) (2010). doi:10.1089/end.2009.0365.

67. Marzano, E.; Piardi, T.; Soler, L.; Diana, M.; Mutter, D.; Marescaux, J.; Pessaux, P.: Augmented reality-guided artery-first pancreatico-duodenectomy. *Journal of Gastrointestinal Surgery* 17(11) (2013), 1980–1983. doi:10.1007/s11605-013-2307-1.

68. Haouchine, N.; Dequidt, J.; Peterlik, I.; Kerrien, E.; Berger, M.-O.; Cotin, S.: Towards an accurate tracking of liver tumors for augmented reality in robotic assisted surgery. In: *Robotics and Automation (ICRA), 2014 IEEE International Conference on*, IEEE, pp. 4121–4126.

69. Pessaux, P.; Diana, M.; Soler, L.; Piardi, T.; Mutter, D.; Marescaux, J.: Towards cybernetic surgery: Robotic and augmented reality-assisted liver segmentectomy. *Langenbeck's Archives of Surgery* 400(3) (2015), 381–385. doi:10.1007/s00423-014-1256-9.

70. Vemuri, A. S.; Wu, J. C.-H.; Liu, K.-C.; Wu, H.-S.: Deformable three-dimensional model architecture for interactive augmented reality in minimally invasive surgery. *Surgical Endoscopy* 26(12) (2012), 3655–3662.

71. Ukimura, O.; Gill, I. S.: Imaging-assisted endoscopic surgery: Cleveland clinic experience. *Journal of Endourology* 22(4) (2008), 803–810. doi:10.1089/end.2007.9823.

72. Konishi, K.; Hashizume, M.; Nakamoto, M.; Kakeji, Y.; Yoshino, I.; Taketomi, A.; Sato, Y.; Tamura, S.; Maehara, Y.: Augmented reality navigation system for endoscopic surgery based on three-dimensional ultrasound and computed tomography: Application to 20 clinical cases. *International Congress Series* 1281 (2005), 537–542. doi:10.1016/j.ics.2005.03.234.

73. Suzuki, N.; Hattori, A.; Hashizume, M.: Benefits of augmented reality function for laparoscopic and endoscopic surgical robot systems. In: *MICCAI Workshop: AMI-ARCS*, New York, 2008, pp. 53–60.

74. Buchs, N. C.; Volonte, F.; Pugin, F.; Toso, C.; Fusaglia, M.; Gavaghan, K.; Majno, P. E.; Peterhans, M.; Weber, S.; Morel, P.: Augmented environments for the targeting of hepatic lesions during image-guided robotic liver surgery. *Journal of Surgical Research* 184(2) (2013). doi:10.1016/j.jss.2013.04.032.

75. Conrad, C.; Fusaglia, M.; Peterhans, M.; Lu, H.; Weber, S.; Gayet, B.: Augmented reality navigation surgery facilitates laparoscopic rescue of failed portal vein embolization. *Journal of the American College of Surgeons* 223 (2016). doi:10.1016/j.jamcollsurg.2016.06.392.

76. Teber, D.; Guven, S.; Simpfendörfer, T.; Baumhauer, M.; Güven, E. O.; Yencilek, F.; Gözen, A. S.; Rassweiler, J.: Augmented reality: A new tool to improve surgical accuracy during laparoscopic partial nephrectomy? Preliminary *in vitro* and *in vivo* results. *European Urology* 56(2) (2009), 332–338. doi:10.1016/j.eururo.2009.05.017.

77. Tsutsumi, N.; Tomikawa, M.; Uemura, M.; Akahoshi, T.; Nagao, Y.; Konishi, K.; Ieiri, S.; Hong, J.; Maehara, Y.; Hashizume, M.: Image-guided laparoscopic surgery in an open MRI operating theater. *Surgical Endoscopy* 27(6) (2013), 2178–2184. doi:10.1007/s00464-012-2737-y.

78. Souzaki, R.; Ieiri, S.; Uemura, M.; Ohuchida, K.; Tomikawa, M.; Kinoshita, Y.; Koga, Y. et al.: An augmented reality navigation system for pediatric oncologic surgery based on preoperative CT and MRI images. *Journal of Pediatric Surgery* 48(12) (2013), 2479–2483. doi:10.1016/j.jpedsurg.2013.08.025.

4 Display Technologies

Ulrich Eck and Tobias Sielhorst

CONTENTS

Visual displays are an essential part of augmented reality (AR) systems that enable the fusion of real and virtual images into a consistent user experience. Different technologies have been proposed over the past decades, which can be grouped into six categories. In this chapter, we discuss the relevant properties of AR displays and present representative milestones for systems in these categories with a focus on medical applications. Furthermore, we discuss the advantages and disadvantages of the concepts that define the six types of AR displays.

4.1 INTRODUCTION

As early as 1938, the Austrian mathematician Steinhaus described the first setup of augmenting imaging data registered to an object [1] with a geometric layout aimed at revealing a bullet inside a patient by visually overlaying a pointer on the position of the invisible bullet. He achieved the alignment of the overlay by construction from any point of view, and its registration worked without any computation. However, the registration procedure is cumbersome and it must be repeated for each patient. Such a view into the patient would enable surgeons to operate much more precisely by displaying spatial information related to the ongoing procedure. Before introducing six fundamental classes of augmentation technology, we define four relevant properties of medical AR displays.

> *Extra Value from Image Fusion:* Fusing registered images into the same display offers the best of two modalities in the same view. An extra advantage provided by this approach could be a better understanding of the image by visualizing an anatomical context that has not been obvious before. A further advantage concerns the surgical workflow. Currently, each imaging

device introduces another display into the operating room, so the staff spends valuable time finding a useful arrangement of the displays. A single display integrating all data would solve this issue. Each imaging device also introduces its own interaction hardware and graphical user interface, but a unified system could replace the inefficient multitude of interaction systems.

Implicit 3D Interaction: Interaction with three-dimensional (3D) data is a cumbersome task with two-dimensional (2D) displays and 2D interfaces [2], and there is no best practice for 3D user interfaces. AR technology facilitates implicit viewpoint generation by matching the viewport of the eye/endoscope to the viewport of virtual objects. Changing the eye position relative to an object is a natural approach for 3D inspection. 3D user interfaces reveal their power only in tasks that cannot be easily reduced to two dimensions because 2D user interfaces benefit from simplification by dimension reduction and the fact that they are widespread. For example, the placement of implant screws may be improved by 3D user interaction, as the work of Traub et al. [3] suggests.

3D Visualization: Many AR systems allow for stereoscopic data representation. Stereo disparity and motion parallax due to viewpoint changes can give a strong spatial impression of structures. Calvano et al. [4] reported on the positive effects of the stereoscopic view provided by a stereo endoscope for in-utero surgery. This enhanced spatial perception may also be useful in other fields.

Improved Hand-Eye Coordination: A differing position and orientation between image acquisition and visualization may interfere with the hand-eye coordination of the operator, which is a typical situation in minimally invasive surgery. Hanna et al. [5] showed that the position of an endoscope display has a significant impact on the performance of a surgeon during a knotting task. Their experiments suggest the best position of the display is to be in front of the operator at the level of his or her hands. Using *in situ* visualization, there is no offset between working space and visualization, and no mental transformation is necessary to convert the viewed information into hand coordinates.

4.2   AUGMENTED OPTICS

We start with devices that allow for *in situ* visualization, which means that the view is registered to the physical space. Operating microscopes and operating binoculars can be augmented by inserting a semitransparent mirror into the optics. The mirror reflects the virtual image into the optical path of the real image. This allows for high optical quality of real images without further eye-to-display calibration, which is one of the major issues of optical see-through augmentation. Research on augmented optics evolved from stereotaxy in brain surgery in the early 1980s. The first augmented microscope was proposed by Roberts et al. [6] and Hatch et al. [7]. It showed a segmented tumor slice of a computed tomography data set in a monocular operating microscope. This system can be said to be the first operational medical

AR system, and its application area was interventional navigation. The accuracy requirement for the system was 1 mm [8] to be in the same range as the thickness of the CT slice. An average error of 3 mm was measured for re-projection of the contours, which is a remarkable result for a first system, although the ultrasonic tracking did not allow for real-time data acquisition. A change in the position of the operating microscope required approximately 20 s to acquire the new position.

In 1995, Edwards et al. [9] presented their augmented stereoscopic operating microscope for neurosurgical interventions. It allowed for multicolor representation of segmented 3D imaging data as wire frame surface models or labeled 3D points. The interactive update rate of 1–2 Hz was limited by the infrared tracking system. The accuracy of 2–5 mm is in the same range as the system introduced by Friets et al. [8]. In 2000, the group reported on an enhanced version [10] with submillimeter accuracy, which was evaluated in phantom studies, as well as clinical studies for maxillo-facial surgery. The new version also allowed for calibration of different focal lengths to support variable zoom level settings during the augmentation. For ophthalmology, Berger and Shin [11] suggest augmenting angiographic images into a biomicroscope. The system used image-based tracking but no external tracking, which is possible because the retina offers a relatively flat surface that is textured with visible blood vessel structures.

Edwards et al. [12] evaluated the effectiveness of an AR system for microscope-assisted ear, nose, and throat surgery and neurosurgery in a clinical trial with 17 cases. They found that AR improved the procedure in about 30% of the cases the confidence of surgeons was improved, specifically, for three cases with accurate (≤1 mm) registration. AR furthermore helped with complicated cases.

Integrating optical coherence tomography into the optical path of operating microscopes enables the acquisition and visualization of highly detailed surface features. Roodaki et al. [13] used it to display the distance between tools and surfaces during ophthalmic surgery. Claus et al. [14] presented a prototype of a digital surgical microscope setup that enabled surgeons to use 3D monitors instead of binoculars to improve their working conditions during microscope-assisted surgeries. Their system provides depth cues, such as convergence, parallax, and accommodation with the help of optomechanical components, such as tunable lenses and laterally moving pupil apertures for image acquisition, which are controlled by tracking the head and gaze of the operating surgeon.

Birkfellner and colleagues developed an augmented operating binocular for maxillo-facial surgery in 2000 [15,16], which enables augmentation by employing variable zoom and focus as well as customizable eye distances. As opposed to the operating microscopes that are mounted on a swivel arm, operating binoculars are worn by the user.

4.3   HMD-BASED AR SYSTEMS

The first head-mounted display (HMD)-based AR system was described by Ivan Sutherland [17] in 1968. A stereoscopic monochrome HMD combined real and virtual images by means of a semitransparent mirror, which also is referred to as optical see-through HMD. The tracking was performed mechanically. Research on this display was not application driven but aimed at the "ultimate display" (as referred to by Sutherland). Bajura et al. [18] reported in 1992 on their video see-through system for the augmentation of ultrasound (US) images. The system used a magnetic tracking system to determine the pose of a US probe and the HMD. The idea of augmenting live video instead of optical image fusion appears counterproductive at first sight, as it reduces image quality and introduces latency for the real view. However, by this means the real view can be controlled electronically, thus resulting in the following advantages:

Fixed Calibration: No eye-to-display calibration is needed, and only the camera-to-tracker transformation needs to be calculated, which may remain fixed.

Arbitrary Merging: Arbitrary functions between virtual and real objects are possible, as opposed to brightening up the real view by virtual objects in optical overlays. Only video overlay allows for opaque virtual objects, dark virtual objects, and correct color representation of virtual objects.

Relative Lag: By delaying the real view until the data from the tracking system is available, the relative lag between real and virtual objects can be eliminated, as described by Bajura and Neumann [19].

Similar Quality: For the real view, the image quality is limited by the display specifications in a similar way as it is for the rendered objects. Because the color spectrum, brightness, resolution, accommodation, and field of view are the same for real and virtual objects, they can be merged in a more sophisticated way than for optical overlays.

Validation of Merged Images: The overlay is not user dependent, as the generation of the augmentation is already performed in the computer, as opposed to the physical overlay of light in the eye. The resulting image of an optical see-through system is formed on the user's retina and can therefore not be captured. Validation is only possible through subjective feedback while users are interacting with the system.

In 1996, in a continuation of the work of [18], State et al. [20] reported on a system that used 10 frames per second (fps) to create output. While this system facilitates hybrid magnetic and optical tracking for higher accuracy and faster performance, current systems can rely on optical tracking to be used exclusively. The continued system has been evaluated in randomized phantom studies in a needle biopsy experiment [21]. As a result, users hit the targets significantly more accurately using AR guidance compared to standard guidance.

In 2000, Sauer et al. [22] presented a video see-through system that allowed for a synchronized view of real and virtual images in real time (i.e. 30 fps). The system ensures video and tracking data to be from exactly the same point of time by triggering both electronically. Thus, the relative lag is reduced to zero without interpolating tracking data. The system uses inside-out optical tracking, which means that the tracking camera is placed on the HMD to track a reference frame rather than the other way around. This way of tracking allows for very low re-projection errors because the orientation of the head can be computed in a numerically more stable way than with outside-in tracking using the same technology [23] (see Figure 4.1).

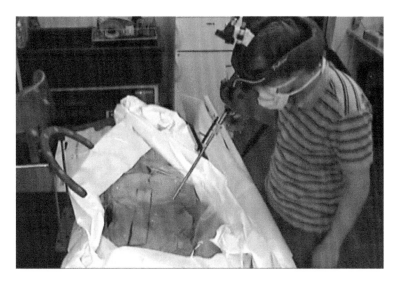

FIGURE 4.1 Video see-through HMD evaluated during cadaver study for image-guided laparoscopic intervention. (From Bichlmeier, C. et al., Contextual anatomic mimesis: Hybrid in-situ visualization method for improving multi-sensory depth perception in medical augmented reality, in *Proceedings of the 6th International Symposium on Mixed and Augmented Reality (ISMAR)*, Nara, Japan, pp. 129–138, November 2007 [24].)

Wright et al. [25] reported in 1995 on optical see-through visualization for medical education. The continuation of the system of Argotti et al. [26] augments anatomical data on a flexible knee joint phantom to teach the dynamic spatial behavior of anatomy. Sielhorst et al. [27] suggested augmentation of recorded expert motions with regard to a simulator phantom to teach medical actions. The system allows for comparative visualization and automatic quantitative comparison of two actions.

Luo and Peli [28] use HMD visualization as an aid for the visually impaired rather than for supporting physicians. They use an optical see-through system to superimpose contour images from an attached camera. The system is meant to help patients with tunnel vision to improve visual search performance.

Rolland and Fuchs [29] discuss in detail the advantages and shortcomings of optical and video see-through technology. Keller et al. [30] also compare the two competing HMD designs with a focus on medical use. They have identified inaccurate eye-to-display calibration to be the biggest show-stopper for optical see-through technology, followed by the inability to block environment light. While video-see-through designs overcome the aforementioned problems, their drawbacks are limited resolution, system complexity, and ergonomics. Detailed review on designs for optical see-through displays is provided by Kress and Starner [31]. The suitability for surgical use was recently tested by Gasques Rodrigues et al. [32].

Due to its small form factor, monocular, optical see-through HMDs have been evaluated as a personal information display for medical practice [33]. The authors found that the display has clear utility for handsfree communication, information retrieval from the hospital system, and internet resources. Tepper et al. [34] found that an untethered, headworn computer with stereoscopic Optical See-Through (OST) display can improve decision making and the surgical workflow during plastic surgery interventions. The device can seamlessly and in a sterile fashion integrate 3D information, such as holograms of virtual surgical plans, 3D models, and digital implants into the surgeon's operative visual field. In contrast to previous research, the authors did not aim to co-locate the anatomical structures with the patient, which avoids complex display calibration and patient registration procedures. With a similar objective, Quian et al. [35] evaluated three state-of-the art OST HMDs for object-anchored virtual 2D displays in regard to text readability, contrast perception, task load, frame rate, and system lag. They argue that the use of HMDs allows surgeons to optimize the arrangement of information displays to best suit the surgical procedure.

4.4   AR WINDOWS

The third type of device that allows for *in situ* visualization is an AR window. Masutani et al. [36] described a system in 1995 with a semitransparent mirror that is placed between the viewer and the augmented object. An autostereoscopic screen displays the virtual objects. However, this reduces the resolution or limits the effective viewing range of the user. On the other hand, no tracking system is necessary in this setup to maintain the registration after it has been established once. The correct alignment is independent of the point of view. Therefore, these autostereoscopic AR windows involve no lag when the viewer is moving. The first system could not compute the integral photography dynamically, and it had to be precomputed for a certain data set. In 2001, Liao et al. [37] proposed a medical AR window based on integral videography that could handle dynamic scenes for a navigation scenario, in which the position of an instrument was supposed to be visualized in the scene. Tran et al. [38] also developed an AR window based on integral videography for oral surgeries. Their system operates nearly in real time with frame rates ranging from 5 fps for complex anatomical model overlays to 80 fps for simple geometries. Blackwell et al. [39] presented an AR window using a semitransparent mirror for merging the real view with virtual images from an ordinary monitor. This technology requires tracked shutter glasses for the correct alignment of augmented objects and stereo vision, but it can handle dynamic images for navigation purposes at a high resolution and update rate.

For *in situ* visualization, AR windows seem to be a perfect match to the operating room at first sight, as current wearable displays cannot be sterilized and are not sufficiently ergonomic to be worn during long surgeries. However, all known AR window designs also introduce trade-offs: auto-stereoscopic displays suffer from poorer image quality in comparison to other display technologies. In principle, they offer a visualization for multiple users. However, this feature introduces another trade-off regarding image quality. Shutter glasses or polarization glasses, as those used in the system introduced by Goebbels et al. [40] weigh less than an HMD but limit the viewing angle of the surgeon and still introduce an additional object in the workflow. Nonautostereoscopic AR windows need to track the position of the user's eye in addition to the position of the patient and the AR window, which introduces another source of error. Wesarg et al. [41] suggest a monoscopic AR window based on a transparent display. The design offers a compact setup, as no mirror is used, and no special glasses are required. However, it cannot display stereoscopic images, and only one eye can see a correct image overlay. Because no mirror is used, the foci of the virtual and real image are at completely different distances.

All AR window designs must take into account distracting reflections from surrounding light sources. Last but not least, the display must be placed between the patient and the viewer, although this can obstruct the physicians' working area.

4.5 AUGMENTED MONITORS AND ENDOSCOPES

In this section, we cluster all systems that augment video images on ordinary monitors.

The point of view in an augmented monitor system is defined by an additional tracked video camera. In 1993, Lorensen et al. [42] published their live video augmentation of segmented MRI data on a monitor.

Sato et al. [43] visualized segmented 3D US images registered to video camera images on a monitor for image guidance of breast cancer surgery. Nicolau et al. [44] described a camera-based AR system using markers that are detected in the camera image. The system aims at minimally invasive liver ablation. Kockro et al. [45] integrated a lipstick-sized video camera into a tracked surgical probe to augment preoperative planning data for neurosurgery guidance and navigation on the video image that is displayed on an LCD screen. They evaluated their system intraoperatively on 12 cases and found that surgeons felt more confident because they could better understand the spatial relations of critical structures.

Augmented monitors do not offer *in situ* visualization, but their strength is that users need not wear an HMD or glasses, and different people can share the visualization at the same time. As a special case, augmenting data into endoscopes does not necessarily introduce additional hardware into the workflow of navigated interventions.

Video endoscopy permits different team members to see the endoscopic view simultaneously. It enables an assistant to position the endoscope while the operating surgeon can use both hands for the procedure. This feature opened the field of endoscopic surgeries. Although endoscopic augmentation seems to be a straightforward step, it has only been developed as recently as the late 1990s by Freysinger et al. [46] for ENT surgery and Shahidi et al. [47] for brain surgery. Scholz et al. [48] presented a navigation system for neurosurgery based on processed images. Shahidi and Scholz used infrared tracking technology and a rigid endoscope, while Freysinger's system used magnetic tracking. To reliably track a flexible endoscope, Feuerstein et al. [49] combined optical and electromagnetic tracking. Their approach combines the accuracy of optical tracking with the ability to track objects inside the patient. Mourgues and Coste-Maniere [50] describe endoscope augmentation in a robotic surgery system in which the tracking is done by the robot's arm, so no additional tracking system is necessary. Figure 4.2 illustrates the concept of augmented endoscopes for robotic surgery.

In recent years, the camera resolution and image quality has been constantly improved, reaching 4K for monoscopic cameras and full HD for stereoscopic systems. Bernhardt et al. [52] provided an overview on the current state of research for endoscopic augmentation. They state two main remaining challenges to bring laparoscopic AR into medical practice. First, registering preoperative and

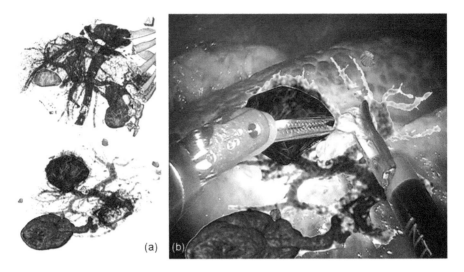

FIGURE 4.2 Augmented endoscope for robotic liver surgery: (a) 3D volume rendering of a hepatic tumor and (b) fusion of 3D, reconstructed images and endoscope image. (From Volonte, F. et al., *J. Hepato-Biliary-Pancreat. Sci.*, 18, 506–509, 2011 [51].)

intraoperative images from multiple modalities with sufficient accuracy is difficult due to deformations between acquisitions and missing correspondences between modalities. Second, maintaining accuracy during the intervention is difficult due to highly complex, dynamic scenes. They argued that the lack of accuracy introduces a clear need for verification; however, most studies only work on synthetic data sets with limited realism.

4.6 AUGMENTED MEDICAL IMAGING

Augmented imaging devices can be defined as imaging devices that allow for an augmentation of their images without a tracking system. The alignment is guaranteed by their geometry. A construction for the overlay of fluoroscopic images on the scene was proposed by Navab et al. [53] in 1999. An ordinary mirror is inserted into the X-ray path of a mobile C-arm. A C-arm is a medically widespread X-ray imaging device with a C-shaped gantry, which makes it possible to place a video camera that records light following the same path as the X-rays. Thus, it is possible to register both images by estimating the homography between them, without spatial knowledge of the objects in the image. The correct camera position is determined once during the construction of the system. The system provides augmented images without continuous X-ray exposure for both the patient and the physician. The overlay is correct unless the patient moves relative to the fluoroscope, in which case a new X-ray image must be taken. The authors evaluated the accuracy and clinical feasibility of the camera-augmented C-arm [54] and showed that the accuracy of the X-ray overlays is approximately 0.5 mm after calibration. They also studied the clinical feasibility for implant placement through cadaver studies and simulated procedures for intramedullary nail locking and pedicle screw placement.

They could significantly reduce the radiation time and dose for these procedures with the augmented imaging device.

In 2000, Masamune et al. [55] proposed an image overlay system that could display CT slices *in situ*. A semitransparent mirror allows for a direct view of the patient as well as a view of the aligned CT slice. The viewer may move freely while the CT slice remains registered without any tracking. The overlaid image is generated by a screen that is placed on top of the imaging plane of the scanner. The semitransparent mirror is placed in the plane that halves the angle between the slice and the screen. The resulting overlay is correct from any point of view up to a similarity transform that must be calibrated during the construction of the system. The system is restricted to a single slice per position of the patient. For any different slice, the patient must be moved on the bed. Fischer et al. [56] extended this principle to magnetic resonance imaging. A similar principle has been applied to create an augmented US echography device. Stetten and Chib [57] proposed the overlay of US images on the patient using a semitransparent mirror and a small screen that is attached to the ultrasound probe. The mirror is placed on the plane that halves the angle between the screen and the B-scan plane of ultrasonic measurements. Similar to the tomographic reflection of CT or MRI slices, it allows for *in situ* visualization without tracking. In addition to real-time images, it allows for arbitrary slice views, as the US probe can be freely moved.

4.7   PROJECTIONS ON THE PATIENT

An AR system can provide *in situ* visualization without looking through an additional device by projecting data directly onto the patient. If the visualization is meant to be on the skin rather than beneath, the user need not be tracked. Therefore, such a visualization can be used for multiple users.

The simplicity of this kind of setup, however, introduces certain limitations as a compromise. Glossop and wang [58] suggested a laser projector that makes trajectories of the laser appear as lines due to the persistence of vision effect. The images are limited to a certain number of bright monochrome lines or dots and non-raster images. The system also includes an infrared laser for interactive patient digitization. Sasama et al. [59] used two lasers for mere guidance. Each of these lasers creates a plane by means of a moving mirror system. The intersection of both planes is used to guide laparoscopic instruments in two ways. The intersecting lines of the laser on the patient mark the spot of interest, such as an incision point. The laser plane scan can also be used to determine an orientation in space. The system manipulates the two laser planes in such a way that their intersecting line defines the desired orientation. If both lasers are projected in parallel to the instrument, the latter has the correct orientation. The system can only guide instruments to points and lines in space, but it cannot show contours or more complex structures.

Volonte et al. [51] projected 3D reconstructions from CT data onto patients for navigation during laparoscopic interventions to highlight regions of interest and marked pathologies. Such image overlays on the patient are beneficial during port placement [60] and needle insertion [61] (see Figure 4.3). A drawback of projections on the patients is that the viewpoint of the surgeon differs from the projector, which

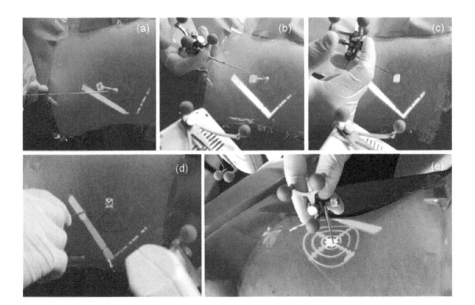

FIGURE 4.3 Percutaneous needle guidance through projections on the patient: (a) tip alignment, (b) shaft alignment, (c) aligned needle at point of puncture, (d) depth guidance, and (e) target visualization. (From Gavaghan, K., *Int. J. Comput. Assist. Radiol. Surg.*, 7, 547–556, 2012 [61].)

limits the correct augmentation in terms of perspective. Furthermore, such systems are not able to display stereoscopic images, which limits depth perception.

4.8 SUMMARY

There is no silver bullet in medical AR visualization and we do not expect there will be one. As AR visualization is meant to make the work of the physician easier, the displaying device must fit seamlessly into the physician's workflow. Therefore, we believe that the best displaying technology is the one that fits best into the environment while conveying the missing pieces of information.

REFERENCES

1. H. Steinhaus. Sur la localisation au moyen des rayons x. *Comptes Rendus de L'Academie des Science*, 206:1473–1475, 1938.
2. D. A. Bowman, E. Kruijff, J. J. LaViola, and I. Poupyrev. *3D User Interfaces: Theory and Practice*, Addison Wesley Longman Publishing, Redwood City, CA, 2004.
3. J. Traub, P. Stefan, S. M. Heining, T. Sielhorst, C. Riquarts, E. Euler, and N. Navab. Hybrid navigation interface for orthopedic and trauma surgery. In *Proceedings of the MICCAI*, Copenhagen, Denmark, pp. 373–380, 2006.
4. C. J. Calvano, M. E. Moran, L. D. Tackett, P. P. Reddy, K. E. Boyle, and M. M. Pankratov. New visualization techniques for in utero surgery: Amnioscopy with a three-dimensional head-mounted display and a computer-controlled endoscope. *Journal of Endourology*, 12(5):407–410, 1998.

5. G. B. Hanna, S. M. Shimi, and A. Cuschieri. Task performance in endoscopic surgery is influenced by location of the image display. *Annals of Surgery*, 227(4):481–484, 1998.

6. D. W. Roberts, J. W. Strohbehn, J. F. Hatch, W. Murray, and H. Kettenberger. A frameless stereotaxic integration of computerized tomographic imaging and the operating microscope. *Journal of Neurosurgery*, 65(4):545–549, 1986.

7. J. F. Hatch, J. W. Strohbehn, and D. W. Roberts. Reference-display system for the integration of CT scanning and the operating microscope. In *Proceedings of the Eleventh Annual Northeast Bioengineering Conference*, Institute of Electrical and Electronics Engineers, New York, 1985.

8. E. M. Friets, J. W. Strohbehn, J. F. Hatch, and D. W. Roberts. A frameless stereotaxic operating microscope for neurosurgery. *IEEE Transactions on Biomedical Engineering*, 36(6):608–617, 1989.

9. P. J. Edwards, D. L. G. Hill, D. J. Hawkes, and A. C. F. Colchester. Neurosurgical guidance using the stereo microscope. In *Proceedings of the Computer Vision, Virtual Reality and Robotics in Medicine*, Springer-Verlag, Berlin, Germany, 1995.

10. A. P. King, P. J. Edwards, C. R. Maurer, Jr., D. A. de Cunha, D. J. Hawkes, D. L. G. Hill, R. P. Gaston et al. Design and evaluation of a system for microscope-assisted guided interventions. *IEEE Transactions on Medical Imaging*, 19(11):1082–1093, 2000.

11. J. W. Berger and D. S. Shin. Computer-vision-enabled augmented reality fundus biomicroscopy. *Ophthalmology*, 106(10):1935–1941, 1999.

12. P. J. Edwards, L. G. Johnson, D. J. Hawkes, M. R. Fenlon, A. J. Strong, and M. J. Gleeson. Clinical experience and perception in stereo augmented reality surgical navigation. In *Proceedings of the MIAR*, Springer-Verlag, Berlin, Germany, pp. 369–376, 2004.

13. H. Roodaki, K. Filippatos, A. Eslami, and N. Navab. Introducing augmented reality to optical coherence tomography in ophthalmic microsurgery. In *Proceedings of the ISMAR*, IEEE, Fukuoka, Japan, pp. 1–6, 2015.

14. D. Claus, C. Reichert, and A. Herkommer. Focus and perspective adaptive digital surgical microscope: Optomechanical design and experimental implementation. *Journal of Biomedical Optics*, 22(5):7–13, 2017.

15. W. Birkfellner, K. Huber, F. Watzinger, M. Figl, F. Wanschitz, R. Hanel, D. Rafolt, R. Ewers, and H. Bergmann. Development of the varioscope AR—A see-through HMD for computer-aided surgery. In *Proceedings of the ISAR*, IEEE Computer Society Press, pp. 54–59, 2000.

16. M. Figl, C. Ede, J. Hummel, F. Wanschitz, R. Ewers, H. Bergmann, and W. Birkfellner. A fully automated calibration method for an optical see-through head-mounted operating microscope with variable zoom and focus. *IEEE Transactions on Medical Imaging*, 24(11):1492–1499, 2005.

17. I. Sutherland. A head-mounted three dimensional display. In *Proceedings of the Fall Joint Computer Conference*, pp. 757–764, 1968.

18. M. Bajura, H. Fuchs, and R. Ohbuchi. Merging virtual objects with the real world: Seeing ultrasound imagery within the patient. In *Proceedings of the Conference on Computer Graphics and Interactive Techniques*, ACM, New York, Vol. 26, pp. 203–210, 1992.

19. M. Bajura and U. Neumann. Dynamic registration correction in video-based augmented reality systems. *IEEE Computer Graphics and Applications*, 15(5):52–60, 1995.

20. A. State, M. A. Livingston, W. F. Garrett, G. Hirota, M. C. Whitton, E. D. Pisano, and H. Fuchs. Technologies for augmented reality systems: Realizing ultrasound-guided needle biopsies. In *Proceedings of the SIGGRAPH'96*, ACM, New York, pp. 439–446, 1996.

21. M. Rosenthal, A. State, J. Lee, G. Hirota, J. Ackerman, K. Keller, E. D. Pisano, M. Jirotek, K. Muller, and H. Fuchs. Augmented reality guidance for needle biopsies: An initial randomized, controlled trial in phantoms. *Medical Image Analysis*, 6(3):313–320, 2002.

22. F. Sauer, F. Wenzel, S. Vogt, Y. Tao, Y. Genc, and A. BaniHashemi. Augmented workspace: Designing an AR testbed. In *Proceedings of the ISAR*, Munich, Germany, pp. 47–53, 2000.

23. W. A. Hoff and T. L. Vincent. Analysis of head pose accuracy in augmented reality. *IEEE Transactions on Visualization and Computer Graphics*, 6(4):319–334, 2000.

24. C. Bichlmeier, F. Wimmer, S. M. Heining, and N. Navab. Contextual anatomic mimesis: Hybrid in-situ visualization method for improving multi-sensory depth perception in medical augmented reality. In *Proceedings of the 6th International Symposium on Mixed and Augmented Reality (ISMAR)*, Nara, Japan, pp. 129–138, November 2007.

25. D. L. Wright, J. P. Rolland, and A. R. Kancherla. Using virtual reality to teach radiographic positioning. *Radiologic Technology*, 66(4):233–238, 1995.

26. Y. Argotti, L. Davis, V. Outters, and J. P. Rolland. Dynamic superimposition of synthetic objects on rigid and simple-deformable real objects. *Computers & Graphics*, 26(6):919–930, 2002.

27. T. Sielhorst, T. Blum, and N. Navab. Synchronizing 3d movements for quantitative comparison and simultaneous visualization of actions. In *Proceedings of the ISMAR*, IEEE Computer Society, Washington, DC, 2005.

28. G. Luo and E. Peli. Use of an augmented-vision device for visual search by patients with tunnel vision. *Investigative Ophthalmology & Visual Science*, 47(9):4152–4159, 2006.

29. J. P. Rolland and H. Fuchs. Optical versus video see-through headmounted displays in medical visualization. *Presence*, 9:287–309, 2000.

30. K. Keller, A. State, and H. Fuchs. Head mounted displays for medical use. *Journal of Display Technology*, 4(4):468–472, 2008.

31. B. Kress and T. Starner. A review of head-mounted displays (HMD) technologies and applications for consumer electronics. In *Proceedings of the SPIE*, 2013.

32. D. Gasques Rodrigues, A. Jain, S. R. Rick, L. Shangley, P. Suresh, and N. Weibel. Exploring mixed reality in specialized surgical environments. In *CHI 2017—Late-Breaking Work*, ACM, New York, pp. 2591–2598, May 2017.

33. O. J. Muensterer, M. Lacher, C. Zoeller, M. Bronstein, and J. Kübler. Google Glass in pediatric surgery: An exploratory study. *International Journal of Surgery*, 12(4):281–289, 2014.

34. O. M. Tepper, H. L. Rudy, A. Lefkowitz, K. A. Weimer, S. M. Marks, C. S. Stern, and E. S. Garfein. Mixed reality with HoloLens: Where virtual reality meets augmented reality in the operating room. *Plastic and Reconstructive Surgery*, 140(5):1066–1070, 2017.

35. L. Qian, A. Barthel, A. Johnson, G. Osgood, P. Kazanzides, N. Navab, and B. Fuerst. Comparison of optical see-through head-mounted displays for surgical interventions with object-anchored 2D-display. *International Journal of Computer Assisted Radiology and Surgery*, 12(6):901–910, 2017.

36. Y. Masutani, M. Iwahara, O. Samuta, Y. Nishi, N. Suzuki, M. Suzuki, T. Dohi, H. Iseki, and K. Takakura. Development of integral photography-based enhanced reality visualization system for surgical support. *Proceedings of the ISCAS*, 95:16–17, 1995.

37. H. Liao, S. Nakajima, M. Iwahara, E. Kobayashi, I. Sakuma, N. Yahagi, and T. Dohi. Intra-operative real-time 3-D information display system based on integral videography. In *Proceedings of the MICCAI*, Springer-Verlag, Berlin, Germany, pp. 392–400, 2001.

38. H. H. Tran, H. Suenaga, K. Kuwana, K. Masamune, T. Dohi, S. Nakajima, and H. Liao. Augmented reality system for oral surgery using 3D auto stereoscopic visualization. In *Proceedings of the MICCAI*, Toronto, Canada, pp. 81–88, 2011.

39. M. Blackwell, C. Nikou, A. M. Di Gioia, and T. Kanade. An image overlay system for medical data visualization. In *Proceedings of the MICCAI*, Springer-Verlag, Berlin, Germany, pp. 232–240, 1998.

40. G. Goebbels, K. Troche, M. Braun, A. Ivanovic, A. Grab, K. von Lübtow, R. Sader, F. Zeilhofer, K. Albrecht, and K. Praxmarer. Arsys–tricorder—Development of an augmented reality system for intraoperative navigation in maxillofacial surgery. In *Proceedings of the ISMAR*, 2003.

41. S. Wesarg, E. A. Firle, B. Schwald, H. Seibert, P. Zogal, and S. Roeddiger. Accuracy of needle implantation in brachytherapy using a medical ar system: A phantom study. In *Proceedings of the SPIE*, Vol. 5367, pp. 341–352, 2004.

42. W. Lorensen, H. Cline, C. Nafis, R. Kikinis, D. Altobelli, L. Gleason, G. E. Co, and N. Y. Schenectady. Enhancing reality in the operating room. In *IEEE Conference on Visualization*, pp. 410–415, 1993.

43. Y. Sato, M. Nakamoto, Y. Tamaki, T. Sasama, I. Sakita, Y. Nakajima, M. Monden, and S. Tamura. Image guidance of breast cancer surgery using 3-d ultrasound images and augmented reality visualization. *IEEE Transactions on Medical Imaging*, 17(5):681–693, 1998.

44. S. Nicolau, X. Pennec, L. Soler, and N. Ayache. An accuracy certified augmented reality system for therapy guidance. In *Proceedings of the 8th European Conference on Computer Vision (ECCV 04)*, Springer-Verlag, Berlin, Germany, pp. 79–91, 2004.

45. R. A. Kockro, Y. T. Tsai, I. Ng, P. Hwang, C. Zhu, K. Agusanto, L. X. Hong, and L. Serra. Dex-ray: Augmented reality neurosurgical navigation with a hand-held video probe. *Neurosurgery*, 65(4):795–808, 2009.

46. W. Freysinger, A. R. Gunkel, and W. F. Thumfart. Image-guided endoscopic ent surgery. *European Archives of Otorhinolaryngology*, 254(7):343–346, 1997.

47. R. Shahidi, B. Wang, M. Epitaux, R. Grzeszczuk, and J. Adler. Volumetric image guidance via a stereotactic endoscope. In *Proceedings of the MICCAI*, Cambridge, MA, pp. 241–252, 1998.

48. M. Scholz, W. Konen, S. Tombrock, B. Fricke, and L. Adams. Development of an endoscopic navigation system based on digital image processing. *Computer Aided Surgery*, 3:134–143, 1998.

49. M. Feuerstein, T. Reichl, J. Vogel, J. Traub, and N. Navab. Magneto-optical tracking of flexible laparoscopic ultrasound: Model-based online detection and correction of magnetic tracking errors. *IEEE Transactions on Medical Imaging*, 28(6):951–967, 2009.

50. F. Mourgues and E. Coste-Maniere. Flexible calibration of actuated stereoscopic endoscope for overlay in robot assisted surgery. In *Proceedings of the MICCAI*, Springer-Verlag, Berlin, Germany, pp. 25–34, 2002.

51. F. Volonte, F. Pugin, P. Bucher, M. Sugimoto, O. Ratib, and P. Morel. Augmented reality and image overlay navigation with OsiriX in laparoscopic and robotic surgery: Not only a matter of fashion. *Journal of Hepato-Biliary-Pancreatic Sciences*, 18(4):506–509, 2011.

52. S. Bernhardt, S. A. Nicolau, L. Soler, and C. Doignon. The status of augmented reality in laparoscopic surgery as of 2016. *Medical Image Analysis*, 37:66–90, 2017.

53. N. Navab, M. Mitschke, and A. Bani-Hashemi. Merging visible and invisible: Two camera-augmented mobile C-arm (CAMC) applications. In *Proceedings of the IEEE and ACM Int'l Workshop on Augmented Reality*, pp. 134–141, 1999.

54. N. Navab, S. M. Heining, and J. Traub. Camera augmented mobile C-arm (CAMC): Calibration, accuracy study, and clinical applications. *IEEE Transactions on Medical Imaging*, 29(7):1412–1423, 2010.

55. K. Masamune, Y. Masutani, S. Nakajima, I. Sakuma, T. Dohi, H. Iseki, and K. Takakura. Three-dimensional slice image overlay system with accurate depth perception for surgery. In *Proceedings of the MICCAI*, Springer-Verlag, Berlin, Germany, pp. 395–402, 2000.

56. G. S. Fischer, A. Deguet, D. Schlattman, L. Fayad, S. J. Zinreich, R. H. Taylor, and G. Fichtinger. Image overlay guidance for MRI arthrography needle insertion. *Computer Aided Surgery*, 12(1):2–4, 2007.

57. G. D. Stetten and V. S. Chib. Overlaying ultrasound images on direct vision. *Journal Ultrasound in Medicine*, 20:235–240, 2001.

58. N. Glossop and Z. Wang. Laser projection augmented reality system for computer assisted surgery. In *Proceedings of the MICCAI*, Springer-Verlag, Berlin, Germany, pp. 239–246, 2003.

59. T. Sasama, T. Ochi, S. Tamura, N. Sugano, Y. Sato, Y. Momoi, T. Koyama et al. A novel laser guidance system for alignment of linear surgical tools: Its principles and performance evaluation as a man-machine system. In *Proceedings of the MICCAI*, Springer-Verlag, Berlin, Germany, pp. 125–132, 2002.

60. M. Sugimoto, H. Yasuda, K. Koda, M. Suzuki, M. Yamazaki, T. Tezuka, C. Kosugi et al. Image overlay navigation by markerless surface registration in gastrointestinal, hepatobiliary and pancreatic surgery. *Journal of Hepato-Biliary-Pancreatic Sciences*, 17(5):629–636, 2010.

61. K. Gavaghan, T. Oliveira-Santos, M. Peterhans, M. Reyes, H. Kim, S. Anderegg, and S. Weber. Evaluation of a portable image overlay projector for the visualisation of surgical navigation data: Phantom studies. *International Journal of Computer Assisted Radiology and Surgery*, 7(4):547–556, 2012.

5 Active Sensorimotor Augmentation in Robotics-Assisted Surgical Systems

Seyed Farokh Atashzar, Michael Naish, and Rajni V. Patel

CONTENTS

5.1 INTRODUCTION

In this chapter, we investigate the concepts of active sensory augmentation and active motor augmentation for robotic surgery. Surgical robots can provide surgeons with supplementary, real-time perceptual information about a surgical procedure (sensory augmentation) to indirectly enhance the quality of surgery. Also, the robots can directly correct and enhance the manipulations generated by the surgeon (motor augmentation) to minimize errors and increase the quality of surgery.

Sensory augmentation has been conducted through visual, auditory, and haptic cueing channels. For example, vision-based sensory augmentation has been used to help surgeons navigate surgical tools with respect to registered preoperative medical images that are partially superimposed with intraoperative information. It should be noted that vision-based and auditory-based sensory augmentation are delivered through passive (not actuated) cueing channels, while kinesthetic and kinematic augmentations are delivered through active motorized components of the system. In general, the goal of sensory augmentation is to provide superior awareness of interaction with tissue during surgery.

In addition to sensory augmentation, active robotic technologies have been used to augment motor control capabilities of surgeons. An example is tremor-cancellation mechatronic devices that are designed to compensate for surgeons' natural hand tremors during delicate microsurgeries. Another example of motor augmentation is workspace down-scaling techniques in master-slave telerobotic surgical systems for reducing the burden of fine motor control on surgeons. In addition to the examples mentioned above, force-enabled virtual guidance (which is an active sensory augmentation scheme) and haptics-based, forbidden-region virtual fixtures (an active motor augmentation scheme) have been used in the literature to provide guidance and avoidance, respectively, based on patient-specific anatomy and surgical trajectories, during robotics-assisted surgeries. In this chapter, the use of active sensorimotor augmentation techniques is investigated for three categories of computerized robotic systems.

5.1.1 Telerobotics-Assisted Surgical (Tele-RAS) Systems

The first category of computerized robotic technologies used for surgical procedures is Tele-RAS, which are composed of two main modules, namely, the Master Robotic Console (MRC) and the Slave Robotic Console (SRC). The MRC is, in fact, the surgeon-side unit with which a surgeon can generate appropriate motion trajectories to be conducted by the SRC on the patient's body. The SRC is a patient-side unit that is primarily designed to accurately follow the movement commands generated by the surgeon. One of the most successful commercialized examples of Tele-RAS systems is the da Vinci Surgical System, which is a minimally-invasive telerobotic system, made by Intuitive Surgical Inc. (Sunnyvale, California, United States). The two consoles of the da Vinci system are connected through a dedicated, bilateral, computerized communication architecture. This computer-mediated connection separates the commands generated by the surgeon and the actions applied on the surgical side and allows for bilateral augmentation of sensorimotor signals. Any trajectory generated by the surgeon can be monitored, processed, and analyzed on–the fly. Tremor filtering and motion scaling are two standard techniques used in Tele-RAS systems to enhance the motor commands of the surgeons [1–3].

5.1.2   Ungrounded Portable Hand-Held Robotics-Assisted Surgical (UPH-RAS) Systems

The second category of computerized robotic technology used for surgical procedures is UPH-RAS. This technology is composed of a light-weight, portable, actuated, hand-held device that does not have a grounded kinematic chain. An example of the use of this technology is to provide a surgeon with vibrotactile cueing signals to augment the perception of the surgeon during procedures such as brachytherapy and needle biopsy [4,5] to help them during tool navigation and to allow them to provide enhanced control of needle deflection. In addition to sensory augmentation, this technology can provide actuation between the point that is held by the surgeon and the point that is in contact with tissue (i.e., serial actuation), which can augment the fine motor control of surgeons. Three examples are provided below.

The first example of the motor augmentation functionality of this technology is compensation for the high-frequency, low-amplitude hand tremor of surgeons during delicate surgical tasks such as vitreoretinal microsurgeries, membrane peeling procedures, and intraocular laser surgeries. In this regard, a successful example is the MICRON system [6–8]. The second example of the motor augmentation functionality of this technology is providing superimposed rotational actuation to compensate for needle bending during insertion into soft tissue for biopsy and brachytherapy procedures [9]. The third example for motor augmentation functionality is retracting the rotary surgical blade in the axial direction when the tool reaches a specified forbidden region, registered with intraoperative maps. This approach has been used in the Navio™ system, from Blue Belt Technologies Inc., Plymouth, MN, USA. The Navio™ system is commercialized for bone resection and preparation for unicondylar knee arthroplasty [10].

5.1.3   Grounded Cooperatively-Actuated Hand-Held Robotics-Assisted Surgical (GCH-RAS) Systems

The third category of computerized robotic technology used for surgical procedures is GCH-RAS systems. This technology is an interactive robotic device that has a grounded kinematic chain. The end-effector of the robot is connected to a surgical tool and provides a sensorized gripping mechanism for the surgeon. The mechanism measures force applied by the surgeon as an indication of the intended motion profile. As a result, the robot can detect the surgeon's intention and can react to the intended motions by providing corrective forces to enhance the surgical outcomes. Consequently, the final motion of the tool will be affected by both the actuation provided by the surgeon and the one provided by the robotic system. The cooperative control architecture of this technology is usually a composite method. It includes

(a) an admittance control technique to convert the measured forces generated by the surgeon to appropriate actions and (b) a corrective algorithm, such as a virtual fixture, to assist the surgeon in following a registered surgical trajectory. This technology realizes a form of intelligent cooperation between the robot and the surgeon and has been reported as a "very convenient and natural [11] form of control."

An example of a GCH-RAS system is the Steady-Hand Robotic system (developed at John Hopkins University), which was designed to provide "smooth, tremor-free and precise motion control and force scaling" in submillimeter surgical tasks [12]. The second generation of the Steady-Hand Robotic system is called Eye-Robot-I and was reported in [13] to make the use more ergonomically convenient for surgeons and to meet accuracy and safety requirements during vitreoretinal surgeries. The manipulator and the force sensing unit of the system were improved in the third generation of the Steady-Hand Robotic system, which was named Eye-Robot-II [14]. The Eye-Robot-II was equipped with a sensitive force sensor and a "guided cooperative control method" that was used to enforce limits of interaction forces and assist the surgeon in "manipulating tissue in the direction of least resistance" during challenging tasks, such as retinal membrane peeling procedures [14].

In addition to microsurgeries, the GCH-RAS systems have been used for orthopedic surgeries to assist with bone milling procedures [15,16]. In this regard, the Makoplasty system (from Stryker, Orlando, FL) [17] is a commercially-available system that is designed for total knee replacement, total hip replacement, and partial knee replacement procedures. In addition, the Acrobot system (from Acrobot Company Ltd., London, UK) is designed for total knee replacement procedures [18]. These robots are based on a "co-manipulation concept," whereby the surgeon provides the needed maneuvers for conducting the milling procedure, while the robot provides a haptics enabled forbidden region to stop the milling tool from penetrating into a predefined three-dimensional (3D) surgical plane. In other words, to preserve the bone tissue and to accurately prepare the surface for the replacement phase of the operation, the robot does not allow the surgeon to mill tissues beyond the predefined surgical plane. With the use of an optical tracking system during surgery, the geometry of the 3D plane is registered with the 3D scans of the patient's anatomy (acquired prior to the operation) to enhance accuracy and safety.

5.2   MOTOR AUGMENTATION

Using robotics-assisted surgical systems, it is possible to enhance and correct motor commands generated by surgeons directly. In this regard, (a) motion scaling (to enhance fine motor control of surgeons), (b) motion filtering (to eliminate the effects of surgeon's hand tremors), (c) motion compensation (to minimize the effects of movements of physiological organs), and (d) motion restriction using haptics-enabled forbidden-region virtual fixtures are several examples of motor augmentation realized by computerized robotic systems for surgical operations.

5.2.1 Motion Filtering and Motion Scaling

Using the filtering scheme, first, the high-frequency components of the motion, which are mainly result from physiological and fatigue-related hand tremors of surgeons, can be estimated. These components can then (a) be excluded from the trajectory that is assigned to the SRC in Tele-RAS systems [1], or (b) be compensated using UPH-RAS systems [6], or (c) be restricted using GCH-RAS systems [12]. Motion filtering can significantly reduce the risk factors associated with a surgeon's hand tremor during delicate surgery.

In addition to tremor cancellation, motion scaling can also be achieved using robotics-assisted surgical systems. Based on this feature, the movements generated by the surgeon can be scaled down for delicate surgical tasks. Motion scaling helps surgeons to use their large, comfortable workspace to conduct fine manipulations in a scaled-down region that includes the surgical site. Using the possibility of movement filtering and scaling, the motion applied to the tissue is smoother and safer. This is a significant need for delicate surgeries such as microsurgeries (e.g., vitreoretinal surgeries and neurosurgeries). It has been shown that motion scaling and tremor filtering are two essential factors that result in enhanced dexterity and can significantly improve the performance of surgeons in the conduction of delicate operations in comparison to manual surgeries [1,2,19].

5.2.1.1 Technical Challenges in Motion Filtering

A technical challenge associated with motion filtering in surgical robotics is to accurately extract the involuntary physiological motions of surgeons while imposing minimum latency for high-quality augmentation of motor precision. Slow filters that cause significant phase shifts cannot be used for appropriately counteracting motions associated with hand tremors and can also affect the quality of visuomotor synchrony. In most of commercialized Tele-RAS systems that operate on relatively large scales, conventional linear low-pass filters have been used to eliminate physiological hand tremor. In this regard, filtering at 6 Hz has been suggested to improve the performance during robotics-assisted surgeries. However, for microsurgeries (such as ophthalmic surgery, vitreoretinal surgery, microvascular surgery, and neurosurgery) conducted by Tele-RAS or UPH-RAS systems, the estimation of and compensation for physiological hand tremor is very challenging because the amplitude of the tremor is comparable with the needed accuracy of the operation. As an example, it has been reported that for telerobotics assisted vitreoretinal surgeries, tip positioning accuracy of 10 μm may be needed [20]. To deal with this issue, adaptive filters have been proposed in the literature. The technique mentioned above utilizes recursive algorithms to adaptively model and extract the physiological hand tremors of surgeons. In this regard, algorithms that function based on a Fourier Linear Combiner (FLC) have attracted a great deal of interest for extracting hand tremors while imposing minimum latency [21,22].

Among the developed FLC-based adaptive filters, a Band-limited Multiple Fourier Linear Combiner (B-MFLC) technique [22] has demonstrated good potential in characterizing physiological hand tremors, particularly for surgical applications. Several variations of BMFLC have been recently proposed in the literature to enhance the performance of the filtering technique further. In this regard, a BMFLC-Kalman filter technique is proposed in [23] to enhance the performance of the filter. In addition, an Enhanced-BMFLC (E-BMFLC) technique has been reported in [24] which is designed to enrich the embedded harmonic model of the filter and manipulate the memory of the algorithm to enhance the accuracy and reduce the sensitivity to parameter tuning, particularly in the presence of quasiperiodic tremors.

In addition to the challenges associated with the design of the filtering scheme, there are several mechatronic challenges with the design of tremor-compensating piezoelectric-based UPH-RAS systems. Designing a lightweight, hand-held, portable surgical device that can sense high-frequency tremors while providing several degrees of freedom in which the tremors can be compensated for has been an active field of research during the last decade [6,7].

5.2.1.2 Technical Challenges in Motion Scaling

In most surgical operations conducted by Tele-RAS systems, a scaling factor of 3:1 or 5:1 has been suggested to enhance the performance of fine motor tasks. However, the limited size of the workspace of the master console imposes a technical challenge. Even if we assume that the accessible workspace of the master console is similar in size to that of the surgical site, scaling down the motions results in a mismatch. In fact, during a scaled-down task, the overall motions generated by the surgeon are larger than the conducted motion at the surgical site. Thus, the surgeon may hit the boundaries of the workspace of the master console during scaled-down operations and cannot move the surgical tool beyond the resulting limits. This issue can potentially make a surgeon unable to conduct tasks in the needed motion range of the surgery. To address this issue, a clutching algorithm has been implemented in most of the commercialized surgical robotic systems. To enable the clutching mechanism, the surgeon should push a clutching foot pedal to temporally disconnect the motion synchrony between the master and the slave consoles. While pushing the pedal, the surgeon can shift and match the achievable workspace of the master console with the needed one at the surgical site. Releasing the clutching pedal results in resuming the motion synchrony in the shifted workspace. This technique has been implemented in commercial systems (such as the da Vinci surgical system). Although using the concept of clutching the issue of workspace limitation has been addressed, this requires a decision between the following choices. The first choice for a surgeon would be to choose a high scaling factor to enhance the accuracy while sacrificing speed and continuity of motions (due to the need for repetitive clutching). The second choice would be to choose a relatively low (or no) scaling factor to produce fast and continuous motions that may not be as accurate as the ones associated with a higher scaling factor. Addressing this problem is an active line of research. An example is the adaptive scheme designed in [25] to enhance the performance of motion scaling by detecting the intention of surgeons (through tracking the gaze motions) and adaptively matching the scaling factor with the size of the *intended* workspace.

5.2.2 PHYSIOLOGICAL MOTION COMPENSATION

Computerized Tele-RAS and UPH-RAS systems have also been equipped with technological means of compensating for physiological cardiac and respiratory motions. The goal is to make the robot synchronized with the motions of the moving organs, while the surgeon focuses on providing relative motions to conduct the surgery [26–28]. Motion compensation is one format of shared autonomy, as the task is divided between a local autonomous control loop and the surgeon. It has been suggested for several procedures, including (a) minimally invasive coronary artery bypass surgery on a beating heart [29–31], intracardiac surgery [32,33], and lung tumor biopsy [34,35].

Image-based motion estimation [30,36] and compensation [27,32] have been frequently suggested in the literature, based on tracking artificial or biological landmarks. A significant challenge with techniques that rely on imaging modalities (such as endoscopic video images and UltraSound (US) images) is the large latency in collecting and processing the data, in comparison with the fast and highly-accelerated motions of the physiological organs [28,31,32,37] (e.g., heart motion has velocities up to 210 mm/s and acceleration up to 3800 mm/s^2 [28]).

To address the latency and enhance the accuracy, adaptive filters for estimation and prediction of organ motions (to be tracked by the robot), together with predictive control techniques (that directly control the robot while compensating for the delay) have been investigated and have shown promising results [26,28,31,32,38,39]. Examples of implemented predictive control techniques are (a) model predictive control [38], (b) Smith predictor-based control [28], and (c) generalized predictive control [26]. In addition, implemented examples of adaptive filters suggested for this application are (a) Kalman filters [32], (b) recursive least-square algorithm [19], and (c) nonlinear adaptive Volterra Lattice prediction algorithm [39]. Data augmentation has also been used to enhance the accuracy while minimizing latencies. In this regard, ElectroCardioGram (ECG)-based data fusion has been reported as an efficient technique, as ECG activities precede and are highly correlated with heart motions [37,40].

Although predictive, adaptive and data augmentation techniques have addressed some of the technical issues, there still exist several practical and technical challenges. The low-frequency update rate and the possibility of faults during image processing are two significant problems. For techniques that use US images, the challenge arises due to a low signal-to-noise ratio [26,32]. In vision-based techniques, there are several sources of faults, such as a blocked field of view (vision occlusion), optical illumination, and surgical smokes [30,41].

To address these issues regarding the use of image-based synchronization, other modalities have been utilized. Sonomicrometry crystal technology is one alternative that has been suggested to track heart motion without relying on images [31,37]. Although using sonomicrometry it is possible to significantly enhance the accuracy in tracking heart motions [32], while avoiding issues such as optical occlusion, there still exist some practical challenges, such as high computational cost, difficulties with real-time implementation, noise from US echoes, and clinical issues with attaching the piezoelectric crystals to the heart.

As an alternative to image-based synchronization, tool-tissue interaction forces have been used in the design of several control algorithms. Two main algorithms that have been investigated in the literature, are (a) force control techniques [42–44], and (b) impedance control techniques [34,35,45]. The basic functionality of force control techniques for robot-tissue synchronization is to ensure the regulation of a small or predefined interaction force (to preserve a controlled contact during motions) between one part of the robotic tool and the moving tissue. This will result in local synchronization of the robot and the tissue. Although the use of force control algorithms to realize motion synchrony is interesting, stability, robustness, and bandwidth of conventional force control techniques can be a challenge [33,43,44]. In this regard, composite control techniques such as fusing the interaction force data with (a) motion data (that may be based on an imaging modality) [33] and (b) soft tissue models [44], have shown improved performance.

As mentioned in the above, impedance control schemes have also been used in the literature for synchronizing surgical robotic systems with moving organs [34,35,45]. The basic functionality is to control the dynamic, interactive behavior of the robot through a predefined mechanical impedance model. In other words, using an impedance control technique, the robot reacts to the measured acting forces (applied by the moving tissue), based on the defined computational impedance model. Thus, if the robot is controlled in a way that reacts rapidly to the interactive forces (through considering a low-amplitude impedance model in the frequency range of the forces), it will be synchronized with the motions of the tissue. Here, there will be a trade-off between the stability of the system and the synchronization performance. It has been shown that the biomechanical characteristics of the tissue can be used to mathematically calculate a minimum allowable impedance of the robot that maximizes the synchrony while preserving the stability [34]. However, this may require an identification procedure to be conducted before the operation.

To summarize, physiological motion compensation is an important line of research. Due to the current interest in the area of intelligent autonomous surgical robotics [46], autonomous compensation for physiological motion is a crucial need [47].

5.2.3 FORBIDDEN-REGION VIRTUAL FIXTURES

Forbidden-Region Virtual Fixtures (FVFs) are active, repulsive geometric constraints; kinesthetically generated by a robotic surgical system; designed based on the fusion of preoperative and intraoperative information; and implemented to enhance the accuracy of surgery by restricting the surgeon from operating on sensitive tissues that are beyond the implemented virtual constraints [15,48,49]. In some articles, FVFs are called "active constraints" [48], as FVFs facilitate the design of "active anatomy-based no-fly-zone constraints" that can directly enhance the performance, accuracy, and safety of surgery by augmenting the motor capabilities of surgeons through preventing damage caused by the robotic tool to tissue [15,50]. Most of the commercially-available examples of surgical robotic systems that are equipped with FVF technology are under the category of GCH-RAS systems. Examples of these are the Makoplasty system (by Stryker, Orlando, FL, USA) [17] designed for total knee replacement, total hip replacement and partial knee replacement procedures. Another example is the Acrobot system (by Acrobot Company Ltd., London, UK) designed for total knee replacement procedures [18]. In addition to GCH-RAS systems, FVF technology has been also used in Tele-RAS research platforms. Examples are FVF-enabled Tele-RAS research platforms [52] to enhance the accuracy and safety in beating heart surgery [52], eye surgery [53], and endoscopic sinus surgery [50].

FVF technology is one format of shared autonomy, as the surgical task can be divided between the surgeon (who conducts the surgery) and the robot (that prevents deviation from the predefined surgical planes). Thus, the manipulation resulting from the use of FVF technology is also called "co-manipulation" in some articles [15]. Due to the specific nature of co-manipulation that keeps the surgeon kinesthetically in charge and in the loop of surgery, besides several proven clinical benefits, this format of shared autonomy has successfully reached the point of commercialization (as mentioned above).

Although FVF technology has been commercially successful for performing robotics-assisted procedures on hard tissues, the situation is not the same for enabling FVF-based surgeries on soft tissues. This is likely due to the complex variable dynamic nature of soft tissue. As a result, FVF technology is still in the research and development phase for procedures involving soft tissue. Some examples of research projects can be found in [52,54,55]. Designing FVF-based technologies for procedures on soft tissue requires further research. Recently, Dynamic Active Constraints (DACs) [54,55] have been suggested, which are specifically designed for addressing some of the issues mentioned above. There are several technical benefits with operation on hard tissues that makes it easier to implement FVF technologies. For hard tissue, the pre-operative images remain very reliable during procedures due to the static nature and minimal deformation. As a result, registration of intra-operative information (such as optical tracking data) and pre-operative information (such as CT scans) is not computationally expensive and is subject to minimal uncertainties.

In addition, it is worth mentioning that in both Tele-RAS and GCH-RAS systems, adding FVF technology results in a haptics-enabled closed interaction loop between the surgeon and the robot [56,57]. It is well known that stability of closed-loop haptics-enabled systems can be degraded by non-passive lags that may be caused by signal discretization, processing lags, and time delays [58–63]. Nonpassive accumulation of interaction mechanical energy and instability in a surgical robotic system can be a significant safety concern. This concern is more severe when complex processing of feedback data (such as the one needed for implementation of DACs) is part of the closed control loop. As a result, this topic is an active line of research, and several controllers and schemes have been designed in the literature to enhance the corresponding safety [15,48,57,64,65].

5.3   SENSORY AUGMENTATION

Computerized robotics-assisted surgical systems can also augment the perceptual awareness of surgeons regarding kinematics and kinesthetics of tool-tissue interaction during surgery. This benefit is more pronounced when a surgeon's access to the surgical site is limited, such as in Minimally Invasive Surgery (MIS) to reduce trauma and in microsurgery because of size constraints. In this section, the existing sensory limitations in MIS are discussed, and the uses of robotic systems in enhancing sensory perception are reviewed.

5.3.1 SENSORY RESTRICTIONS IN MINIMALLY INVASIVE SURGERY

Although there are proven clinical benefits associated with MIS, such as reduction in trauma, risk of infection, and blood loss, together with faster recovery and cosmetic benefits, this type of surgical procedure results in several sensory restrictions for surgeons, primarily due to the limited and indirect access. The three significant sensory restrictions caused by MIS are as follows: (a) degraded hand-eye coordination [66], (b) lack of depth perception [67], and (c) insufficient or inaccurate haptic feedback [68]. Haptic feedback provides key information that cannot be obtained through other sensing modalities. This includes (a) the physical characteristics of tissue (such as the texture, stiffness, size, and location of tumors), (b) the amount of force being exerted on tissue during surgery, and (c) the state of surgical tool manipulation (to avoid issues such as needle slippage and suture breakage). Thus, the sense of touch is important in reducing surgical errors, tissue damage, and operating times. However, the manual tools currently used in MIS are not adequate for providing haptic sensation to surgeons [68,69].

5.3.2 SENSORY ENHANCEMENT IN ROBOTICS-ASSISTED SURGERY

While issues regarding limited dexterity [1], depth perception [70], and hand-eye coordination [71,72] have been well addressed in commercialized robotics-assisted surgical systems, such as the da Vinci system [11,73], currently the development of haptic technology for RAMIS is still in a research stage. However, promising results and systems have been reported [3,74–77].

5.3.2.1 Depth Perception and Hand-Eye Coordination in Robotics-Assisted Surgery

The da Vinci surgical system overcomes several sensory restrictions caused by indirect manipulation in MIS. The system provides an immersive, high-quality 3D stereo visualization that enables depth perception, while not requiring a head-mounted display. Specific attention has been given to the design of a high-definition, 3D visualization system and a stereo endoscope to provide the surgeon with a true, natural, and convenient immersive experience. The surgeon's console is ergonomically designed to enable the surgeon to have a comfortable posture during surgery, while providing intuitive control of the tools and the camera. Through real-time computation and control of the forward and inverse kinematics, the motions of the surgeon's hands are directly tracked by the motions of the tool inside the patient's body. As a result, issues related to indirect mirrored manipulation in MIS are addressed. The surgical instruments used in the da Vinci system are articulated and provide the surgeon with an intuitive, natural feel of manual maneuvering. In addition, the designed posture and the location of the surgeon's console are implemented in a way that the 3D stereoscopic display is located exactly above the coordinates in which the surgeon's hands are acting. As a result, when the surgeon watches the high-quality, 3D video of the tools through the displays, extrapolating the line-of-sight of the surgeon's eyes beyond the display crosses the coordinates of the surgeon's hands. The features mentioned above resolve the visual-motor misalignment issue and the hand-eye coordination problem. As a result, the robot equips the surgeon with an intuitive, natural feel of direct operation, with all possible degrees of motions inside the patient's body and without being cognitively loaded by restrictions that have been traditionally imposed by manual MIS [1,11,72,73,78].

5.3.2.2   Haptics in Robotics-Assisted Surgery

Several studies have shown the importance of haptics for many surgical procedures. However, this sensory input is significantly affected by MIS. Also, in microsurgeries, the magnitude of forces is often too small to be adequately felt by the surgeon. The sensory restriction can be addressed using sensorized robotics-assisted surgical systems. Small and accurate sensors can be mounted in or on surgical instruments that are inserted inside the patient's body, to measure the interaction forces between the tips of the tools and tissue. Measured forces can be filtered, processed, and amplified and then sent to the surgeon's console, which is equipped with accurate actuators. The actuators can apply the processed forces through force tracking control loops so that the surgeon's hand can directly feel the interaction forces. Besides directly providing haptic feedback [77], the measured forces may be provided by other indirect means of sensory modalities, such as visualization [79,80], sonification [75], and cutaneous tactile feedback (e.g., skin stretch) [81,82].

The concept above has been studied under the topic of haptics-enabled Tele-RAS, and there are several platforms equipped with haptics technology, most of which are designed for research use. Examples can be found in [74,83]. To address the challenge of small-amplitude forces in microsurgeries, ultra-accurate small force sensors are used that can measure milli-Newton to micro-Newton forces, to be amplified, visualized, sonified, and provided to clinicians using (a) the Tele-RAS system (e.g., for cell injection and cell manipulation [84–86]), and (b) GCH-RAS systems (e.g., for Vitreoretinal surgeries [12–14]). Examples of ultra-accurate small force sensors are those designed based on optical Fiber Bragg Grating (FBG) technology [87], and polyvinylidene fluoride piezopolymer technology [88,89].

The effectiveness of haptic feedback has been validated in several research projects based on the da Vinci surgical robotic system [75,90,91]. In addition, there are several studies that have identified significant clinical benefits of haptic feedback for robotic surgery, such as (a) reducing the average and the peak values of forces applied to the tissue and the resulting tissue damage [90,92,93]; (b) enhancing the quality of knot tying, reducing the frequency of suture breakage during surgery, enhancing force consistency [79,80]; and (c) enabling haptics-based tumor localization [94]. Despite the benefits mentioned above, there still exist several challenges [74,76] that have resulted in a lack of enabling force feedback in most commercialized surgical robotic systems. This has been considered as a significant drawback of commercially-available Tele-RAS technologies [73,78]. The main problems to be addressed in this regard are the (a) stability of bilateral teleoperation and (b) the difficulties in developing cost-effective, force-sensorized instrumentation.

5.3.2.3   Stability Challenge for Haptics in Robotics-Assisted Surgery

Enabling direct force feedback in any telerobotic architecture results in a closed-loop control system, whose stability is not guaranteed. For a haptics-enabled telerobotic system with ideal force fidelity, the stability of the closed-loop interaction will be marginal. This means that small time delays, data losses, and signal discretization can all result in instability. An unstable interaction can significantly degrade the safety of a surgical robotic system and is not acceptable. Resolving this issue for haptics-enabled telerobotic systems is an active area of research. Two promising solutions have been proposed in the literature. The first suggestion is to design and implement efficient stabilizing control algorithms that can guarantee the stability of the system while minimizing the resulting distortion of system transparency in force generation. Several stabilizers have been suggested, such as Wave Variable Control (WVC) techniques [95–97], Time-Domain Passivity Control (TDPC) techniques [59,61,98,99], and Small-gain Control schemes [63,100]. The second solution to resolve the stability issue is to substitute [75,79,80,82], or augment (partly-substitute) [101], direct kinesthetic force feedback using other sensory modalities (such as visual, auditory, and cutaneous tactile feedback) for an indirect demonstration of interaction forces to surgeons. In this way, the gain of the closed control loop can be reduced (in the case of augmentation), or the loop may be completely opened (in the case of substitution) to guarantee system stability.

5.3.2.4   Instrumentation for Haptics in Robotics-Assisted Surgery

Measuring interaction forces during robotics-assisted surgery is a significant challenge, especially when the force sensor is deployed inside a patient's body to maximize the quality of measurements while minimizing the effects of environmental disturbances [102]. A major problem is the limited available size and space to be used for mounting the force sensing system. For this purpose, the miniaturized sensors should be fabricated in a way that can be embedded on/in the surgical tools and deployed inside the patient's body while being capable of measuring relatively high surgical interaction forces.

To deploy a sensorized device inside the patient's body, and deal with the challenges associated with the limited size and space, the sensor should be designed in a way that is sterilizable and biocompatible [69,94,102,103]. This can potentially increase the cost of fabrication and manufacturing process, instrumentation and can also reduce the possible technological options for implementing a clinically-practical sensorized tool, to be used inside a human body. The problem is even more challenging when there is a need to have a disposable and limited-use device. In this regard, optical force sensing technologies (such as FBG sensors) have been investigated as a possible promising option. Optical force sensing allows for placing all electronic components and wiring outside the patient's body to address some of the issues mentioned above while realizing the measurement of multidirectional forces with high accuracy and resolution [104–106].

5.3.2.5   Force-Enabled Virtual Guidance in Robotics-Assisted Surgery

Unlike enabling the use of actual force feedback, realizing software-generated virtual forces (e.g., [107,108]) is not subject to instrumentation challenges, because of the omission of the need to sensorize the robots. In this regard, Force-enabled Virtual Guidance (FVG) and FVF are two possible formats of virtual force fields used for robotics-assisted surgical systems. Similar to the concept of FVFs, introduced in Section 5.2.3, FVG techniques provide surgeons with some formats of haptic feedback, applied by surgical robotic systems, and designed based on intraoperative and preoperative information. FVG techniques are also cited as guiding virtual fixtures in the literature. Although there are similarities in the engineering designs of FVG and FVF techniques, there are several distinct differences between FVF and FVG schemes (from the sensorimotor augmentation point of view).

In general, FVF techniques generate strong repulsive forces to deter surgeons from penetrating into forbidden regions. In other words, FVF techniques do not require cognitive processing of force-enabled sensory feedback by surgeons to correct the trajectory, as the robot directly corrects for the potential and existing inaccuracies by the generation of kinesthetically impenetrable and inaccessible regions. In addition, the ultimate purpose of FVFs is to enhance the quality of surgery, by simplifying the motor control task and reducing possible damage to a protected region. However, FVG techniques usually provide guiding forces and in some cases are used for training purposes. The force fields of FVG techniques are mainly designed such that they encourage the user to (a) follow a specific path (which is time-independent), or (b) follow a specific trajectory (which is time-dependent), or (c) move toward a specific static/dynamic target. In most of the existing examples, the force fields generated by FVG techniques are in the format of attractive forces (that encourages particular motions), though the force fields may be combined with some repulsive, regional forces to encourage staying on/within a specific trajectory/region. As a result, FVG encourages the user to perform some specific movements (rather than imposing or forbidding movements), by providing haptic cues (rather than "nofly" zones). Using FVG, a surgeon would cognitively process sensory cues and try to respond accordingly by correcting motor outputs. As a result, the robot provides cueing signals for the surgeon, and it is the surgeon who corrects the motions. Thus, in contrast to techniques that implement FVFs, most of the existing FVG techniques do not realize a shared autonomy framework, while they may provide an autonomous sensory cueing framework. In some applications, FVF and FVG are fused and embedded into one control algorithm, such as in [50], for both anatomical obstacle avoidance and trajectory control assistance. In [48], a comprehensive survey is provided regarding different designs and formats of software-based virtual force fields that can be used for FVG and FVF techniques. Examples of FVG techniques can be found in [109] for contactless laser surgery, in [50,110] for sinus surgery, and in [108] for microsurgery.

In addition to the above, the use of haptics-enabled virtual guidance has been studied widely for robot-mediated training of general dynamic motor skills [111–113].

Motivated by this, and taking advantage of computerized, haptics-enabled, dual-user telerobotic systems [114], the concept of FVG has been recently suggested for the training of novice robotic surgeons [64,115,116]. It has been shown that using FVG-based, dual-user telerobotic systems, it is possible to provide kinesthetic cueing for a novice surgeon (who is holding a second master console) in real time. The cueing is to push the novice surgeon toward the correct trajectory during surgery, which is calculated based on real-time measurements collected from an expert surgeon located at the first master console, who is conducting and supervising the task. As a result, during a collaborative surgical training task, the expert surgeon can kin-esthetically supervise, guide, and correct the trainee and can also demonstrate the current trajectory of surgery. It has been shown that the intensity of the applied guidance force field can be designed such that it correlates with the sensorimotor skills of the novice surgeon. In addition, using a tunable authority factor, the participation of the novice surgeon (the trainee) in conducting the surgical task can be adaptively tuned [64,115,116].

5.4　CONCLUDING REMARKS

Using computerized, robotics-assisted surgical systems, it is now possible to augment the sensory and motor skills of surgeons during various surgical tasks, from macro to micro scales. Robots have made it possible for surgeons to conduct surgeries with an enhanced and augmented level of sensory awareness, despite the physical limitations that are clinically imposed to minimize surgical trauma. Robots have also enabled surgeons to conduct tasks with accuracies beyond the natural competence of humans. As a result, robots are able to provide new opportunities to relax several sensorimotor issues and restrictions, such as: visuomotor misalignment and poor ergonomics in MIS, natural hand tremors of surgeons, imprecise micro-manipulation, lack of depth perception in MIS, lack of haptic guidance, inability to perceive micro-forces, and the lack of articulated actuation in MIS. The ultimate goal of this technology has been to enhance the quality of surgery and the predictability of the outcomes. During the last two decades, performance, benefits, and efficacy of commercialized surgical robotic systems and several research platforms have been studied and validated in extensive clinical studies. In this chapter, we introduced sensorimotor augmentation techniques achieved using computerized, robotics-assisted surgical systems. Different categories, technologies, and techniques, together with the relevant literature, were examined, and potential challenges and unresolved research problems were discussed.

REFERENCES

1. K. Moorthy, Y. Munz, A. Dosis et al., Dexterity enhancement with robotic surgery, *Surgical Endoscopy and Other Interventional Techniques*, vol. 18, no. 5, pp. 790–795, 2004.
2. S. M. Prasad, S. M. Prasad, H. S. Maniar et al., Surgical robotics: Impact of motion scaling on task performance, *Journal of the American College of Surgeons*, vol. 199, no. 6, pp. 863–868, 2004.

3. B. T. Bethea, A. M. Okamura, M. Kitagawa et al., Application of haptic feedback to robotic surgery, *Journal of Laparoendoscopic & Advanced Surgical Techniques*, vol. 14, no. 3, pp. 191–195, 2004.

4. C. Rossa, J. Fong, N. Usmani et al., Multiactuator haptic feedback on the wrist for needle steering guidance in brachytherapy, *IEEE Robotics and Automation Letters*, vol. 1, no. 2, pp. 852–859, 2016.

5. M. Raitor, J. M. Walker, A. M. Okamura, and H. Culbertson, Wrap: Wearable, restricted-aperture pneumatics for haptic guidance, in *IEEE International Conference on Robotics and Automation*, 2017, pp. 427–432.

6. S. Yang, R. A. MacLachlan, and C. N. Riviere, Manipulator design and operation of a six-degree-of-freedom handheld tremorcanceling microsurgical instrument, *IEEE/ASME Transactions on Mechatronics*, vol. 20, no. 2, pp. 761–772, 2015.

7. R. A. MacLachlan, B. C. Becker, J. C. Tabares et al., Micron: An actively stabilized handheld tool for microsurgery, *IEEE Transactions on Robotics*, vol. 28, no. 1, pp. 195–212, 2012.

8. T. Wells, S. Yang, R. MacLachlan et al., Hybrid position/force control of an active handheld micromanipulator for membrane peeling, *The International Journal of Medical Robotics and Computer Assisted Surgery*, vol. 12, no. 1, pp. 85–95, 2016.

9. C. Rossa, N. Usmani, R. Sloboda, and M. Tavakoli, A hand-held assistant for semiautomated percutaneous needle steering, *IEEE Transactions on Biomedical Engineering*, vol. 64, no. 3, pp. 637–648, 2017.

10. J. H. Lonner, J. R. Smith, F. Picard et al., High degree of accuracy of a novel image-free handheld robot for unicondylar knee arthroplasty in a cadaveric study, *Clinical Orthopaedics and Related Research*, vol. 473, no. 1, pp. 206–212, 2015.

11. R. H. Taylor, A. Menciassi, G. Fichtinger et al., Medical robotics and computer-integrated surgery, in *Springer Handbook of Robotics*, Cham, Switzerland: Springer, 2016, pp. 1657–1684.

12. R. Taylor, P. Jensen, L. Whitcomb et al., A steady-hand robotic system for microsurgical augmentation, *The International Journal of Robotics Research*, vol. 18, no. 12, pp. 1201–1210, 1999.

13. B. Mitchell, J. Koo, I. Iordachita et al., Development and application of a new steady-hand manipulator for retinal surgery, in *IEEE International Conference on Robotics and Automation*, 2007, pp. 623–629.

14. A. Uneri, M. A. Balicki, J. Handa et al., New steady-hand eye robot with micro-force sensing for vitreoretinal surgery, in *IEEE RAS and EMBS International Conference on Biomedical Robotics and Biomechatronics (BioRob)*, 2010, pp. 814–819.

15. M.-A. Vitrani, C. Poquet, and G. Morel, Applying virtual fixtures to the distal end of a minimally invasive surgery instrument, *IEEE Transactions on Robotics*, vol. 33, no. 1, pp. 114–123, 2017.

16. J.-D. Chang, I.-S. Kim, A. M. Bhardwaj, and R. N. Badami, The evolution of computer-assisted total hip arthroplasty and relevant applications, *Hip & Pelvis*, vol. 29, no. 1, pp. 1–14, 2017.

17. D. H. Nawabi, M. A. Conditt, A. S. Ranawat et al., Haptically guided robotic technology in total hip arthroplasty: A cadaveric investigation, *Proceedings of the Institution of Mechanical Engineers, Part H: Journal of Engineering in Medicine*, vol. 227, no. 3, pp. 302–309, 2013.

18. M. Jakopec, F. R. y Baena, S. J. Harris et al., The hands-on orthopaedic robot "acrobot": Early clinical trials of total knee replacement surgery, *IEEE Transactions on Robotics and Automation*, vol. 19, no. 5, pp. 902–911, 2003.

19. C.-C. Abbou, A. Hoznek, L. Salomon et al., Laparoscopic radical prostatectomy with a remote controlled robot, *The Journal of Urology*, vol. 165, no. 6, pp. 1964–1966, 2001.

20. S. Charles, Dexterity enhancement for surgery, in *Computer Integrated Surgery: Technology and Clinical Applications*, pp. 467–471, 1996.
21. C. N. Riviere, R. S. Rader, and N. V. Thakor, Adaptive cancelling of physiological tremor for improved precision in microsurgery, *IEEE Transactions on Biomedical Engineering*, vol. 45, no. 7, pp. 839–846, 1998.
22. K. Veluvolu, W. Latt, and W. Ang, Double adaptive bandlimited multiple Fourier linear combiner for real-time estimation/filtering of physiological tremor, *Biomedical Signal Processing and Control*, vol. 5, no. 1, pp. 37–44, 2010.
23. K. C. Veluvolu and W. T. Ang, Estimation of physiological tremor from accelerometers for real-time applications, *Sensors*, vol. 11, no. 3, pp. 3020–3036, 2011.
24. S. F. Atashzar, M. Shahbazi, O. Samotus et al., Characterization of upper-limb pathological tremors: Application to design of an augmented haptic rehabilitation system, *IEEE Journal of Selected Topics in Signal Processing*, vol. 10, no. 5, pp. 888–903, 2016.
25. G. Gras, K. Leibrandt, P. Wisanuvej et al., Implicit gaze-assisted adaptive motion scaling for highly articulated instrument manipulation, in *IEEE International Conference on Robotics and Automation*, 2017, pp. 4233–4239.
26. M. Bowthorpe and M. Tavakoli, Generalized predictive control of a surgical robot for beating-heart surgery under delayed and slowly-sampled ultrasound image data, *IEEE Robotics and Automation Letters*, vol. 1, no. 2, pp. 892–899, 2016.
27. R. Konietschke, D. Zerbato, R. Richa et al., Integration of new features for telerobotic surgery into the MiroSurge system, *Applied Bionics and Biomechanics*, vol. 8, no. 2, pp. 253–265, 2011.
28. M. Bowthorpe, M. Tavakoli, H. Becher, and R. Howe, Smith predictor-based robot control for ultrasound-guided teleoperated beating-heart surgery, *IEEE Journal of Biomedical and Health Informatics*, vol. 18, no. 1, pp. 157–166, 2014.
29. A. Ruszkowski, C. Schneider, O. Mohareri, and S. Salcudean, Bimanual teleoperation with heart motion compensation on the da Vinci research kit: Implementation and preliminary experiments, in *IEEE International Conference on Robotics and Automation*, 2016, pp. 4101–4108.
30. R. Richa, A. P. Bo, and P. Poignet, Towards robust 3D visual tracking for motion compensation in beating heart surgery, *Medical Image Analysis*, vol. 15, no. 3, pp. 302–315, 2011.
31. E. E. Tuna, T. J. Franke, and O. Bebek et al., Heart motion prediction based on adaptive estimation algorithms for robotic-assisted beating heart surgery, *IEEE Transactions on Robotics*, vol. 29, no. 1, pp. 261–276, 2013.
32. S. G. Yuen, D. T. Kettler, P. M. Novotny et al., Robotic motion compensation for beating heart intracardiac surgery, *The International Journal of Robotics Research*, vol. 28, no. 10, pp. 1355–1372, 2009.
33. S. G. Yuen, D. P. Perrin, N. V. Vasilyev et al., Force tracking with feed-forward motion estimation for beating heart surgery, *IEEE Transactions on Robotics*, vol. 26, no. 5, pp. 888–896, 2010.
34. S. F. Atashzar, I. Khalaji, M. Shahbazi et al., Robot-assisted lung motion compensation during needle insertion, in *IEEE International Conference on Robotics and Automation*, 2013, pp. 1682–1687.
35. Y. J. Kim, J. H. Seo, H. R. Kim, and K. G. Kim, Impedance and admittance control for respiratory-motion compensation during robotic needle insertion—a preliminary test, *The International Journal of Medical Robotics and Computer Assisted Surgery*, vol. 34, no. 4, p. e1795, 2017.
36. W.-K. Wong, B. Yang, C. Liu, and P. Poignet, A quasi-spherical triangle-based approach for efficient 3-d soft-tissue motion tracking, *IEEE/ASME Transactions on Mechatronics*, vol. 18, no. 5, pp. 1472–1484, 2013.

37. O. Bebek and M. C. Cavusoglu, Intelligent control algorithms for robotic-assisted beating heart surgery, *IEEE Transactions on Robotics*, vol. 23, no. 3, pp. 468–480, 2007.

38. G. J. Vrooijink, A. Denasi, J. G. Grandjean, and S. Misra, Model predictive control of a robotically actuated delivery sheath for beating heart compensation, *The International Journal of Robotics Research*, vol. 36, no. 2, pp. 193–209, 2017.

39. F. Liang, Y. Yu, H. Wang, and X. Meng, Heart motion prediction in robotic-assisted beating heart surgery: A nonlinear fast adaptive approach, *International Journal of Advanced Robotic Systems*, vol. 10, no. 1, p. 82, 2013.

40. T. Ortmaier, M. Groger, D. H. Boehm et al., Motion estimation in beating heart surgery, *IEEE Transactions on Biomedical Engineering*, vol. 52, no. 10, pp. 1729–1740, 2005.

41. H. Mohamadipanah, M. Andalibi, and L. Hoberock, Robust automatic feature tracking on beating human hearts for minimally invasive cabg surgery, *Journal of Medical Devices*, vol. 10, no. 4, pp. 041010–1–8, 2016.

42. B. Cagneau, N. Zemiti, D. Bellot, and G. Morel, Physiological motion compensation in robotized surgery using force feedback control, in *IEEE International Conference on Robotics and Automation*, 2007, pp. 1881–1886.

43. J. M. Florez, D. Bellot, and G. Morel, LWPR-model based predictive force control for serial comanipulation in beating heart surgery, in *IEEE/ASME International Conference on Advanced Intelligent Mechatronics (AIM)*, 2011, pp. 320–326.

44. P. Moreira, N. Zemiti, C. Liu, and P. Poignet, Viscoelastic model based force control for soft tissue interaction and its application in physiological motion compensation, *Computer Methods and Programs in Biomedicine*, vol. 116, no. 2, pp. 52–67, 2014.

45. J. M. Florez, J. Szewczyk, and G. Morel, An impedance control strategy for a hand-held instrument to compensate for physiological motion, in *IEEE International Conference on Robotics and Automation*, 2012, pp. 1952–1957.

46. G.-Z. Yang, J. Cambias, K. Cleary et al., Medical robotics—regulatory, ethical, and legal considerations for increasing levels of autonomy, *Science Robotics*, vol. 2, no. 4, 2017.

47. V. Patel, S. Krishnan, A. Goncalves et al., Using intermittent synchronization to compensate for rhythmic body motion during autonomous surgical cutting and debridement, *arXiv preprint arXiv:1712.02917*, 2017.

48. S. Bowyer, B. L. Davies, and F. Y. Baena, Active constraints/virtual fixtures: A survey, *IEEE Transactions on Robotics*, vol. 30, no. 1, pp. 138–157, 2014.

49. R. A. Beasley and R. D. Howe, Increasing accuracy in image-guided robotic surgery through tip tracking and model-based flexion correction, *IEEE Transactions on Robotics*, vol. 25, no. 2, pp. 292–302, 2009.

50. M. Li, M. Ishii, and R. H. Taylor, Spatial motion constraints using virtual fixtures generated by anatomy, *IEEE Transactions on Robotics*, vol. 23, no. 1, pp. 4–19, 2007.

51. S. Nia Kosari, F. Ryden, T. S. Lendvay et al., Forbidden region virtual fixtures from streaming point clouds, *Advanced Robotics*, vol. 28, no. 22, pp. 1507–1518, 2014.

52. J. Ren, R. Patel, K. McIsaac et al., Dynamic 3-d virtual fixtures for minimally invasive beating heart procedures, *IEEE Transactions on Medical Imaging*, vol. 27, no. 8, pp. 1061–1070, 2008.

53. J. J. Abbott, G. D. Hager, and A. M. Okamura, Steady-hand teleoperation with virtual fixtures, in *The 12th IEEE International Workshop on Robot and Human Interactive Communication*, 2003, pp. 145–151.

54. K.-W. Kwok, K. H. Tsoi, V. Vitiello et al., Dimensionality reduction in controlling articulated snake robot for endoscopy under dynamic active constraints, *IEEE Transactions on Robotics*, vol. 29, no. 1, pp. 15–31, 2013.

55. S. Bowyer and F. Y. Baena, Deformation invariant bounding spheres for dynamic active constraints in surgery, *Proceedings of the Institution of Mechanical Engineers, Part H: Journal of Engineering in Medicine*, vol. 228, no. 4, pp. 350–361, 2014.

56. J. G. Petersen, S. A. Bowyer, and F. R. Y. Baena, Mass and friction optimization for natural motion in hands-on robotic surgery, *IEEE Transactions on Robotics*, vol. 32, no. 1, pp. 201–213, 2016.

57. S. A. Bowyer and F. R. Y. Baena, Dissipative control for physical human–robot interaction, *IEEE Transactions on Robotics*, vol. 31, no. 6, pp. 1281–1293, 2015.

58. K. Hashtrudi-Zaad and S. E. Salcudean, Analysis of control architectures for teleoperation systems with impedance/admittance master and slave manipulators, *The International Journal of Robotics Research*, vol. 20, no. 6, pp. 419–445, 2001.

59. J.-H. Ryu, C. Preusche, B. Hannaford, and G. Hirzinger, Time domain passivity control with reference energy following, *IEEE Transactions on Control Systems Technology*, vol. 13, no. 5, pp. 737–742, 2005.

60. A. Haddadi, K. Razi, and K. Hashtrudi-Zaad, Operator dynamics consideration for less conservative coupled stability condition in bilateral teleoperation, *IEEE/ASME Transactions on Mechatronics*, vol. 20, no. 5, pp. 2463–2475, 2015.

61. S. F. Atashzar, M. Shahbazi, M. Tavakoli, and R. V. Patel, A grasp-based passivity signature for haptics-enabled human-robot interaction: Application to design of a new safety mechanism for robotic rehabilitation, *The International Journal of Robotics Research*, vol. 36, no. 5–7, pp. 778–799, 2017.

62. M. Shahbazi, S. F. Atashzar, M. Tavakoli, and R. V. Patel, Position-force domain passivity of human arm in telerobotics systems, *IEEE/ASME Transactions on Mechatronics*, vol. 23, no. 2, pp. 552–562, 2018.

63. S. F. Atashzar, I. G. Polushin, and R. V. Patel, A small-gain approach for nonpassive bilateral telerobotic rehabilitation: Stability analysis and controller synthesis, *IEEE Transactions on Robotics*, vol. 33, no. 1, pp. 49–66, 2017.

64. M. Shahbazi, S. F. Atashzar, and R. V. Patel, A dual-user teleoperated system with virtual fixtures for robotic surgical training, in *2013 IEEE International Conference on Robotics and Automation*, May 2013, pp. 3639–3644.

65. J. J. Abbott and A. M. Okamura, Stable forbidden-region virtual fixtures for bilateral telemanipulation, *Journal of Dynamic Systems, Measurement, & Control*, vol. 128, no. 1, pp. 53–64, 2006.

66. B. Wentink, Eye-hand coordination in laparoscopy-an overview of experiments and supporting aids, *Minimally Invasive Therapy & Allied Technologies*, vol. 10, no. 3, pp. 155–162, 2001.

67. S. Sorensen, M. Savran, L. Konge, and F. Bjerrum, Three dimensional versus two dimensional vision in laparoscopy: A systematic review, *Surgical Endoscopy*, vol. 30, no. 1, pp. 11–23, 2016.

68. E. Westebring-Van Der Putten, R. Goossens, J. Jakimowicz, and J. Dankelman, Haptics in minimally invasive surgery—a review, *Minimally Invasive Therapy & Allied Technologies*, vol. 17, no. 1, pp. 3–16, 2008.

69. A. Trejos, R. Patel, and M. Naish, Force sensing and its application in minimally invasive surgery and therapy: A survey, *Proceedings of the Institution of Mechanical Engineers, Part C: Journal of Mechanical Engineering Science*, vol. 224, no. 7, pp. 1435–1454, 2010.

70. J. C. Byrn, S. Schluender, C. M. Divino et al., Three-dimensional imaging improves surgical performance for both novice and experienced operators using the da Vinci robot system, *The American Journal of Surgery*, vol. 193, no. 4, pp. 519–522, 2007.

71. Y. Gao, S. Wang, J. Li et al., Modeling and evaluation of hand-eye coordination of surgical robotic system on task performance, *The International Journal of Medical Robotics and Computer Assisted Surgery*, vol. 13, no. 4, p. 1829, 2017.

72. G. S. Guthart and J. K. Salisbury, The Intuitive telesurgery system: overview and application, in *IEEE International Conference on Robotics and Automation*, vol. 1, 2000, pp. 618–621.

73. V. Vitiello, S.-L. Lee, T. P. Cundy, and G.-Z. Yang, Emerging robotic platforms for minimally invasive surgery, *IEEE Reviews in Biomedical Engineering*, vol. 6, pp. 111–126, 2013.

74. N. Enayati, E. De Momi, and G. Ferrigno, Haptics in robotassisted surgery: Challenges and benefits, *IEEE Reviews in Biomedical Engineering*, vol. 9, pp. 49–65, 2016.

75. M. Kitagawa, D. Dokko, A. M. Okamura, and D. D. Yuh, Effect of sensory substitution on suture-manipulation forces for robotic surgical systems, *The Journal of Thoracic and Cardiovascular Surgery*, vol. 129, no. 1, pp. 151–158, 2005.

76. A. M. Okamura, Methods for haptic feedback in teleoperated robot-assisted surgery, *Industrial Robot: An International Journal*, vol. 31, no. 6, pp. 499–508, 2004.

77. M. Tavakoli, R. V. Patel, M. Moallem, and A. Aziminejad, *Haptics for Teleoperated Surgical Robotic Systems*, World Scientific, Hackensack, NJ, 2008.

78. C. Freschi, V. Ferrari, F. Melfi et al., Technical review of the da Vinci surgical telemanipulator, *The International Journal of Medical Robotics and Computer Assisted Surgery*, vol. 9, no. 4, pp. 396–406, 2013.

79. C. E. Reiley, T. Akinbiyi, D. Burschka et al., Effects of visual force feedback on robot-assisted surgical task performance, *The Journal of Thoracic and Cardiovascular Surgery*, vol. 135, no. 1, pp. 196–202, 2008.

80. A. Talasaz, A. L. Trejos, and R. V. Patel, The role of direct and visual force feedback in suturing using a 7-DOF dual-arm teleoperated system, *IEEE Transactions on Haptics*, vol. 10, no. 2, pp. 276–287, 2017.

81. Z. Quek, S. Schorr, I. Nisky et al., Sensory substitution and augmentation using 3-degree-of-freedom skin deformation feedback, *IEEE Transactions on Haptics*, vol. 8, no. 2, pp. 209–221, 2015.

82. S. B. Schorr, Z. F. Quek, and I. Nisky et al., Tactor-induced skin stretch as a sensory substitution method in teleoperated palpation, *IEEE Transactions on Human-Machine Systems*, vol. 45, no. 6, pp. 714–726, 2015.

83. M. Tavakoli, A. Aziminejad, R. Patel, and M. Moallem, Methods and mechanisms for contact feedback in a robot-assisted minimally invasive environment, *Surgical Endoscopy and Other Interventional Techniques*, vol. 20, no. 10, pp. 1570–1579, 2006.

84. S. Faroque, B. Horan, H. Adam et al., Haptic technology for micro-robotic cell injection training systemsa review, *Intelligent Automation & Soft Computing*, vol. 22, no. 3, pp. 509–523, 2016.

85. A. Pillarisetti, M. Pekarev, A. D. Brooks, and J. P. Desai, Evaluating the effect of force feedback in cell injection, *IEEE Transactions on Automation Science and Engineering*, vol. 4, no. 3, pp. 322–331, 2007.

86. M. Zareinejad, S. Rezaei, A. Abdullah, and S. Shiry Ghidary, Development of a piezo-actuated micro-teleoperation system for cell manipulation, *The International Journal of Medical Robotics and Computer Assisted Surgery*, vol. 5, no. 1, pp. 66–76, 2009.

87. K. O. Hill and G. Meltz, Fiber Bragg Grating technology fundamentals and overview, *Journal of Lightwave Technology*, vol. 15, no. 8, pp. 1263–1276, 1997.

88. D.-H. Kim, B. Kim, and H. Kang, Development of a piezoelectric polymer-based sensorized microgripper for microassembly and micromanipulation, *Microsystem Technologies*, vol. 10, no. 4, pp. 275–280, 2004.

89. Y. Wang, J. Zheng, G. Ren et al., A flexible piezoelectric force sensor based on pvdf fabrics, *Smart Materials and Structures*, vol. 20, no. 4, p. 045009, 2011.

90. C. R. Wottawa, B. Genovese, B. N. Nowroozi et al., Evaluating tactile feedback in robotic surgery for potential clinical application using an animal model, *Surgical Endoscopy*, vol. 30, no. 8, pp. 3198–3209, 2016.

91. T. N. Judkins, D. Oleynikov, and N. Stergiou, Real-time augmented feedback benefits robotic laparoscopic training, *Studies in Health Technology and Informatics*, vol. 119, p. 243, 2005.

92. C. R. Wagner, N. Stylopoulos, and R. D. Howe, The role of force feedback in surgery: Analysis of blunt dissection, in *Symposium on Haptic Interfaces for Virtual Environment and Teleoperator Systems*, IEEE Computer Society, Los Alamitos, CA, 2002, pp. 68–74.

93. T. Ortmaier, B. Deml, B. Kubler et al., *Robot Assisted Force Feedback Surgery*, 2007.

94. A. S. Naidu, R. V. Patel, and M. D. Naish, Low-cost disposable tactile sensors for palpation in minimally invasive surgery, *IEEE/ASME Transactions on Mechatronics*, vol. 22, no. 1, pp. 127–137, 2017.

95. G. Niemeyer and J. Slotine, Stable adaptive teleoperation, *IEEE Journal of Oceanic Engineering*, vol. 16, no. 1, pp. 152–162, 1991.

96. Y. Ye and P. X. Liu, Improving trajectory tracking in wave-variable-based teleoperation, *IEEE/ASME Transactions on Mechatronics*, vol. 15, no. 2, pp. 321–326, 2010.

97. M. Shahbazi, H. A. Talebi, and R. V. Patel, Networked dual-user teleoperation with time-varying authority adjustment: A wave variable approach, in *IEEE/ASME International Conference on Advanced Intelligent Mechatronics (AIM)*, 2014, pp. 415–420.

98. J.-H. Ryu, D.-S. Kwon, and B. Hannaford, Stable teleoperation with time-domain passivity control, *IEEE Transactions on Robotics and Automation*, vol. 20, no. 2, pp. 365–373, 2004.

99. S. F. Atashzar, M. Shahbazi, M. Tavakoli, and R. V. Patel, A passivity-based approach for stable patient-robot interaction in haptics-enabled rehabilitation systems: Modulated time-domain passivity control, *IEEE Transactions on Control Systems Technology*, vol. 25, no. 3, pp. 991–1006, 2017.

100. I. G. Polushin, A. Takhmar, and R. V. Patel, Projection-based force-reflection algorithms with frequency separation for bilateral teleoperation, *IEEE/ASME Transactions on Mechatronics*, vol. 20, no. 1, pp. 143–154, 2015.

101. Z. Quek, S. Schorr, I. Nisky et al., Augmentation of stiffness perception with a 1-degree-of-freedom skin stretch device, *IEEE Transactions on Human-Machine Systems*, vol. 44, no. 6, pp. 731–742, 2014.

102. P. Puangmali, K. Althoefer, L. D. Seneviratne et al., State-ofthe-art in force and tactile sensing for minimally invasive surgery, *IEEE Sensors Journal*, vol. 8, no. 4, pp. 371–381, 2008.

103. V. Arabagi, O. Felfoul, A. H. Gosline et al., Biocompatible pressure sensing skins for minimally invasive surgical instruments, *IEEE Sensors Journal*, vol. 16, no. 5, pp. 1294–1303, 2016.

104. S. C. Ryu and P. E. Dupont, FBG-based shape sensing tubes for continuum robots, in *IEEE International Conference on Robotics and Automation*, 2014, pp. 3531–3537.

105. R. Haslinger, P. Leyendecker, and U. Seibold, A fiberoptic force-torque-sensor for minimally invasive robotic surgery, in *IEEE International Conference on Robotics and Automation*, 2013, pp. 4390–4395.

106. M. S. Muller, L. Hoffmann, T. Christopher Buck, and A. Walter Koch, Fiber bragg grating-based force-torque sensor with six degrees of freedom, *International Journal of Optomechatronics*, vol. 3, no. 3, pp. 201–214, 2009.

107. L. B. Rosenberg, Virtual fixtures: Perceptual tools for telerobotic manipulation, in *IEEE Virtual Reality Annual International Symposium*, 1993, pp. 76–82.

108. A. Bettini, P. Marayong, S. Lang et al., Vision-assisted control for manipulation using virtual fixtures, *IEEE Transactions on Robotics*, vol. 20, no. 6, pp. 953–966, 2004.

109. E. Olivieri, G. Barresi, D. G. Caldwell, and L. S. Mattos, Haptic feedback for control and active constraints in contactless laser surgery: Concept, implementation and evaluation, *IEEE Transactions on Haptics*, vol. 11, no. 2, pp. 241–254, 2018.

110. M. Li and R. H. Taylor, Spatial motion constraints in medical robot using virtual fixtures generated by anatomy, in *IEEE International Conference on Robotics and Automation*, vol. 2, 2004, pp. 1270–1275.

111. R. Sigrist, G. Rauter, R. Riener, and P. Wolf, Augmented visual, auditory, haptic, and multimodal feedback in motor learning: A review, *Psychonomic Bulletin & Review*, vol. 20, no. 1, pp. 21–53, 2013.
112. D. Powell and M. K. O'Malley, The task-dependent efficacy of shared-control haptic guidance paradigms, *IEEE Transactions on Haptics*, vol. 5, no. 3, pp. 208–219, 2012.
113. J. C. Huegel and M. K. O'Malley, Progressive haptic and visual guidance for training in a virtual dynamic task, in *IEEE Haptics Symposium*, 2010, pp. 343–350.
114. M. Shahbazi, S. F. Atashzar, H. A. Talebi, and R. V. Patel, Novel cooperative tele-operation framework: Multi-master/single-slave system, *IEEE/ASME Transactions on Mechatronics*, vol. 20, no. 4, pp. 1668–1679, 2015.
115. M. Shahbazi, S. F. Atashzar, C. Ward et al., Multimodal sensorimotor integration for expert-in-the-loop telerobotic surgical training, *IEEE Transactions on Robotic*, 2018.
116. M. Shahbazi, S. F. Atashzar, H. A. Talebi, and R. V. Patel, An expertise-oriented training framework for robotics-assisted surgery, in *IEEE International Conference on Robotics and Automation*, May 2014, pp. 5902–5907.

6 Visual Perception and Human–Computer Interaction in Surgical Augmented and Virtual Reality Environments

Roy Eagleson and Sandrine de Ribaupierre

CONTENTS

6.1 INTRODUCTION

Augmented and virtual reality (AR/VR) is like a double-edged sword: displays can be compelling and powerful, yet when certain design principles are violated, they can be confusing and unusable. This chapter explores some of the reasons for ambiguity and poor usability from the perspective of human–computer interaction, which necessitates a design process that is informed by basic scientific results from the overlapping domains of perception, action, and cognition (cf. Figure 6.1). We also examine some of these fundamental concerns for general AR and then focus on the implications of AR for particular applications in surgical planning, guidance, and targeting using some specific case studies drawn from published papers on the use of AR for neurosurgery.

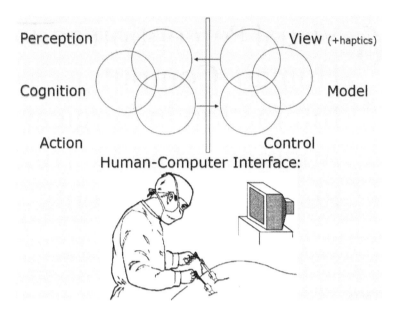

FIGURE 6.1 Schematic overview of the flow of information in a general human–computer interface, stressing the symmetry between the software engineering pattern of "Model, View, and Control (MVC)" with the main human capacities of "Perception, Action, and Cognition."

6.2 PERCEPTION, ACTION, AND COGNITION IN HUMAN–COMPUTER INTERFACE DESIGN

When several imaging modalities are combined from across disparate sources onto one screen using an AR presentation, the resulting scene dynamics and translucency effects open up a number of empirical questions. To begin answering these questions, we must first establish the classical distinction between "bottom-up" and "top-down" perception (roughly equivalent to data-driven processes versus model-driven processes—or, more formally, the distinction between deductive versus inductive reasoning). Computational theories of bottom-up perceptual integration (cf. Barrow and Tenenbaum, 1981; Marr, 1982; Terzopoulos, 1986; Cavanagh, 1987; Bulthoff and Mallot, 1990), along with top-down models of perception (Gregory, 1970; Ullman, 1989), exist in the literature. Illusions in bottom-up perception are classical and contrast with top-down processes, which are knowledge-driven, yet can also lead to illusions, such as the formation of subjective contours in stereoscopic presentation, thus leading to inconsistencies between structure-from-motion, texture gradients, and occlusion boundaries. These perceptual effects inform us that display design needs careful consideration of the special capacities and surprising constraints of the human perceptual, motor, and cognitive subsystems (Eagleson and Peters, 2008).

The design of an interactive AR display is, in principal, no different from the development of any user interface in the domain of human–computer interface design. On the other hand, the resulting user experience of three-dimensional (3D), immersive AR/VR interfaces is strikingly different from that of one based on the classical, two-dimensional (2D) "desktop metaphor." The predominant 2D GUI toolkits include APIs such as Microsoft's Windows.System.Forms, Oracle's Swing APIs (which are extended from the Java AWT by Sun Microsystems), the Android View classes, or HTML input tags on JavaScript frameworks. By using APIs such as these, standardized GUIs can be composed by instantiating objects derived from the classes in these libraries and by arranging them within the display according to the designed layout. Although many VR/AR developers "roll their own" libraries, 3D widgets and toolkit frameworks for 3D GUIs do exist: VRML and VTK are early examples, while Leap Motion provides a new "ButtonBuilder" API compatible with Unity3D (Figure 6.2).

From a perceptual-motor standpoint, the user interactions with these interfaces (whether they are 2D or 3D) will always be restricted to a surprisingly simple taxonomy of four fundamental types:

1. Selection interactions (such as button presses, checkboxes, or menu-item selections)
2. Values set on quantifiers (generally sliders or scrollbars)
3. Position interactions (which are a pair of values, [x, y], on 2D interfaces (or, more recently, changes in position, such as swiping motions)
4. Text-based interactions (generally typed on keyboards, though other text-based interactions also exist)

This is a fundamental list. There are no other types of interactions in HCI (Foley and Van Dam, 1982) or even in general human–machine interfaces. This is a surprising result because all "outputs" from a human are restricted to motor system action.

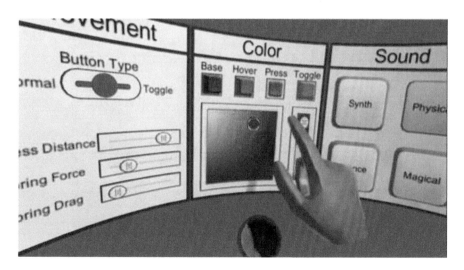

FIGURE 6.2 GUIs can be implemented within AR/VR displays with classical GUI interaction items that afford selection, quantification, positioning, and text.

The only way information can flow outwards from a human is by activating muscle (this is as true for mouse-and-keyboard events as it is for gestures in 3D). Text-based interactions are move-and-press on keyboards (or even speech-based interfaces, which we will not discuss in this chapter) that are resolved into strings of text, but even in this special case, the lung and vocal cord functionality ultimately depend on muscle actuation.

Accordingly, all GUI-based interactions are movement-based. The user changes the position of the cursor to form a virtual collision with an object, such as a button. A "selection" is then merely a special type of movement in which the motion is made against a target object, such as a key on a keyboard or a mouse-button. In the user's physical space, these interactions are "collision" events between the fingertip and the physical input device. Buttons move at first in response to a downclick force, but then after the downclick event occurs, the button quickly stops moving in response to the force of the fingertip and becomes an isometric device (it stops moving and resists the fingertip force with an equal but opposite static force). This may seem an unusually pedantic description of something as fundamental as a simple button click interaction, but the story changes completely when considering "virtual buttons" in 3D immersive environments. The lack of the static force makes such virtual selections quite different from the perspective of the user experience (Figure 6.3).

From the standpoint of the flow of information from a human to a computer on a 2D GUI, what results is a sequence of move-and-click primitives—although the move-and-click interactions are peppered from time-to-time with a downclick-drag-upclick,

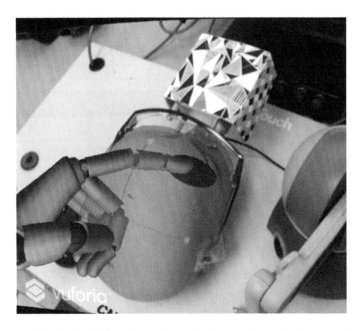

FIGURE 6.3   Within AR/VR interfaces, "selection" interactions arise from virtual collisions between a tooltip (or fingertip) and the iterative object (in this case, an ellipsoid representing a target) within the 3D virtual workspace.

seemingly just to spice things up with a drag-and-drop interaction (this is so common that it has its own Wikipedia entry: https://en.wikipedia.org/wiki/Point_and_click)

From the perspective of the computer software being executed as a program, the instantiation of objects from class libraries merely adds entries to a dynamic table in memory. However, from the perspective of the user's environment, visual representations of these objects are rendered on the display and are readily perceived and recognized by the user as having certain affordances (to use Gibson's 1977 term). From the user's perspective, these virtual objects rendered on the display can be perceived at specific locations (where), recognized (what), and understood as tools for performing tasks in accordance with the user's goals, beliefs, and expectations (i.e., knowledge understanding, reasoning, and planning are accomplished by the cognitive system) (Figure 6.4).

Two fundamental observations can be identified and aligned with Norman's principles to minimize the user interface: the "gulf of execution" and "the gulf of evaluation" (cf. Norman, 1986):

(P1 **"Execution"**) The Principle of "Movement and Selection" Interaction for Task Execution: The flow of control from human-to-computer will consist of only two types: (i) movement in the n-dimensional workspace and (ii) selection interactions with components that are object-based (usually cursor-to-object virtual collisions, but also including object-to-object collisions involving virtual tools other than the cursor or the user's own body motions). Accordingly, maximizing the product of speed and accuracy of these interactions forms the basis for the optimality of user interactions.

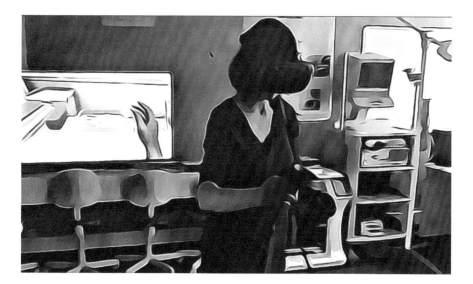

FIGURE 6.4   The user experience within a virtual environment follows the same HCI loop-of-control as characterized in Figure 6.1 for graphical user interfaces. (Courtesy of the Jannin Lab, Rennes, France.)

(P2 "**Evaluation**") The Principle of the User's Perception-Based Evaluation: The user evaluates the state of his/her progress in executing a task using his/her perceptual system to update his/her situational assessment based on the position and shape of the object, and, accordingly, the rendering of these objects to convey position and shape must respect the special capacities and constraints of the human perceptual system (which, perhaps surprisingly, is subject to errors when inconsistent perceptual cues are mixed). Accordingly, maximizing the product of speed and accuracy to evaluate the state of an item—its type ("what") or its position ("where")—forms the basis for the optimality of the rendering of the display.

Some additional comments can be made here to extend the results obtained from HCI for 2D GUIs to 3D AR/VR interfaces (upon which time we can consider APIs for instantiating 3D interfaces):

P1(i): For interactions that are movement-based, it will be important to respect the need for "Stimulus-Response (SR)" compatibility. On a classical GUI, the mode of movement-based interaction using a mouse-and-cursor (including touchpad-and-cursor) have separate and distinct spaces for the input and outputs. We can contrast this with the "direct manipulation" mode (cf. Norman, 1986), such as touchscreen displays, in which the input and output spaces are co-registered.

P1(ii): For interactions that are selection-based, such events are discrete collisions that are triggered once the user has moved a cursor to a GUI object. The trigger may be a discrete downclick-and-upclick composite event or by positioning the cursor to be coincident with a feature on the virtual interaction object (such as when a cascaded submenu is launched when the cursor is dragged through the side border of a menu item, or in the case of 3D virtual interfaces, when a 3D cursor has been placed coincident with a virtual button). In all such cases, the event will be associated with an object that has already been instantiated in the workspace.

6.3 HUMAN PERCEPTION CONSIDERATIONS DURING SYSTEM DESIGN

When considering the perceptual aspects of objects that are rendered in the users 2D or 3D visual workspaces, the user will perceive two particular aspects: (i) perception of the object's position ("where") and (ii) recognition and understanding of its state or identity ("what").

P2(i): The perception of the position and the orientation of objects (including cursors) in the workspace (typically this will be the perceived absolute position of the object, but in certain cases, the user may only perceive the relative position with respect to other objects, in terms of spatial relations such as "in front of" or "beside").

P2(ii): The perception of the state of objects, such as "clicked," "selected," "with focus," "hovered," "active," etc., using colors, icons, text, or textures that can be used by the interface designer to allow the user to evaluate the objects' current state must appear as "affordances" of these objects.

These four overarching design principles can be summarized in Table 6.1.

By characterizing the attributes of the objects in the display in this manner, we can reflect on the principle that the rendering of objects must consider the special perceptual capacities and constraints of the sensory channels that carry the information that feeds the cognitive and action systems with information about the location, configuration, state, and identity of objects in the user's environment. To be sure, in the case of 2D GUIs, the rendering of the positions of objects is relatively straightforward, and, as APIs for 2D GUI have matured considerably, these rendered objects are typically free of perceptual illusions, so long as guidelines for clean layouts are followed. Put coarsely, the interface layout should not be so complicated as to disturb the user with busy patterns or flickering indicators. Put in more principled terms, the layout should be designed in a way that avoids illusory parametric choices in their rendering, such as context-based illusions (cf. Müller-Lyer, 1889; Ponzo, 1912), isoluminant color palettes, poor contrast between borders of overlapping items, or illusions that call into question whether the absolute or relative positions of objects are based on violations of the co-constraints of the separate channels carrying information about the position and orientation of objects. Traps and pitfalls abound when rendering 3D virtual and augmented environments by the unintentional violation of the constraints between the separate but interacting perceptual channels that convey information about the position and orientation of objects (i.e., "where" they are) (Figures 6.5 and 6.6).

Similarly, there are special capacities and constraints on perceptual channels carrying information about the state and identity of objects (i.e., "what" they are). To be sure, for 2D GUIs, the perception of something as simple as the state of a button (i.e., whether it has been pressed or not) relies on the functionality associated with the shape-from-shading perceptual channel (i.e., the seemingly hardwired perceptual constraint that is an intrinsic expectation that objects are always

---

TABLE 6.1

Four Overarching Design Principles

Design Principle	Metric Space (Position/Orientation)	Discrete Categories (State/Identity)
User Interactions: (Task Execution)	P1(i) Movement events in space require SR compatibility	P1(ii) Selection events are bound to objects designed to have "Affordances"
Displayed to User: (Scene Evaluation)	P2(i) Perception of spatial relations must not be impaired by incompatible spatial information	P2(ii) Perception of Affordances or state of object must be conveyed using appropriate icon or recognizable item

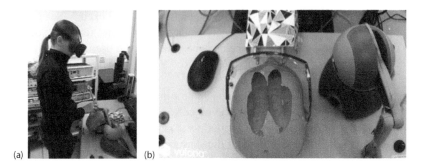

FIGURE 6.5 Tabletop simulator setups and generic configuration using phantom-tracked pointer and neurosurgical Endoscopic Third Ventriculostomy (ETV) configuration using skull phantom: (a) tracked pointer tool and AR goggles display; (b) Graphically-rendered ventricles within AR visualization mode.

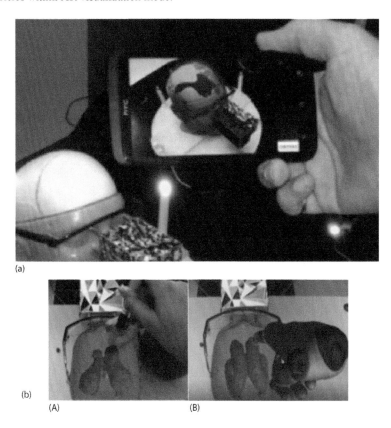

FIGURE 6.6 When the display can move through the workspace (a), the induced motion can resolve ambiguities associated with inconsistent depth cues across perceptual channels; however, it is generally very difficult to resolve depth when pointing within an immersive display (b-left: "A"). In these cases, AR may need to be replaced with a VR representation (b-right: "B").

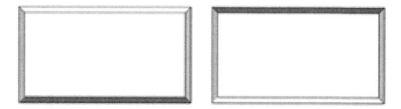

FIGURE 6.7   Illustration of the simple shading cues that can give rise to a pushbutton's affordances—the states "unclicked" and "clicked." If you turn this page upside-down, the sense of these two states will flip (the "unclicked" will always be on the left, in either case).

"lit from above"). In the two rendered buttons in Figure 6.7, the button on the left is perceived as being "unclicked," and that on the right is perceived as "clicked." However, if the page is turned upside-down, these two buttons will be perceived in exactly the opposite state (later, this will be extended to a discussion regarding similar 3D illusions involving the shape, color, and texture of objects that may be used to depict their state). Keeping this in mind, we can discuss the dichotomy of "perception of location" and "perception of shape" as dissociable perceptual channels (cf. Loomis et al., 2002).

For the purpose of this chapter, we can distil from the vast literature on perception the following visual information processing modes that are used in real time to transform the input images to perceptions of the shape, orientation, and position of objects in a 3D scene:

- Shape from contour and object boundaries
- Shape from shading (and shadow)
- Shape from motion (including kinetic depth effects and motion parallax)
- Shape from stereo disparity
- Shape from texture
- Depth from contour occlusions (including line termination effects)
- Depth from lightness and translucency
- Depth from accommodation (lens-based focusing)
- Depth from familiar or expected size and perspective cues

None of these perceptual modes of processing is particularly good at producing "absolute" metrics but instead seem to be able to produce metrics of the depth to objects, which are framed relative to other objects (Pfautz, 2002). When visual information is available, these channels can rapidly produce relative spatial descriptors about the 3D relations between objects in the scene. One of the most frequent sources of frustration in the design of virtual and augmented reality interfaces is the failure of a display to produce "absolute" depth percepts, even while following prescribed guidelines for the use of computer graphic APIs to depict 3D scenes (Figure 6.8).

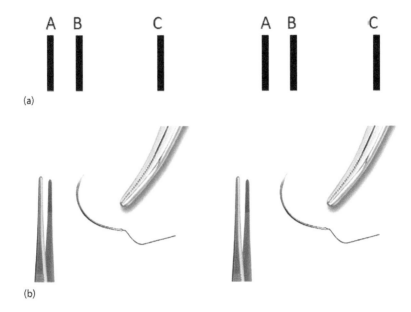

(a)

(b)

FIGURE 6.8 When you fuse these stereo pairs, [geometrical objects in pair (a), or surgical objects in pair (b)] relative depth information is compelling, but it is not an "absolute depth" percept. If you attempt to touch any of the objects using your fingertip, you will fail to experience the 3D scene and your fingertip in the same workspace.

6.4   THE ROLE OF THE SENSORY-MOTOR SYSTEM

Interactive, 3D, immersive AR/VR environments, by their nature, invite the user's motor system response within the environment. Sensory-motor control, for the most part, involves feedback-based dynamics. Human control does not seem to require "absolute" coordinates for control but instead can guide interactions based on the relative spatial, relational information provided by the sensory system. However, by the nature of the production of the final motor system output, all relative inputs must be resolved into a single controlled output. Consequently, any inconsistent or incomplete sensory estimates must somehow be reconciled. In some cases, inconsistent input channels can be ignored but in most cases will lead to errors in the output, or worse, to a breakdown of the entire task, or in many cases, headaches or serious "simulator sickness."

With regards to the overall conversion of "relative" locations of the workspace objects, cursor, user tools, and fingertips to the reference frame of motor control, we can acknowledge the amazingly adaptive nature of the human perceptual-motor system. It is extremely adept in its ability to calibrate (and dynamically recalibrate) the mapping between the spatial reference frame of the sensory inputs to the reference frame of the configuration, kinematics, and dynamical control space of the motor and action system. On the other hand, there is a fairly tight "sweet spot" in terms of the S-R compatibility that must exist between these two spaces. Humans cannot adapt to completely arbitrary remapping of the input and output space. Put more frankly, "stimulus-response compatibility" should not be violated in the design of human–computer interfaces, especially not in the case of 3D immersive environments.

As with all adaptive processes, the system must begin with some model for the transformation between the input and output reference frames, and for human sensory-motor control, the starting point comes in the form of the tacit expectations that the cognitive system has, in addition to the hard-wired perceptual-motor controllers. The bottom line, in terms of the user experience with immersive environments, is that the user typically explores the input–output space with exploratory movements, free-ranging gestures in the environment, and wildly explorative head movements in an attempt to calibrate their sensory-motor reference frames as a precursor to any performance of tasks at hand.

This initial exploratory calibration phase is often repeated each time the user begins a new task. Due to the extremely adaptive nature of the human system, attaining a precompiled adaptation to an environment typically requires a lot of exposure and use of the system. This has an impact on the usability evaluation of such a system. For objective evaluations of user performance, it is often difficult to tease apart the difference between "learning effects" and "practice effects." Unfortunately, in many published reports, the combined impact of these two effects has not been acknowledged, let alone teased apart. There are a few notable exceptions, and we include a short review of these (with references for the interested reader to consult).

6.5 LITERATURE AND EMPIRICAL STUDIES THAT SUPPORT THIS CRITICAL REVIEW

A number of studies support the view that AR/VR displays can be impacted by the special capacities and constraints of the human perceptual system and therefore require experimental testing and verification through controlled empirical methodologies. Here, we provide an overview of the empirical studies of the constraints on AR for medical applications.

In Sielhorst et al. (2006), although the display was programmed "correctly" in terms of the perspective rendering for the display in terms of the graphical API, "the physician often perceives the spatial position of the visualization to be closer or further due to virtual/real overlay." This observation was subsequently revisited for non-medical AR environments, for example, by Jones et al. (2008) who note that "[a] large number of previous studies have shown that egocentric depth perception tends to be underestimated in virtual reality (VR)—objects appear smaller and farther away than they should.... A much smaller number of studies have investigated how depth perception operates [in AR]." Previous studies have examined closed-loop versus open-loop reaching and grasping in virtual environments (Hu et al., 1999) and have shown not only how depth estimation, but also grip size are affected in dissociable ways when reaching and grasping objects in a virtual/augmented environment. These studies were conducted shortly after the initial introduction of AR for medical applications, which faced initial technical challenges and pioneered the need for a critical examination of perceptual effects (cf. Bajura et al., 1992; Lorensen et al., 1993; Grimson et al., 1995; Edwards et al., 1996; Fuchs et al., 1996; Hu et al., 1999). Swan et al. (2006) introduced a technique to measure the "fundamental problem in optical, see-through augmented reality (AR) ... characterizing how it affects the perception of spatial layout and depth.... protocols for measuring egocentric depth judgments in both virtual and augmented environments, and discusses the well-known problem of depth underestimation." Bichlmeier and Navab (2006) draw attention to the difficulty of interacting directly within an augmented scene. The "non-photorealistic" augmentation of scenes (which deliberately manipulate depth cues graphically to overcome some of these known perceptual effects and related shortcomings) has been attempted specifically for medical applications (cf. Lerotic et al., 2007). Studies on the perceptual-motor interactions in AR, specifically for medical applications have been conducted more recently (Klatzky et al., 2008; Meng et al., 2013). The effect on depth cues by specific cues for the occlusion of objects in an augmented scene was highlighted in Dey and Sandor (2014).

Having examined the fundamental concerns for AR considered in general terms, we now focus on some particular applications that will be feasible for the use of AR in neurosurgery in the near future.

6.6   CASES STUDIES AND EXAMPLE FROM THE LITERATURE: AUGMENTED AND VIRTUAL REALITY ENVIRONMENTS FOR NEUROSURGICAL PLANNING

We conclude by examining a number of success stories in the use of AR/VR in the domain of neurosurgery and conclude with some observations about the constraints placed on these systems (which we believe is what affords them their success).

Over the last two decades, an increasing number of research and commercial systems have surfaced for neurosurgical applications. While VR can mainly be used for training only, AR can be used from training to planning and/or navigating in the operating room. We concentrate here on the visual perception and human–computer interaction aspects of computer graphics for augmenting the display, without an extensive review of either modality in neurosurgery. The first successful commercial system was the addition of AR to the microscope. It was first described in Edwards et al. (1996), and the first commercial microscope was described in Haase (1999). The advantage of the microscope is that the focal point where the surgeon is looking and working is known and therefore can be accurately followed in depth, in addition to the (x, y) coordinates that are known by tracking the microscope with neuronavigation. The image can then be either reflected in the lenses and seen when looking through the microscope in the surgical scene or drawn on top of the camera's image from the microscope on the screen. This has been implemented by most of the surgical microscope companies collaborating with the neuronavigation systems. The usability and impact of such systems have mostly been studied through case series, with a few papers examining the clinical impact of the AR display. For example, in the case of vascular surgery, a team has determined that in clipping cerebral aneurysms, AR may have impacted 16.7% of the surgeries in facilitating the positioning of the clip (Cabrilo et al., 2014).

Other cases of vascular neurosurgery in which AR has been used successfully is the display of segmented arterio-venous malformations on the navigation system for training purposes (Kersten-Oertel et al., 2012). In both examples, as the image is displayed onto a screen, there are fewer issues with depth perception; however, there remains the problem of brain shift during the procedure, as the images are not updated with intraoperative information.

Other research teams have been using a tablet to fuse the operating scene or the head of the patient to their segmented world, thus creating a portable AR world (Deng et al., 2014; Kramers et al., 2014). While in the clinical setting it is difficult to know how much the AR systems actually impact the surgery, they can be better evaluated in a training environment.

AR has been evaluated for the training of tumor resection planning (Abhari et al., 2015) with regard to perceptual and spatial reasoning skills. Trainees and experts were instructed to plan a surgery and their selection of entry point and angle of approach and avoidance of eloquent areas were evaluated using a conventional imaging display (seeing the MRI and segmented tumor in the three different planes), an orthogonal display, a 3D VR display, and AR through a head-mounted display on a mannequin head. Significant improvement in performance was seen in the AR setting.

A few systems have examined the accuracy of registration of the image but have not accounted for the accuracy of targeting when a surgeon is using the system. The perception of depth is hard to evaluate in most systems (cf. Sielhorst et al., 2006), and therefore the human factor has not been taken into account when most publications are reporting on accuracy measures of the AR display. For example, the use of the tablet for AR display was published in Deng et al. (2014), but while there was a good accuracy of registration, there was no assessment of depth accuracy or actual targeting by the surgeon. Another example was published in Mahvash and Besharati Tabrizi (2013, 2015) with the direct projection of a tumor on the scalp of a mannequin. They found a good correlation with neuronavigation, but the accuracy in depth was not evaluated.

A recent study looking at depth perception showed that using AR with an actual stylet caused the user to make mistakes in the perception of depth (while the plane in the X and Y axes was relatively accurate, cf. Eagleson et al., 2015), but that inserting a virtual hand instead helped depth perception and therefore the accuracy, as the relative depth cues provided by AR are typically not strong enough when inserting a real object into the view (Wright et al., 2017) For reference, see Figure 6.6 of this chapter.

Neurosurgeons make use of their perceptual and spatial reasoning skills when they make judgements involving anatomical structures and their context. Classically, these are based on 2D, preoperative images, presented on a flat panel with axial, sagittal, and coronal views. To study the facilitation afforded by VR and AR immersive displays of surface-based and 3D, volumetric, biomedical visualization, it is important to develop methodologies to operationalize objective metrics of performance in tasks involving the perception of and spatial reasoning regarding anatomical structures.

6.7 CONCLUSIONS

AR/VR technologies offer a novel visualization modality with an exciting potential for medical visualization and clinical guidance. User acceptance of novel interfaces is always slow, and it is uncertain whether this is due to a tradition of slow acceptance of new technologies in the medical domain, regulatory hurdles, or intrinsic usability issues that may be rooted in problems associated with constraints on the human perceptual system. The chapter has attempted to isolate the core principles, which should not be violated in the design of human computer interfaces, and has contextualized them in the constraints that arise in immersive, 3D visualization and the targeting and navigation phases of a broad class of clinical workspaces. A few examples within the neurosurgical world in which AR has been accepted and is used clinically, as well as examples that may be more difficult to translate into the clinical world, were highlighted. It would appear that the feasibility of developing AR- and VR-based interfaces is greater when the workspace is constrained, such as for AR-enhanced microsurgery. One last point to keep in mind when designing such systems is that other factors, such as brain shift and registration inaccuracies in all dimensions (particularly in depth, as it is harder to visualize the error as a surgeon), must be taken into account for such a system to be useful. Even relatively accurate AR systems constrained to AR-enhanced microsurgery have not shown a large difference in patient outcomes when studied.

REFERENCES

Abhari K, Baxter J, Chen E, Khan A, Peters T, de Ribaupierre S, and Eagleson R (2015) Training for planning tumour resection: Augmented reality and human factors. *IEEE Transactions on Biomedical Engineering*, 62(6), 1466–1477.

Bajura M, Fuchs H, and Ohbuchi R (1992) Merging virtual objects with the real world: Seeing ultrasound imagery within the patient. In *Computer Graphics (SIGGRAPH '92 Proceedings)*, Vol. 26, pp. 203–210.

Barrow H and Tenenbaum J (1981) Interpreting line drawings as three-dimensional surfaces. *Artificial Intelligence*, 17, 75–116.

Besharati Tabrizi L and Mahvash M (2015) Augmented reality-guided neurosurgery: Accuracy and intraoperative application of an image projection technique. *Journal of Neurosurgery*, 123(1), 206–211.

Bichlmeier C and Navab N (2006) Virtual window for improved depth perception in medical AR. *Conference on Augmented Reality in Medicine*.

Bulthoff H and Mallot H (1990) Integration of stereo, shading, and texture. In *A.I. and the Eye*, Blake A and Troscianko T (Eds.). Chichester, UK: John Wiley & Sons.

Cabrilo I, Bijlenga P and Schaller K (2014) Augmented reality in the surgery of cerebral aneurysms: A technical report. *Neurosurgery*, 10(Suppl 2), 252–260; discussion 260–261.

Cavanagh P (1987) Reconstructing the third dimension: Interactions between color, texture, motion, binocular disparity, and shape. *Journal of Computer Vision, Graphics, and Image Processing*, 37, 171–195.

Deng W, Li F, Wang M and Song Z (2014) Easy-to-use augmented reality neuronavigation using a wireless tablet PC. *Stereotactic Functional Neurosurgery*, 92(1), 17–24.

Dey A and Sandor C (2014) Lessons learned: Evaluating visualizations for occluded objects in handheld augmented reality. *International Journal of Human-Computer Studies*, 72, 704–716.

Eagleson R and Peters T (2008) Perceptual capacities and constraints in augmented reality biomedical displays. *Australasian Physical & Engineering Sciences in Medicine*, 31(4), 371.

Eagleson R, Wucherer P, Stefan P, Duschko Y, de Ribaupierre S, Vollmar C, Fallavollita P and Navab N (2015) Collaborative table-top VR display for neurosurgical planning. *IEEE Virtual Reality Conference*, Arles Camargue, France, March 23–27.

Edwards P, Hawkes D, Hill D, Jewell D, Spink R, Strong A and Gleeson M (1996) Augmentation of reality in the stereo operating microscope for otolaryngology and neurosurgical guidance. *Journal of Image-Guided Surgery*, 1(3), 172–178.

Foley J and Van Dam A (1982) *Fundamentals of Interactive Computer Graphics.* Boston, MA: Addison-Wesley.

Fuchs H, State A, Pisano E, Garrett W, Hirota G, Livingston M, Whitton M and Pizer S (1996) Towards performing ultrasound-guided needle biopsies from within a head-mounted display. In *Visualization in Biomedical Computing 1996*, pp. 591–600.

Gibson J (1977) The theory of affordances. In *Perceiving, Acting, and Knowing*, Shaw R and Bransford J (Eds.). Hillsdale, NJ: Lawrence Erlbaum.

Gregory R (1970) *The Intelligent Eye.* London, UK: Weidenfeld & Nicolson.

Grimson W, Ettinger G, White S, Gleason P, Lozano-Perez T, Wells W and Kikinis R (1995) Evaluating and validating an automated registration system for enhanced reality visualization in surgery. In *Proceedings of Computer Vision, Virtual Reality, and Robotics in Medicine '95 (CVRMed '95)*.

Haase J (1999) Image-guided neurosurgery/neuronavigation: The SurgiScope reflections on a theme. *Journal of Minimally Invasive Neurosurgery*, 42(2), 53–59.

Hu Y, Eagleson R and Goodale M (1999) Human visual servoing for reaching and grasping: The role of 3D geometric features. *IEEE International Conference on Robotics and Automation*, 4, 3209–3216.

Jones A, Swan JE, Singh G and Kolstad E (2008) The effects of virtual reality, augmented reality, and motion parallax on egocentric depth perception. *IEEE Virtual Reality Conference*, p. 267.

Kersten-Oertel M, Chen SS, Drouin S, Sinclair DS and Collins DL (2012) Augmented reality visualization for guidance in neurovascular surgery. *Studies in Health Technology Information*, 173, 225–229.

Klatzky RL, Wu B, Shelton D and Stetten G (2008) Effectiveness of augmented-reality visualization vs. cognitive mediation for learning actions in near space. *ACM Transactions on Applied Perception*, 5(1), 1–23.

Kramers M, Armstrong R, Bakhshmand S, Fenster A, de Ribaupierre S and Eagleson R (2014) Evaluation of a mobile augmented reality application for image guidance of neurosurgical interventions. *Studies in Health Technology Information*, 196, 204–208.

Lerotic M, Chung A, Mylonas G and Yang G (2007) pq-space based non-photorealistic rendering for augmented reality. In *Medical Image Computing and Computer-Assisted Intervention – MICCAI 2007*. Lecture Notes in Computer Science, Ayache N, Ourselin S and Maeder A (Eds.), Vol. 4792. Berlin, Germany: Springer.

Loomis J, Philbeck J and Zahorik P (2002) Dissociation between location and shape in visual space. *Journal of Experimental Psychology and Human Perceptual Performance*, 28(5), 1202–1212.

Lorensen W, Cline H, Naris C, Kikinis R, Altobelli D and Gleason L (1993) Enhancing reality in the operating room. In *Proceedings of IEEE Visualization '93*.

Mahvash M and Besharati Tabrizi L (2013) A novel augmented reality system of image projection for image-guided neurosurgery. *Acta Neurochirurgica*, 155, 943–947.

Marr D (1982) *Vision: A Computational Investigation into the Human Representation and Processing of Visual Information.* New York: Freeman.

Meng M, Fallavollita P, Blum T, Eck U, Sandor C, Weidert S, Waschke J and Navab N (2013) Kinect for interactive AR anatomy learning. *IEEE International Symposium on Mixed and Augmented Reality (ISMAR)*, pp. 277–278.

Müller-Lyer F (1889) Optische Urtheilstäuschungen. *Archiv für Anatomie und Physiologie, Physiologische Abteilung*, 2, 263–270.

Norman D (1986) *User Centered System Design: New Perspectives on Human-computer Interaction.* Boca Raton, FL: CRC Press.

Pfautz J (2002) Depth perception in computer graphics. University of Cambridge, Technical Report UCAM-CL-TR-546.

Ponzo M (1912) Rapport entre quelques illusions visualles de contraste angulair et l'appreciation de grandeur des astres a l'horizon. *Archives Italiennes de Biologie*, 58, 327–329.

Sielhorst T, Bichlmeier C, Heining S and Navab N (2006) Depth perception – A major issue in medical AR: Evaluation study by twenty surgeons. In *Medical Image Computing and Computer-Assisted Intervention – MICCAI 2006*. Lecture Notes in Computer Science, Larsen R, Nielsen M and Sporring J (Eds.), Vol. 4190. Berlin, Germany: Springer.

Swan JE, Livingston M, Smallman H, Brown D, Baillot Y, Gabbard J and Hix D (2006) A perceptual matching technique for depth judgments in optical, see-through augmented reality. In *Proceedings of IEEE Virtual Reality Conference*, pp. 19–26.

Terzopoulos D (1986) Integrating visual information from multiple sources. In *From Pixels to Predicates*, Pentland AP (Ed.). Norwood, NJ: Ablex, pp. 111–142.

Ullman S (1989) *High-level Vision: Object Recognition and Visual Cognition*. Cambridge, MA: MIT Press.

Wright T, de Ribaupierre S and Eagleson R (2017) Design and evaluation of an augmented reality simulator using leap motion. *Healthcare Technology Letters*, 4(5), 210–215.

7 Interaction in Augmented Reality Image-Guided Surgery

Simon Drouin, D. L. Collins, and M. Kersten-Oertel

CONTENTS

7.1 INTRODUCTION

The goal of augmented reality (AR) in image-guided interventions is to allow surgeons to access navigation information during a procedure without shifting their attention away from the operative field. To be effective, augmentation should provide the right information at the right time, avoid distracting the surgeons, and provide an unambiguous and perceptually sound representation of the preoperative plans, guidance information, and anatomy under the visible surface of the patient. In this chapter, we argue that to reach these goals, it is necessary to systematically consider user interaction in the design of new surgical AR methods.

User interaction design falls under the domain of human–computer interaction and describes the design of interactions between users and their products. The goal of interaction design is to develop methods that allow users to achieve their objectives in the best way possible. Some of the elements developers need to consider when designing interactions include the visual representations of the data, the hardware device that should be used (e.g., mouse), the physical space in which the user will interact with the system, and the behaviors of the user (i.e., how they perform actions and operate the system). To date, there has been little focus on designing effective and usable interactions in image-guided surgery (IGS), and in particular in AR image-guided surgery, despite an important relationship between AR and interaction.

To illustrate the codependency of user interaction and AR, we classify interactive AR techniques into three categories: *control, task simplification*, and *enhancing perception*. Interactions for the purpose of *control,* as the name suggests, are intended to manipulate or command the IGS system itself. This may involve simple tasks, such as loading anatomical volumes or plans; enabling functions such as registration and segmentation; and changing visualization parameters. The purpose of *task simplification* interactions is to simplify and enable tasks to be executed more easily, more naturally, more quickly, and/or more precisely. Examples of this include easier localization of anatomy and more accurate targeting. Lastly, *enhancing perception* interactions refer to the use of interaction to improve perception of the anatomy, surgical plans, and, in general, the data visualized on the IGS system. Examples in this area include interactions that allow a user to view occluded objects and understand spatial relationships between data.

The remainder of this chapter is organized as follows. First, we establish the basis that supports our claim about the importance of considering interaction when designing AR visualization tools. Next, in Section 7.3, we review the literature on AR in IGS that pertains to some form of user interaction. Finally, in Section 7.4, we look at possible areas of focus for the future.

7.2   ON THE NECESSITY TO CONSIDER INTERACTION

AR and interaction complement each other in different ways, depending on the aspect of the system that is considered or the specific task that is addressed. In this section, we examine how the codependency of AR and interaction unfolds in light of our categorization of AR methods into *control* of the system, *task simplification*, and *enhancing perception*.

7.2.1   CONTROL

Interaction may be used simply to manipulate or *control* an IGS system and its parameters, for example, to allow the surgeon to control the type of visualization and the displayed content at a given point in time. Such control by the surgeon is important, as AR has been shown to be a source of distraction during an operation (Dixon et al. 2013). This effect can be mitigated by ensuring that the display always reflects what is needed by the surgeon. Although research in the area of surgical process modeling, such as the studies conducted by Jannin et al. (2003), Lalys and Jannin (2014), and Forestier et al. (2013), may help to automatically show the right information at the right time, automatic systems may never be able to predict the surgeon's needs all the time (Dergachyova et al. 2016). For this reason, it is important to give the surgeon control over the IGS system and specifically the AR view, allowing them to control what, how, and when content is displayed.

One of the promises of AR in IGS is to allow the surgeon to access navigation information without shifting attention from the operating field. In this chapter, we argue that this promise cannot be completely fulfilled unless the surgeon is able to also control the display without looking away.

7.2.2 Task Simplification

One of the goals of IGS systems is to *simplify tasks* such as positioning and orienting surgical tools relative to a target. This form of interaction, when performed with a conventional IGS system, involves a dissociation of the frames of references of the visual and motor systems of the user (Masia et al. 2009). Such dissociation has received much attention in the field of experimental psychology (Harris 1965) and is known to cause an important degradation in the performance of a subject during different motor tasks, such as aiming and reaching, particularly when frames of references are rotated relative to each other (Abeele and Bock 2001), which is often the case in surgery. In task simplification procedures, interaction with the IGS system is improved by the use of AR, which provides the important service of aligning the frames of reference of the visual and motor system.

7.2.3 Enhancing Perception through User Interaction

One of the most frequently reported problems of current medical AR systems is the degradation of depth perception that occurs when combining real and virtual elements. We argue that interaction can help to compensate for this loss of depth perception.

In his book about human visual perception, Gregory (1977) writes, "Perception is not determined simply by the stimulus patterns; rather it is a dynamic searching for the best interpretation of the available data." This quote highlights how visual perception is essentially a dynamic process through which different pictorial cues are fused by the brain to build a complete representation of the 3D world that is consistent with all cues (Landy et al. 1995). Some of these cues are dynamic by nature. For example, the well-studied motion parallax depth cue (Buckthought et al. 2014), which is generated by head movement relative to the environment, is one such cue where the brain integrates optical flow on the retina over time. Other cues are usually labelled as "static" because they can provide information based on the stimulus patterns captured at a single time point. However, it is often the case that integration over time produces a more complete description of the environment (Johnston et al. 1994).

In the field of cognitive science, researchers have long studied the interaction between visual and motor systems in the human brain. Wexler and van Boxtel (2005) have reviewed how an observer's motor actions influence his or her visual perception of the three-dimensional (3D) environment. Several results reported by Wexler support the importance of considering interaction when designing visualization tools. For example, observers can recognize objects more easily from a novel point of view if the change of point of view is the result of self-motion, rather than if the object itself was moved (Simons et al. 2002). This is an important consideration for IGS interaction design, as often it is not the surgeon but another member of the surgical team who interacts with the system, which therefore may cause a disruption in understanding the anatomical data. Harman et al. (1999) showed that "observers who actively rotated novel, three-dimensional objects on a computer screen later showed more efficient visual recognition than observers who passively viewed the exact same sequence of images of these virtual objects." Anticipatory mechanisms in the brain are thought to foresee the sensory consequences of motor actions and thus facilitate recognition (Wexler and van Boxtel 2005). For example, blindfolded subjects who are led to a new location can point to objects in their environment more easily than when they imagine walking the same path (Rieser et al. 1986) or when they are shown the corresponding optic flow (Klatzky et al. 1998). Regarding motion parallax, Wexler shows that the same optical flow can lead to different perceptions of 3D shapes depending on whether the motion is generated by the observer or the object itself. Knill (2005) showed that the brain changes how it integrates visual cues based not only on the information content of the stimuli but also on the task for which the information is used. Marotta et al. (1995) showed that monocular observers generate more head movement during reaching tasks to better utilize retinal motion cues.

It is important to understand how AR visualization differs from natural vision and where interaction may help. Drascic and Milgram (1996) review perceptual issues in AR and argue that in an AR environment, technological limitations remain such that certain depth cues commonly used in natural vision are absent, or worse, contradict each other, leading to a distorted perception of depth for the user. However, they show that as more cues are present and are congruent with each other, accurate depth perception can be restored.

In Bingham and Pagano (1998), the authors argue that the study of *definite distance perception* requires a perception-action approach. The reason is that definite distance perception entails calibration, which is a task-specific action that provides feedback to the visual system about the environment. They show that calibration can eliminate underestimation of distance generated by restriction of the visual field. In Altenhoff et al. (2012), it was reported that the typical underestimation of distances under virtual environment navigation can be compensated by submitting users to a calibration session, in which a reaching task is performed with haptics and visual feedback.

7.3 LITERATURE REVIEW

Surprisingly, interaction has not received a lot of attention from the IGS research community. Few publications address the topic of surgeon interaction with IGS systems and even fewer of interacting with visualized data to enhance perceptibility. In their review of AR visualization for IGS, Kersten-Oertel et al. (2013) note that interaction has been limited to allowing the end-user "to rotate and translate objects, to navigate through the virtual scene, to use cutting planes, to toggle components, turn visibility on and off, and to change the opacity and color of objects." Further, the authors found that the types of hardware that are most often used for manipulating data and interacting with the IGS system are the keyboard and mouse. In the following section, we give examples of how interaction has been explored in the context of IGS (rather than presenting a comprehensive review).

7.3.1 CONTROL

The classical keyboard and mouse interaction paradigm is not suitable for interactions between surgeons and surgical augmented environments (Navab et al. 2007; Bichlmeier et al. 2009). A major constraint for interaction, owing to the operating room (OR) environment, is the sterile boundary; when the surgeon is scrubbed, they would need to break asepsis to use the input devices to manipulate the images and system. Therefore, typically it is not the end-user of the IGS system (i.e., the surgeon) who interacts with the system but rather a technician or member of the surgical team receiving verbal instructions from the surgeon. This type of indirect communication is often slow and prone to errors and misunderstandings resulting from verbal ambiguities (Onceanu and Stewart 2011). To overcome these issues, a number of research groups have begun to study natural user interfaces that can interpret human action without direct contact. In AR IGS systems, voice interfaces, gesture-based interfaces, and tracked surgical tools have been explored to control the IGS system.

7.3.1.1 Voice

Few groups have explored the use of voice-based interaction within the OR. One exception is the work by Sudra et al. (2007), who allowed both speech- and gesture-based interaction within the context of an endoscopic robotic system. Their interaction methods allowed the surgeon to use speech or gestures to switch between visualization methods: for example, to change parameters or to turn annotation information on and off. The difficulties of voice interfaces include the challenges of a noisy OR and that voice may not be suitable for manipulation of continuous parameters (Mewes et al. 2017). However, combining voice-based interfaces with gestures may overcome the limitations and shortcomings of both of these types of interactions.

7.3.1.2 Gesture-Based Interaction

A number of groups have explored the possibility of using gestures to allow the surgeon to interact with the IGS system directly while remaining sterile. In a gesture-based interface, a set of motions or configurations of the hands or body are recognized by the system as commands. Wen et al. (2014) developed a gesture-based system for their AR needle guidance system for tumor ablation; three hand gestures are recognized: rotation, translation and point selection (Figure 7.1). A Kinect depth sensor (Microsoft Corp., Redmond, WA) is then used to recognize gestures that enable manipulation of the 3D view.

Kocev and his colleagues developed an interface method for projector-based AR through which the interface of a traditional navigation system is projected on the sterile draping close to the operating field. A Microsoft Kinect was then used to recognize gestures that enabled manipulation of the 3D view (Kocev et al. 2014).

Numerous other groups have explored the use of gesture-based interaction in traditional IGS. For example, Gratzel et al. (2004) proposed a paradigm to replace the use of a mouse in conventional navigation systems with a computer vision-based gesture recognition system that provides similar functionality, and Kirmizibayrak et al. (2011) compared the use of a gesture-based interaction system

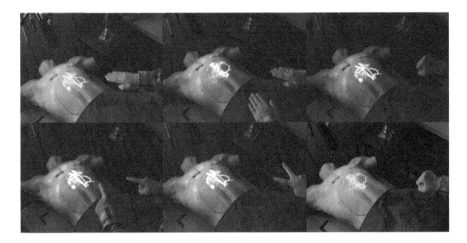

FIGURE 7.1   Gesture-based control of a projected AR navigation system. (From Wen, R. et al., *Comput. Methods Programs Biomed.*, 116, 68–80, 2014.)

with traditional mouse interaction. Although it does not use AR, their system is used for types of interaction that are often found in AR, such as the manipulation of a Magic Lens (Bier et al. 1993), which enables focus and context visualization of multiple volumetric medical datasets. The authors found the Magic Lens gesture interface was faster compared to the mouse but had higher variance. In a similar study with 30 physicians and senior medical students, Wipfli et al. (2016) compared three different interaction modes for image manipulation in the surgical domain: gestures (using Microsoft Kinect), verbal instructions given to a third party, and the mouse. They found that efficiency and user satisfaction were best when using the mouse, followed by gesture-controlled and verbal instructions. Not surprisingly, in their study the mouse outperformed the gesture-based interface, as it was a more familiar tool. For more information about touchless or gesture-based interfaces in surgical environments, the reader is referred to Mewes et al. (2017).

7.3.1.3   Surgical Tool

Another solution to enable the surgeon to interact directly with the IGS system is to make use of the surgical tools within the OR, typically accomplished by providing a way for the surgeon to use the tracked surgical probe. The advantage of using a surgical tool as an interaction solution is that it requires no (or limited) additional hardware in an already crowded OR yet allows the surgeon to have direct control over the IGS system. Examples of this include the work by Salb et al. (2003), who allowed the end-user to interact with a virtual graphical interface through a head-mounted display (HMD) using a tracked Polaris surgical probe. Fischer et al. (2005) use an AR menu that provides selectable menu items and allows interaction using the surgical probe to define points and freely draw shapes in 3D, while Katić et al. (2010) use an AR system that allows the end-user to interact with the system via a 3D pointer with integrated buttons.

In a non-AR IGS system, Onceanu and Stewart (2011) built a joystick-like interaction tool for the OR using a base in which a tracked surgical pointer can be inserted, rotated, and used to click. When comparing their input device with a mouse and verbal communication, the authors found that, although faster than both dictation and the joystick, the mouse was not significantly more accurate. Their results, similar to those of others who have compared novel interaction methods to the mouse and keyboard, suggest that metrics other than accuracy and speed are needed to enable a viable comparison that considers the constraints of the OR.

7.3.2 SIMPLIFYING TASKS

Many surgical procedures require aligning objects or surfaces in 3D, and the solution that is most commonly proposed is to reduce the problem to a two-dimensional (2D) alignment task, which is much simpler to execute. The most common example involves aligning a tool to an axis. Diotte et al. (2015) simplify the interlocking of intramedullary nails by tracking colored markers attached to the drill used to perform the procedure. The drill can then be aligned with overlaid targets and an x-ray image acquired from the same point of view (Figure 7.2a). Herrlich et al. (2017) simplify the needle insertion task by adding a small display to the needle-guiding tool showing a 2D representation of the alignment of the needle with the desired path. Seitel et al. (2016) produce an AR view for percutaneous needle insertion based on a combined color and depth (RGBD) image where the depth information in the image enables registration of the preoperative patient surface and needle plan with the image. A representation of the planned needle path can be superimposed on the image to serve as a guide to accurately position the real needle (Figure 7.2b). State et al. (1996) overlay a 3D representation of an ultrasound (US) image plane with live video of the operating field to guide a needle biopsy. The real part of the image shows the needle insertion point and orientation, while the US image augmentation allows the surgeon to see the target tumor and the

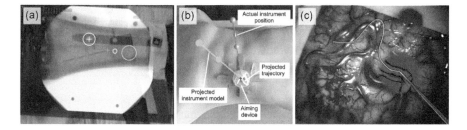

FIGURE 7.2 (a) AR view for interlocking of intramedullary nails: overlay of live video, x-ray, and alignment targets. (From Diotte, B. et al., *IEEE Trans. Med. Imaging*, 34, 487–495, 2015.) (b) AR view for percutaneous needle insertion showing real instrument and alignment target. (From Seitel, A. et al., *Int. J. Comput. Assist. Radiol. Surg.*, 11, 107–117, 2016.) (c) Tracing of virtual blood vessels using the surgical pointer. Trace is then used for registration correction. (From Drouin, S. et al., Interaction-based registration correction for improved augmented reality overlay in neurosurgery, in *Augmented Environments for Computer-Assisted Interventions*, Lecture Notes in Computer Science, Vol. 9365, pp. 21–29, 2015.)

part of the needle that has already been inserted. The fact that both the real needle and the target are displayed in the same 3D context facilitates aiming.

Another very common 3D alignment problem in medical imaging is the registration of the patient with preoperative images and plans. Drouin et al. (2015) propose an AR-based interface to correct the initial patient misregistration in neurosurgical interventions. The interface allows the surgeon to identify corresponding real and virtual anatomical features on the AR view using the tracked pointer typically available in most navigation systems (Figure 7.2c). The registration correction is achieved by automatic alignment of the marked features. An additional advantage of such a method is that it allows the surgeon to visually assess the accuracy of the registration through the AR view. A simpler, but similar, method was presented by Kantelhardt et al. (2015), through which the outlines of pre-segmented brain structures are superimposed on a microscope image of the patient, allowing surgeons to manually modify the initial patient registration to align the outlines with the live video. Cutolo et al. (2015) propose an AR-based interface to help with the manual alignment of non-tracked rigid bodies that need to be accurately positioned on the patient. The rigid bodies can be positioned by aligning virtual points in the AR view with physical landmarks on the object.

AR interaction can also facilitate the localization of a surgical target. Rong Wen et al. (2017) proposed a tablet-based AR system for surgical tool navigation. They evaluated the proposed system and showed that the tablet-based visual guidance system could assist surgeons in locating internal organs, with errors between 1.74 and 2.96 mm, while Shamir et al. (2011) proposed an AR system to explore the safest path for the insertion of straight tools in image-guided keyhole surgery. Their system virtually overlays risk data on a physical model of the patient to facilitate identification of risk-free paths. Shimamura et al. (2013) proposed to use a tracked, handheld display to visualize a slice of the patient's preoperative volume parallel to the display surface. The cutting plane-patient intersection is shown on the skin surface by projecting a laser line from the side of the tablet. As a final example, Bajura et al. (1992) use AR to guide the acquisition of US images. Many other tasks could be simplified by the use of AR, and the body of work on task simplification in conventional image-guidance systems should be thoroughly investigated to find the examples that benefit from adaptation to AR.

7.3.3 ENHANCING PERCEPTION

As demonstrated above, visual perception in augmented environments can be distorted by the absence of specific depth cues or inconsistencies between various depth cues resulting from the combination of real and virtual graphical objects. Perhaps the most important of these cues is occlusion. Inconsistent occlusion patterns in an image take precedence over other depth cues and lead to an incorrect perception. The most common example is found in AR views in which a real video image of a patient is overlaid on a virtual representation of the underlying anatomy. In this case, a naive alpha-blending between real and virtual components of the image produces the perception that virtual components are floating above the surface of the patient, as illustrated in Figure 7.3a.

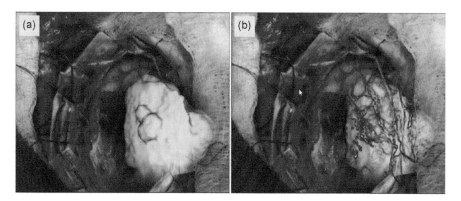

FIGURE 7.3 Example of a medical AR image where (a) the virtual element seems to be floating above the surface for lack of occlusion cues and (b) with occlusion cues restored, the virtual object is perceived to be located behind the surface. (From Kersten-Oertel, M. et al., *Int. J. Comput. Assist. Radiol. Surg.*, 10, 1823–1836, 2015.)

One of the typical approaches to help the visual system solve the occlusion in an AR scene is the virtual window (or Magic Lens) (Bier et al. 1993). Bichlmeier et al. (2007a) cut a virtual window out of the real image by intersecting a 3D model of the patient's skin surface with a user-defined cuboid. The motion of the HMD generates motion parallax and texture accretion/deletion cues to improve perceived relative depth between the surface and the surgical target. The approach was refined in Bichlmeier et al. (2007b) (Figure 7.4b), where the virtual window position is modified according to line of sight of the HMD, and the opacity of the real image inside the window is modulated by the angle between the skin surface and viewing direction as well as the curvature of the skin surface and distance to

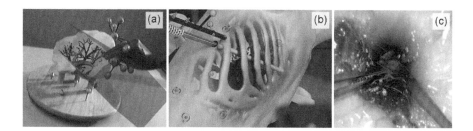

FIGURE 7.4 Different methods using the concept of a virtual window. (a) A tracked virtual cuboid cutout. (From Mendez, E. et al., Interactive context-driven visualization tools for augmented reality, in *IEEE/ACM International Symposium on Mixed and Augmented Reality*, pp. 209–218, IEEE, 2006.) (b) Virtual window based on HMD pose and surface properties. (From Bichlmeier, C. et al., Contextual anatomic mimesis hybrid in-situ visualization method for improving multi-sensory depth perception in medical augmented reality, in *IEEE/ACM International Symposium on Mixed and Augmented Reality*, pp. 1–10, IEEE, 2007; Courtesy of Christoph Bichlmeier.) (c) Force feedback-generated virtual window. (From Gras, G. et al., Visual Force Feedback for Hand-Held Microsurgical Instruments, in *Medical Image Computing and Computer-Assisted Intervention – MICCAI 2015*, Vol. 9349, pp. 480–487, 2015.)

the center of the window. Mendez et al. (2006) propose controlling the pose of a virtual 3D surface using an optical tracker tool. The intersection of the 3D surface with the presegmented organ surfaces is used to create a window where internal organ structures, such as blood vessels, are revealed (c.f., Figure 7.4a). Kalkofen et al. (2009) allow users to manipulate the position of a circular virtual lens, where the virtual window is not simply an area where the real image is semitransparent but instead allows for the application of programmable compositing schemes for the different elements in the scene. Different compositing inside the region covered by the virtual window reveals structures of interest while maintaining contextual information. Gras et al. (2015) (Figure 7.4c) proposed to use a tracked surgical dissector equipped with a force-torque sensor to interact with the AR view. Its location and the measurement of the force applied to the tissues are used to modulate the size of a virtual window, and the pq space method of Lerotic et al. (2007) is used to produce realistic occlusion patterns inside the virtual window. Furthermore, Gras and colleagues used force feedback information to distort a virtual model of the organs below the surface, providing a motion cue that improves depth perception even more.

Researchers address the concept of a virtual window in different ways. While Gras et al. (2015), Mendez et al. (2006), and Kalkofen et al. (2009) rely on the user to manipulate the location of the window, Bichlmeier et al. (2007b) use the motion of an HMD, and Bichlmeier et al. (2007a) use a static virtual window and rely entirely on the relative motion of an HMD to create the depth enhancing effect.

Even when employing a concept such as the virtual window, AR may still suffer from occlusion inconsistencies. For example, if an object such as a scalpel is manipulated above the virtual window, the part of the object intersecting the window will be occluded. Kutter et al. (2008) partially solve the problem by tracking the surgeon's hand in the live video stream to produce an occlusion mask for the virtual content of an AR view. Pauly et al. (2015) propose a similar but more general approach that can track arbitrary objects that occlude the operative field from an RGBD camera data using a random forest approach.

One interesting strategy to enhance perception in AR is to create bridges between real and virtual parts of an image to mitigate the influence of depth inconsistencies on perception. Choi et al. (2015) dynamically trace a line in the AR view connecting a tracked surgical pointer and the closest surface, while Lawonn et al. (2017) draw anchor lines between 3D rendered blood vessels and the internal surface of an interactively manipulated cylindrical cut-out region to allow users to get insight about the relative depth of different vessels.

A trivial approach to interaction that improves perception is to turn the visibility of virtual objects on and off. Choi et al. (2015) demonstrate that providing the possibility for a surgeon to interactively switch the view between AR and VR can improve the ability to reach a surgical target for spine surgery. These authors suggest that this is explained by a better depth perception in VR mode while the AR mode remains useful to provide context and be aware of the surface of the operating field. Bork et al. (2015) encode the distance of virtual objects to a tracked pointer in an AR scene by modulating their opacity following the temporal propagation of a spherical region of interest around the tip of the pointer. The progression of the region is also reflected in

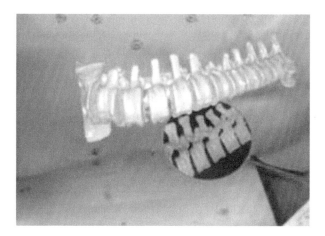

FIGURE 7.5   Example of the virtual mirror. (From Bichlmeier, C. et al., *IEEE Trans. Med. Imaging*, 28, 1498–510, 2009; Courtesy of Christoph Bichlmeier.)

an auditory display where a regular sound marks predefined steps of the progression, and a distinct sound marks the intersection of the region with virtual objects.

Controlling the point of view used to generate an AR image can greatly improve the perception. For all HMD-based systems, the feature is built-in, but the point of view is restricted by the surgeon's ability to move around the patient, which may be limited in a cluttered operating room or constrained by the use of a microscope. Shamir et al. (2006) propose to generate an AR view using a handheld tracked camera that enables fast exploration of the anatomy from various angles. Similarly, Kockro et al. (2009) employ a camera-equipped tracked surgical pointer in the OR to produce the augmented reality image. An alternative to interacting with the point of view is to use the virtual mirror, a concept inspired by a dentist's mirror, proposed by Bichlmeier et al. (2009). The interaction of the user with a tracked tool controls the 3D pose of a virtual mirror rendered in the AR scene and provides the ability to see behind 3D objects (c.f. Figure 7.5). Wieczorek et al. (2011) registered a preoperative 3D CT with an intraoperative x-ray, wherein depth information in the CT enabled the extrapolation of an x-ray image for a restricted range of depths. Various depth enhancement methods are proposed based on this principle. For example, tracked tools can be used to interactively manipulate a virtual plane used to "erase" parts of the x-ray beyond the plane.

7.4   DISCUSSION AND FUTURE DIRECTIONS

The development of novel interaction methods has been underrepresented in the AR IGS research community, with the majority of research focusing on the development of hardware, accurate and robust AR calibration techniques, and AR visualization methods. Yet, well-designed interaction techniques have the potential to simplify tasks, allow for more intuitive methods to control the IGS system and improve the surgical workflow, and enhance the perception of the guidance images and AR visualizations.

In terms of looking at interaction for *control*, some research groups have explored the use of touchless interaction, which has several advantages. These include the fact that the surgeon does not need to rely on someone else to interact with the system, which results in fewer misunderstandings between the surgeon and the person interacting with the IGS system. Further, this should lead to improved surgical workflows. Although there has been some research in this area, more work is needed to allow the surgeon to have easy, intuitive, and direct control over the IGS system.

Although not fully explored in the IGS literature, tangible user interfaces are another approach that may represent a novel solution to interactions for control in the surgical domain. Tangible user interfaces, which allow for the use of physical objects as a direct input mechanism for interaction with graphical representations, first became prominent with the work of Ishii and Ullmer (1997), and there have only been a handful of papers that have explored this type of interaction in medical imaging. Eck et al. (2016) developed a system for the preoperative planning phases of volume exploration and trajectory planning that uses a tracked handle to manipulate a preoperative volume and a force feedback stylus to re-slice the volume along an arbitrary plane. Hinckley et al. (1997) employed a tracked prop (plane or stylus), and a tracked head phantom, to explore an MRI by slicing the volume along the tracked prop axis. This field has yet to be fully explored in the IGS domain; however, one can envision what could be done in an OR, where more and more objects and devices will be modeled and tracked in real-time, and therefore may be used for interaction.

While there has been some work in terms of *task simplification*, we believe there is much potential for further research, particularly in terms of allowing the surgeon to use their knowledge to interact within the surgical field of view to account for inaccuracies of the system (such as brain shift, registration error, etc.), such as the work by Drouin et al. (2015). This would allow IGS systems to maintain accuracy and be used longer throughout surgery.

One of the main problems with AR in IGS is that the visualizations continue to be limited in terms of spatial and depth perception. Although this may be a minor issue in other domains, where labels and virtual elements may float above the real world, for IGS this is of utmost importance. Better depth perception of virtual elements between virtual anatomy and the surgical field of view and spatial relationships between these elements is needed for accurate guidance. By coupling interaction with visualization, it may be possible to enhance perception to allow for accurate localization of anatomy, and this will lead to a greater presence of AR in clinical practice.

REFERENCES

Abeele, S., and O. Bock. 2001. Mechanisms for Sensorimotor Adaptation to Rotated Visual Input. *Experimental Brain Research* 139, no. 2: 248–253.

Altenhoff, B.M., P.E. Napieralski, L.O. Long, J.W. Bertrand, C.C. Pagano, S.V. Babu, and T.A. Davis. 2012. Effects of Calibration to Visual and Haptic Feedback on near-Field Depth Perception in an Immersive Virtual Environment. In *Proceedings of the ACM Symposium on Applied Perception - SAP'12*, Vol. 71. New York: ACM Press.

Bajura, M., H. Fuchs, and R. Ohbuchi. 1992. Merging Virtual Objects with the Real World: Seeing Ultrasound Imagery within the Patient. *Computer Graphics* 26, no. 2: 203–210.

Bichlmeier, C., S.M. Heining, M. Feuerstein, and N. Navab. 2009. The Virtual Mirror: A New Interaction Paradigm for Augmented Reality Environments. *IEEE Transactions on Medical Imaging* 28, no. 9: 1498–1510.

Bichlmeier, C., T. Sielhorst, S.M. Heining, and N. Navab. 2007a. Improving Depth Perception in Medical AR A Virtual Vision Panel to the Inside of the Patient. In *Bildverarbeitung Für Die Medizin*, pp. 217–221. Berlin, Heidelberg: Springer.

Bichlmeier, C., F. Wimmer, S.M. Heining, and N. Navab. 2007b. Contextual Anatomic Mimesis Hybrid In-Situ Visualization Method for Improving Multi-Sensory Depth Perception in Medical Augmented Reality. In *IEEE/ACM International Symposium on Mixed and Augmented Reality*, pp. 1–10. IEEE.

Bier, E.A., M.C. Stone, K. Pier, W. Buxton, and T.D. DeRose. 1993. Toolglass and Magic Lenses. In *Proceedings of the 20th Annual Conference on Computer Graphics and Interactive Techniques - SIGGRAPH'93*, pp. 73–80. New York: ACM Press.

Bingham, G.P., and C.C. Pagano. 1998. The Necessity of a Perception-Action Approach to Definite Distance Perception: Monocular Distance Perception to Guide Reaching. *Journal of Experimental Psychology: Human Perception and Performance* 24, no. 1: 145–168.

Bork, F., B. Fuerst, and C. Graumann. 2015. Auditory and Visio-Temporal Distance Coding for 3-Dimensional Perception in Medical Augmented Reality. In *ISMAR 2015*.

Buckthought, A., A. Yoonessi, and C.L. Baker. 2014. Dynamic Perspective Cues Enhance Depth from Motion Parallax. *Journal of Vision* 14, no. 10: 734.

Choi, H., B. Cho, K. Masamune, M. Hashizume, and J. Hong. 2015. An Effective Visualization Technique for Depth Perception in Augmented Reality-Based Surgical Navigation. *The International Journal of Medical Robotics + Computer Assisted Surgery: MRCAS* (May 5).

Cutolo, F., G. Badiali, and V. Ferrari. 2015. Human-PnP: Ergonomic AR Interaction Paradigm for Manual Placement of Rigid Bodies. In *AE-CAI 2015, LNCS*, ed. C.A. Linte, Z. Yaniv, and P. Fallavollita, Vol. 9365, pp. 50–60. Cham, Switzerland: Springer.

Dergachyova, O., D. Bouget, A. Huaulmé, X. Morandi, and P. Jannin. 2016. Automatic Data-Driven Real-Time Segmentation and Recognition of Surgical Workflow. *International Journal of Computer Assisted Radiology and Surgery* 11, no. 6: 1081–1089.

Diotte, B., P. Fallavollita, L. Wang, S. Weidert, E. Euler, P. Thaller, and N. Navab. 2015. Multi-Modal Intra-Operative Navigation During Distal Locking of Intramedullary Nails. *IEEE Transactions on Medical Imaging* 34, no. 2: 487–495.

Dixon, B.J., M.J. Daly, H. Chan, A.D. Vescan, I.J. Witterick, and J.C. Irish. 2013. Surgeons Blinded by Enhanced Navigation: The Effect of Augmented Reality on Attention. *Surgical Endoscopy* 27, no. 2: 454–461.

Drascic, D., and P. Milgram. 1996. Perceptual Issues in Augmented Reality. In *SPIE Stereoscopic Displays and Virtual Reality Systems III*, pp. 123–134.

Drouin, S., M. Kersten-Oertel, and D.L. Collins. 2015. Interaction-Based Registration Correction for Improved Augmented Reality Overlay in Neurosurgery. In *Augmented Environments for Computer-Assisted Interventions*, Lecture Notes in Computer Science, Vol. 9365, pp. 21–29.

Eck, U., P. Stefan, H. Laga, C. Sandor, P. Fallavollita, and N. Navab. 2016. Exploring Visuo-Haptic Augmented Reality User Interfaces for Stereo-Tactic Neurosurgery Planning. In *Proceedings of the 7th International Conference on Medical Imaging and Virtual Reality, MIAR 2016*, pp. 208–220.

Fischer, J., J. Fischer, D. Bartz, and W. Straßer. 2005. Intuitive and Lightweight User Interaction for Medical Augmented Reality. In *Vision, Modeling and Visualization*, pp. 375–382.

Forestier, G., F. Lalys, L. Riffaud, D. Louis Collins, J. Meixensberger, S.N. Wassef, T. Neumuth, B. Goulet, and P. Jannin. 2013. Multi-Site Study of Surgical Practice in Neurosurgery Based on Surgical Process Models. *Journal of Biomedical Informatics* 46, no. 5: 822–829.

Gras, G., H.J. Marcus, C.J. Payne, and P. Pratt. 2015. Visual Force Feedback for Hand-Held Microsurgical Instruments. In *Medical Image Computing and Computer-Assisted Intervention – MICCAI 2015*, Vol. 9349, pp. 480–487.

Gratzel, C., T. Fong, S. Grange, and C. Baur. 2004. A Non-Contact Mouse for Surgeon-Computer Interaction. *Technology & Health Care* 12, no. 3: 245–257.

Gregory, R.L. 1977. *Eye and Brain, the Psychology of Seeing*, 3rd ed. London, UK: Weidenfeld & Nicolson.

Harman, K.L., G.K. Humphrey, and M.A. Goodale. 1999. Active Manual Control of Object Views Facilitates Visual Recognition. *Current Biology* 9, no. 22: 1315–1318.

Harris, C.S. 1965. Perceptual Adaptation to Inverted, Reversed, and Displaced Vision. *Psychological Review* 72, no. 6: 419–444.

Herrlich, M., P. Tavakol, D. Black, D. Wenig, C. Rieder, R. Malaka, and R. Kikinis. 2017. Instrument-Mounted Displays for Reducing Cognitive Load During Surgical Navigation. *International Journal of Computer Assisted Radiology and Surgery* 12, no. 9: 1599–1605.

Hinckley, K., R. Pausch, J. Hunter Downs, D. Proffitt, and N.F. Kassell. 1997. The Props-Based Interface for Neurosurgical Visualization. *Studies in Health Technology and Informatics*, vol. 39: 552–562.

Ishii, H., and B. Ullmer. 1997. Tangible Bits. In *Proceedings of the SIGCHI conference on Human factors in computing systems - CHI '97*, pp. 234–241.

Jannin, P., M. Raimbault, X. Morandi, L. Riffaud, and B. Gibaud. 2003. Model of Surgical Procedures for Multimodal Image-Guided Neurosurgery. *Computer Aided Surgery* 8, no. 2: 98–106.

Johnston, E.B., B.G. Cumming, and M.S. Landy. 1994. Integration of Stereopsis and Motion Shape Cues. *Vision Research* 34, no. 17: 2259–2275.

Kalkofen, D., E. Mendez, and D. Schmalstieg. 2009. Comprehensible Visualization for Augmented Reality. *IEEE Transactions on Visualization and Computer Graphics* 15, no. 2: 193–204.

Kantelhardt, S.R., A. Gutenberg, A. Neulen, N. Keric, M. Renovanz, and A. Giese. 2015. Video-Assisted Navigation for Adjustment of Image-Guidance Accuracy to Slight Brain Shift. *Neurosurgery* 11, no. 4: 1–8.

Katić, D., G. Sudra, S. Speidel, G. Castrillon-Oberndorfer, G. Eggers, and R. Dillmann. 2010. Knowledge-Based Situation Interpretation for Context-Aware Augmented Reality in Dental Implant Surgery. In *Medical Imaging and Augmented Reality, MIAR 2010*, pp. 531–540. Berlin, Germany: Springer.

Kersten-Oertel, M., I. Gerard, S. Drouin, K. Mok, D. Sirhan, D.S. Sinclair, and D.L. Collins. 2015. Augmented Reality in Neurovascular Surgery: Feasibility and First Uses in the Operating Room. *International Journal of Computer Assisted Radiology and Surgery* 10, no. 11: 1823–1836.

Kersten-Oertel, M., P. Jannin, and D.L. Collins. 2013. The State of the Art of Visualization in Mixed Reality Image Guided Surgery. *Computerized Medical Imaging and Graphics* 37, no. 2: 98–112.

Kirmizibayrak, C., N. Radeva, M. Wakid, J. Philbeck, J. Sibert, and J. Hahn. 2011. Evaluation of Gesture Based Interfaces for Medical Volume Visualization Tasks. In *Proceedings of the 10th International Conference on Virtual Reality Continuum and Its Applications in Industry - VRCAI'11*, Vol. 69. New York: ACM Press.

Klatzky, R.L., J.M. Loomis, A.C. Beall, S.S. Chance, and R.G. Golledge. 1998. Spatial Updating of Self-Position and Orientation During Real, Imagined, and Virtual Locomotion. *Psychological Science* 9, no. 4: 293–298.

Knill, D.C. 2005. Reaching for Visual Cues to Depth: The Brain Combines Depth Cues Differently for Motor Control and Perception. *Journal of Vision* 5, no. 2: 2.

Kocev, B., F. Ritter, and L. Linsen. 2014. Projector-Based Surgeon–computer Interaction on Deformable Surfaces. *International Journal of Computer Assisted Radiology and Surgery* 9, no. 2: 301–312.

Kockro, R.A., Y.T. Tsai, I. Ng, P. Hwang, C. Zhu, K. Agusanto, L.X. Hong, and L. Serra. 2009. Dex-Ray: Augmented Reality Neurosurgical Navigation with a Handheld Video Probe. *Neurosurgery* 65, no. 4: 795–808.

Kutter, O., A. Aichert, C. Bichlmeier, J. Traub, S.M. Heining, B. Ockert, E. Euler, N. Navab, and S. Michael. 2008. Real-Time Volume Rendering for High Quality Visualization in Augmented Reality. In *International Workshop on Augmented Environments for Medical Imaging Including Augmented Reality in Computer-Aided Surgery*.

Lalys, F., and P. Jannin. 2014. Surgical Process Modelling: A Review. *International Journal of Computer Assisted Radiology and Surgery* 9, no. 3: 495–511.

Landy, M.S., L.T. Maloney, E.B. Johnston, and M. Young. 1995. Measurement and Modeling of Depth Cue Combination: In Defense of Weak Fusion. *Vision Research* 35, no. 3: 389–412.

Lawonn, K., M. Luz, and C. Hansen. 2017. Improving Spatial Perception of Vascular Models Using Supporting Anchors and Illustrative Visualization. *Computers & Graphics* 63: 37–49.

Lerotic, M., A.J. Chung, G. Mylonas, and G.-Z. Yang. 2007. Pq-Space Based Non-Photorealistic Rendering for Augmented Reality. *International Conference on Medical Image Computing and Computer-Assisted Intervention* 10, no. Pt 2: 102–109.

Marotta, J.J., T.S. Perrot, D. Nicolle, P. Servos, and M.A. Goodale. 1995. Adapting to Monocular Vision: Grasping with One Eye. *Experimental Brain Research* 104, no. 1: 107–114.

Masia, L., M. Casadio, G. Sandini, and P. Morasso. 2009. Eye-Hand Coordination during Dynamic Visuomotor Rotations. *PloS One* 4, no. 9: e7004.

Mendez, E., D. Kalkofen, and D. Schmalstieg. 2006. Interactive Context-Driven Visualization Tools for Augmented Reality. In *IEEE/ACM International Symposium on Mixed and Augmented Reality*, pp. 209–218. IEEE.

Mewes, A., B. Hensen, F. Wacker, and C. Hansen. 2017. Touchless Interaction with Software in Interventional Radiology and Surgery: A Systematic Literature Review. *International Journal of Computer Assisted Radiology and Surgery* 12, no. 2: 291–305.

Navab, N., J. Traub, T. Sielhorst, M. Feuerstein, and C. Bichlmeier. 2007. Action- and Workflow-Driven Augmented Reality for Computer-Aided Medical Procedures. *IEEE Computer Graphics and Applications* 27, no. 5: 10–14.

Onceanu, D., and A.J. Stewart. 2011. Direct Surgeon Control of the Computer in the Operating Room. In *Medical Image Computing and Computer-Assisted Intervention*, pp. 121–128. Berlin, Germany: Springer.

Pauly, O., B. Diotte, P. Fallavollita, S. Weidert, E. Euler, and N. Navab. 2015. Machine Learning-Based Augmented Reality for Improved Surgical Scene Understanding. *Computerized Medical Imaging and Graphics* 41: 55–60.

Rieser, J.J., D.A. Guth, and E.W. Hill. 1986. Sensitivity to Perspective Structure While Wa/King without Vision. *Perception* 15, no. 1: 173–188.

Rong Wen, C.-B. Chng, and C.-K. Chui. 2017. Augmented Reality Guidance with Multimodality Imaging Data and Depth-Perceived Interaction for Robot-Assisted Surgery. *Robotics* 6, no. 2: 13.

Salb, T., J. Brief, T. Welzel, B. Giesler, S. Hassfeld, J. Muehling, and R. Dillmann. 2003. INPRES (Intraoperative Presentation of Surgical Planning and Simulation Results): Augmented Reality for Craniofacial Surgery. In *SPIE Electronic Imaging: Stereoscopic Displays and Virtual Reality Systems*, ed. A.J. Woods, M.T. Bolas, J.O. Merritt, and S.A. Benton, Vol. 453. International Society for Optics and Photonics.

Seitel, A., N. Bellemann, M. Hafezi, A.M. Franz, M. Servatius, A. Saffari, T. Kilgus et al. 2016. Towards Markerless Navigation for Percutaneous Needle Insertions. *International Journal of Computer Assisted Radiology and Surgery* 11, no. 1: 107–117.

Shamir, R., L. Joskowicz, and Y. Shoshan. 2006. An Augmented Reality Guidance Probe and Method for Image-Guided Surgical Navigation. In *5th International Symposium on Robotics and Automation*, pp. 1–6.

Shamir, R.R., M. Horn, T. Blum, J.H. Mehrkens, Y. Shoshan, L. Joskowicz, and N. Navab. 2011. Trajectory Planning with Augmented Reality for Improved Risk Assessment in Image-Guided Keyhole Neurosurgery. In *IEEE International Symposium on Biomedical Imaging: From Nano to Macro*, pp. 1873–1876.

Shimamura, S., M. Kanegae, Y. Uema, M. Inami, T. Hayashida, H. Saito, and M. Sugimoto. 2013. Virtual Slicer: Development of Interactive Visualizer for Tomographic Medical Images Based on Position and Orientation of Handheld Device. In *2013 International Conference on Cyberworlds*, pp. 383–383. IEEE.

Simons, D.J., R.F. Wang, and D. Roddenberry. 2002. Object Recognition Is Mediated by Extraretinal Information. *Perception & Psychophysics* 64, no. 4: 521–530.

State, A., M.A. Livingston, W.F. Garrett, G. Hirota, M.C. Whitton, E.D. Pisano, and H. Fuchs. 1996. Technologies for Augmented Reality Systems. In *Proceedings of the 23rd Annual Conference on Computer Graphics and Interactive Techniques - SIGGRAPH'96*, pp. 439–446. New York: ACM Press.

Sudra, G., S. Speidel, D. Fritz, B.P. Müller-Stich, C. Gutt, and R. Dillmann. 2007. MEDIASSIST: Medical Assistance for Intraoperative Skill Transfer in Minimally Invasive Surgery Using Augmented Reality. In *SPIE Medical Imaging 2007*, ed. K.R. Cleary and M.I. Miga. International Society for Optics and Photonics.

Wen, R., W.L. Tay, B.P. Nguyen, C.B. Chng, and C.K. Chui. 2014. Hand Gesture Guided Robot-Assisted Surgery Based on a Direct Augmented Reality Interface. *Computer Methods and Programs in Biomedicine* 116, no. 2: 68–80.

Wexler, M., and J.J.A. van Boxtel. 2005. Depth Perception by the Active Observer. *Trends in Cognitive Sciences* 9, no. 9: 431–438.

Wieczorek, M., A. Aichert, P. Fallavollita, O. Kutter, A. Ahmadi, L. Wang, and N. Navab. 2011. Interactive 3D Visualization of a Single-View X-Ray Image. In *Medical Image Computing and Computer-Assisted Intervention – MICCAI 2011 SE - 10*, Lecture Notes in Computer Science. ed. G. Fichtinger, A. Martel, and T. Peters, Vol. 6891, pp. 73–80. Berlin, Germany: Springer.

Wipfli, R., V. Dubois-Ferrière, S. Budry, P. Hoffmeyer, C. Lovis, J. Wobbrock, and W. Schlegel. 2016. Gesture-Controlled Image Management for Operating Room: A Randomized Crossover Study to Compare Interaction Using Gestures, Mouse, and Third Person Relaying. Ed. Peter M.A. van Ooijen. *PLoS One* 11, no. 4: e0153596.

8 Cognitive Oriented Design and Assessment of Augmented Reality in Medicine

Pierre Jannin and Thierry Morineau

CONTENTS

8.1 INTRODUCTION

Mixed and Augmented Reality (AR) is a technology that aims to augment the perception of reality by adding computer-generated information. Such technology has been applied for medical procedures (especially surgery) the past 20 years to help physicians understand and perform procedures, as well as for training. However, as outlined in different review papers, AR has not yet reached its full potential usefulness and implementation in the medical workflow. Many reasons for this have been expressed; one is that the AR system design approach is mainly technology driven, resulting in the need to develop relevant and clinically valuable AR applications. Another reason is the lack of relevant assessments of proposed AR systems to validate their benefits in all aspects of medical care (Kersten-Oertel et al. 2013; Khor et al. 2016).

In the main ontological approaches to describe an AR system, much emphasis has been placed on the display. In Gabbard and Hix (1997), the main AR components included (1) real and virtual media representation; (2) interaction as input to the AR system; and (3) display technology and methods as outputs of the system. More recently, Kersten and colleagues (2012) went a step further by adding concepts related to data and the scenario. The main AR components were classified as (1) view-related components (i.e., perception location, display, and interaction); (2) data (including patient-specific raw imaging data or clinical data, knowledge, and derived data); and (3) visualization processing, including rendering and data transformation. The concepts of scenario and steps were included in their model in an informal way.

Mixed and AR is considered a man/machine interface that provides the physician with input into his/her perception component of the perception/decision/action loop. This input comprises two main components: what is represented (i.e., the data) and the way the data are represented. There are different types of AR data that have been identified in previous AR frameworks, including raw, analyzed, derived, and prior knowledge data, in AR, all of these data are transformed into visualized data, which are then rendered (i.e., viewed) by the viewing component. The latter is characterized by the location where the AR view is perceived, the display system used for perception, and the additional interaction tools that may help optimize perception by modification of the view. However, by eluding the understanding stage into the perception/decision/action loop, AR design and assessment are constrained to be part of (and restricted by) the perception component.

In this chapter, we propose a paradigm shift for AR that may facilitate design and assessment for improving the dissemination of AR systems in medical applications. We suggest a cognitive-oriented approach for both the optimal design and assessment of AR systems. This approach is based on two main statements: (1) ensuring proper definition and modeling of medical objective(s) and (2) considering understanding as the main motivation for AR.

8.1.1 HYPOTHESIS

We propose to consider the use of AR in a medical procedure as a tool to help the physician realize the goal of that procedure. We first suggest that AR design in medicine is concerned with the use of AR technology to achieve this goal. Second, we propose to express this goal as the state(s) of the work domain that must be reached by the clinician.

To the usual perception/decision/action/validation paradigm, we suggest adding a cognition component concerning understanding (Figure 8.1), as a crucial stage before decision-making and validation. "Understanding" emphasizes the cognitive task involved after perception and before decision and validation. By adding this stage, we shift the objective for AR design from perception to understanding. Assuming that the medical objective is to reach a final state for the work domain, we define AR as a system to provide the physician with an optimal understanding of the state(s) of the work domain through perception, which may be visual, haptic, audible, or olfactory. We propose to rely on cognitive engineering as a framework to describe the work domain and to map the objective with technology.

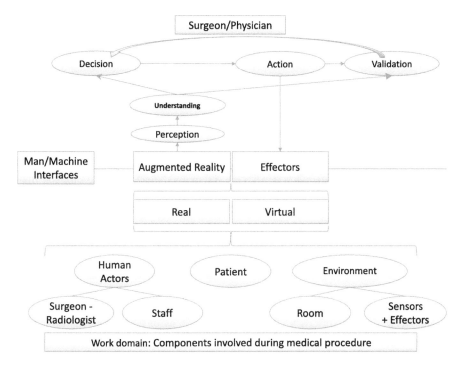

FIGURE 8.1 Mixed and Augmented Reality: a system to assist physicians in perception, understanding, decision, action and validation processes.

8.2 COGNITIVE-ORIENTED DESIGN FOR AR IN MEDICINE

In the next sections, we propose an approach to design AR as the specifications of the following:

- What are the *objectives* of the medical procedure?
- What is the optimal *support* (i.e., data, information, and knowledge) helping to reach this objective?
- What is the optimal *representation* mode to perceive this support?

8.2.1 OBJECTIVE AND CORRESPONDING SUPPORT

For AR design, we suggest the objective(s) of a medical procedure be defined as the state(s) of the work domain that must be reached by the clinician. To realize the medical objective(s), a sequential combination of perception, understanding, decision, and action tasks are performed. Whereas decision and action tasks are performed by the clinician without involvement of the AR system, AR should augment the perception of data, information, and knowledge to help understanding. Understanding includes both the pre- and post-conditions of the objective(s). Pre-conditions include assumptions about the state of the work domain that facilitate making the next decision and performing the next action. Post-conditions include verification of the state of the work domain after performance of the action to check the success of the performed action—the stage we call validation. We assume that, if understanding is optimal, the conditions are optimal for reasoning and decision making.

To represent the work domain states, we propose to use the abstraction hierarchy (AH) model from the work domain analysis (WDA) approach (Hajdukiewicz et al. 2001). WDA is an approach used in cognitive engineering to represent and model work domains. The WDA produces work domain models with two dimensions: a structural dimension—the part-whole hierarchy (PWH) and a functional dimension—the abstraction hierarchy (AH). The PWH outlines the hierarchical structural organization of the domain, aggregating structural components into less detailed objects. This dimension copes with the management of the complexity that derives from biological systems. Components are grouped together to form a structure with the top corresponding to the whole work domain. In medicine, the anatomy is described hierarchically thanks to the PWH, however, in this chapter, we will not address this dimension. Most relevant contributions to the PWH dimension can be found in ontological representations, such as the foundational model of anatomy (Rosse and Mejino 2003). The AH and PWH dimensions can be displayed at the same time through a matrix with AH levels in lines and PWH levels in columns. This matrix constitutes a work domain model, both in structure and content.

The AH describes work domains through a hierarchy of functions structured by a "means-ends" relationship (Table 8.1). In this hierarchy, the lower levels of functions are means to reach the higher levels, and, conversely, the higher levels are the reasons explaining why the lower functional levels are available. An AH is composed of five levels of work domain functions: *functional purposes*, *abstract functions*, *generalized functions*, *physical functions*, and *physical forms*.

> *Functional purposes* correspond to the general objectives of the medical procedure. A medical procedure is driven and motivated by general objectives represented at this level, such as tumor removal, aneurysm clipping, or radiation therapy. The general objectives can be broken down into an additional hierarchy of functional subjectives. In surgery, for instance, the general objectives are divided into (1) functions for structure identification; (2) functions related to the access to the target(s) through crossable structures; (3) strategies to preserve and avoid structures; and (4) interventional functions, such as those to extract, reach, stimulate, repair, or replace.
>
> *Abstract functions* (also called domain values) are the principles by which the functional purposes operate. The abstract functions describe how the work domain is understood with respect to the objectives or subjectives to be performed. Abstract functions include strategies, reasoning, and logic-related functions and main rules.
>
> *Generalized functions* (also called domain functions or processes) describe the properties of the domain, which are conditions for validating principles.
>
> *Physical functions* correspond to the information required to verify properties.
>
> *Physical forms* correspond to the actual physical parameters from which information is derived. Physical functions are defined independently of the manner in which they are physically perceived.

TABLE 8.1

The AH as a Functional Work Domain Model (e.g., in surgery)

AH Level	Definition	Examples in Neurosurgery			
Functional purposes	Objectives	Structure/tissue identification	Crossable medium	Tissue preservation or avoidance	Intervention
Abstract functions	Integration of information, strategies, reasoning, understanding	Environmental compliancy, neurophysiological balances, neural plasticity, certainty, precision, exhaustivity	Possible trajectories, trade-off "exploration/risk," trade-off "path progression/risk"	Strategies to avoid tissues, life risks incurred	Trade-off "full extraction/risk," extraction strategies
Generalized functions	Known properties validating principles	Chemical reactivity, pressure on/of environment, impact of pathological entity, state evolution of pathology, patient anamnesis, brain position/surgeon, conditions of imaging acquisition	Distance between entities, anatomical landmarks	Technical conditions to preserve tissues	Circumstances in which extraction, exclusion, stimulation, removing, and rebuilding are feasible
Physical functions	Information needed to verify properties	Entity names, boundaries between entities, anatomical structures	Obstacles, entry point, target point	Preservation of anatomical structures and functional areas	Direction of action during extraction, proportion to extract, proportion of extracted lesion
Physical forms	Data	Forms, density, elasticity, plasticity, solidity, adhesion, color, size, volume			

The AH assumes that the higher the perceived levels are, the better the understanding of the work domain.

8.3 PROPOSAL

We propose to design AR as a system that is able to provide virtual augmentation at the higher levels of the AH, thus allowing a better understanding of the work domain.

The following methodology is proposed to assist the design process of AR systems in medicine. The first step in the design process is to identify the functional purposes of the targeted clinical application. This can be achieved by soliciting knowledge through a "think aloud" interview while asking surgeons to describe the medical procedure with possible alternatives. First, cognitive conflict identification, consisting of identifying all time points in the procedure when a critical decision/action will be taken, is performed. From this, the most important identified conflicts are selected. These conflicts are expressed as *functional purposes* (i.e., objectives). Second, from this selection, the corresponding controls (i.e., mitigations) are identified as *abstract functions*. One possibility for helping to identify abstract functions is to rely on the Skill, Rule, Knowledge, Assistance (*SRKA*) *extended coding* (Morineau et al. 2009) extension from (Rassmussen 1993). *Skill*-based control is coded as the implementation of a perceptual or motor process, respectively divided into *perceptual-* and *motor skill*-based controls. *Rule*-based control corresponds to a conditional control of the conflict. If some conditions are satisfied, then an operation can be performed. *Knowledge*-based control refers to concepts or reasoning relying on an understanding of the conflict foundations. *Assistance*-based control involves the use of external resources for conflict regulation, such as patient images or surgical staff advice. Then, for these identified abstract functions, the designer of the AR system selects one or several on which he/she wants to focus and uses them as objectives. For each of them, a further hierarchical analysis consists of identifying corresponding generalized functions as related properties. If such properties can be computed or estimated from available digital data and represented, then they are integrated in the AR system. If not, then the sublevel is considered a physical function. Similarly, if such information can be computed or estimated from available digital data and represented, then it is integrated in the AR system. If not, the final sublevel is considered a physical form. Similarly, if such data can be computed or estimated and represented, then they are integrated in the AR system (Figure 8.2).

8.3.1 PERCEPTION

After identification of the objective(s) and corresponding support(s) for each support, the designer must select the optimal representation mode to perceive this support. Whereas AR has been mainly addressed using visual perception, there is a recent body of work providing other representation modes as well. For instance, in Matinfar et al. (2017) and Black et al. (2017), the authors suggest AR by means of auditory augmentation. In fact, any type of augmentation targeting the human senses is feasible (such as visual, haptic, auditory, and olfactory).

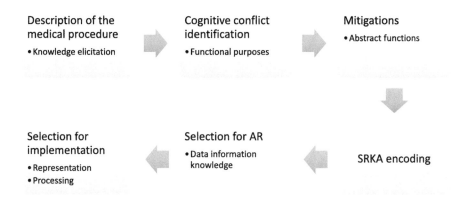

FIGURE 8.2 Proposal for a cognitive based approach to design Mixed and Augmented Reality Systems in Medicine.

For the usual visual augmentation, there is an important emerging body of work that attempts to study representation paradigms, which can be distinguished by means of the following:

- *Point of view*: Is it an ego- or exocentric point of view?
- *Overlay*: Which processing method should be used to overlay real and virtual worlds?
- *Interaction*: What are the user interactions between both real and virtual worlds within the AR system?
- *Animation*: What kind of dynamic representation is employed (such as a blinking object representation)?

Designing AR consists of completion of the form in Table 8.2, including specifying the objectives at two levels, as well as their corresponding support at three possible levels and the way they are computed and represented.

TABLE 8.2

Design Form for AR Based on Work Domain Analysis

	Objectives
Functional purpose	
Abstract function	
	Corresponding Support
Generalized function	Involved properties
	How is it computed? From information to properties
	How is it represented?
Physical function	Involved information
	How is it computed? From data to information
	How is it represented?
Physical form	Data
	How is it represented?

8.4   MIXED AND AUGMENTED REALITY ASSESSMENT

8.4.1   Validation

Validation is about demonstrating that the system does what it is intended to do. If AR is designed to provide an optimal understanding of the work domain, validation will mainly consist of demonstrating that AR improves the understanding of the work domain as implemented above. While to date, validation has mainly been addressed by studying the impact on perception, this chapter emphasizes understanding the scene following its perception. We therefore recommend performing validation as a study involving a representative population of users, covering the diversity of possible users in term of skills, age, technology usage, gender, and other possible characteristics, as well as under special conditions such as fatigue and stress. For each session, we recommend evaluating the level of understanding of the work domain. This may be estimated using questionnaires such as that presented in Morineau et al. (2013), in which the questionnaire spans the whole AH of the corresponding work domain within the questions.

8.4.2   Assessment Metrics

In addition to the above validation, AR designers would like to study the impact of their system on decision and action, and several metrics can be studied. Metrics may be related to four main categories (Figure 8.3). The first concerns the user who wears the AR system (e.g., head-mounted system). The system has a direct impact on the user

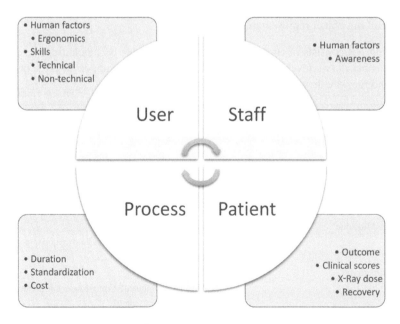

FIGURE 8.3   Four categories of assessment metrics for Mixed and Augmented Reality Systems in Medicine.

through human factors, such as the ergonomics of the system (e.g., comfort of use). The system also may directly impact the user's technical skills (such as dexterity, tremor) and nontechnical skills (such as situation awareness, stress, or risk anticipation). The system may affect the whole medical team by providing them with enhanced situation awareness as well as impact human factors. Although it is known that the success of the procedure is mainly defined with regards to its objective, the procedure followed to reach the objective may be of interest and serves as a metric for AR system assessment, such as minimal duration, minimal energy, minimal workspace, cost, repeatability, or standardization. Finally, the system hopefully may influence the patient by affecting clinical scores, time in the operating room, or time for recovery (Figure 8.3).

8.4.3 ASSESSMENT STUDY CONDITIONS

It is crucial when performing AR evaluation studies to follow the usual guidelines for ensuring proper reporting and understanding of the results. In Jannin and Korb (2008), the importance of clear design and reporting of the study conditions was described in the context of the assessment of image-guided intervention systems. Being able to fully describe the conditions in which the evaluation studies have been performed is crucial for developing a proper understanding of the results and any possible bias (Figure 8.4). This includes the characteristics of the operators who used the AR system during evaluation, the location in which the study was performed, as well as the corresponding setup, the mimicked medical process, and the type of data manipulated during the study. The degree of realism of all these conditions during the studies strongly affects the findings and their relevance (Figure 8.4).

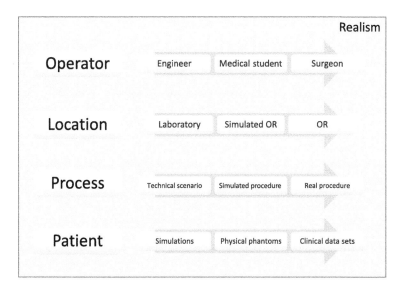

FIGURE 8.4 Assessment study conditions for Mixed and Augmented Reality Systems in Medicine. Left to right: from low to high clinical realism and full to no control of the conditions.

8.5 DISCUSSION

In this chapter, we proposed addressing AR design using a new paradigm based on cognitive engineering. We are convinced that this approach will allow for the development of clinically relevant systems in which emphasis is placed on understanding rather than on perception. However, we believe that this approach is complementary to those previously proposed, and correct perception is still mandatory to help understanding. Reliance on functional work domain analysis will ensure proper understanding of the main functional concepts (including data, information, and knowledge) that are involved in the decision-making process of clinical applications. The main interest of the proposed framework is that it is independent from the way the task is performed.

In this quest for optimal perception, it is also important to note that objective and corresponding support are user-independent, whereas representation and perception are user-dependent. Different users will be sensitive to different representations according to their specialty, skill level, and psychological characteristics. In Jannin et al. (2010), we demonstrated that higher levels of abstraction were understood for expert surgeons with a two-dimensional representation mode of a brain scene than with a three-dimensional mode, with the inverse being true for more novice observers. This is important to consider when designing and assessing AR systems.

The main difficulties in the assessment of AR technology are in being able to compare performances with and without the use of the AR system, assuming that there will be a statistically significant difference in performances due to the use of the AR system, which is never easy to reach or to demonstrate.

REFERENCES

Black, D., Hansen, C., Nabavi, A., Kikinis, R., and Hahn, H. 2017. A survey of auditory display in image-guided interventions. *Int J Comput Assist Radiol Surg* 12(10):1665–1676.

Gabbard, J. L., and Hix, D. 1997. A taxonomy of usability characteristics in virtual environments. http://csgrad.cs.vt.edu/jgabbard/ve/taxonomy/ (accessed December 2017).

Hajdukiewicz, J. R., Vicente, K. J., Doyle, D. J., Milgram, P., and Burns, C. M. 2001. Modeling a medical environment: An ontology for integrated medical informatics design. *Int J Med Inform* 62(1):79–99. doi: S1386-5056(01)00128-9.

Jannin, P., and Korb, W. 2008. Assessment in image guided interventions. In *Image-Guided Interventions: Technology and Applications*, edited by TM. Peters and K. Cleary, pp. 531–549. Berlin, Germany: Springer.

Jannin, P., Le Moellic, N., Morineau, T., and Morandi, X. 2010. Assessment of medical imaging based on work domain analysis. In *International Conference of Computer Assisted Radiology and Surgery*, Geneva (CH), Switzerland.

Kersten-Oertel, M., Jannin, P., and Collins, D. L. 2012. DVV: A taxonomy for mixed reality visualization in image guided surgery. *IEEE Trans Vis Comput Graph* 18(2):332–352. doi:10.1109/TVCG.2011.50.

Kersten-Oertel, M., Jannin, P., and Collins, D. L. 2013. The state of the art of visualization in mixed reality image guided surgery. *Comput Med Imaging Graph* 37(2):98–112. doi:10.1016/j.compmedimag.2013.01.009.

Khor, W.S., Baker, B., Amin, K., Chan, A., Patel, K., and Wong, J. 2016. Augmented and virtual reality in surgery—The digital surgical environment: applications, limitations and legal pitfalls. *Ann Transl Med* 23(4):454.

Matinfar, S., Nasseri, A., Eck, U., Roodaki, A., Lohmann, C., Maier, M., and Navab, N. 2017. Surgical soundtracks: Towards automatic musical augmentation of surgical procedures *International Conference on Medical Image Computing and Computer Assisted Interventions (MICCAI)*, Quebec, Canada, September 2017.

Morineau, T., Morandi, X., Le Moellic, N., Diabira, S., Riffaud, L., Haegelen, C., Henaux, P. L., and Jannin, P. 2009. Decision making during preoperative surgical planning. *Hum Factors* 51(1):67–77.

Morineau, T., Morandi, X., Le Moellic, N., and Jannin, P. 2013. A cognitive engineering framework for the specification of information requirements in medical imaging: Application in image-guided neurosurgery. *Int J Comput Assist Radiol Surg* 8(2):291–300. doi:10.1007/s11548-012-0781-7.

Rassmussen, J. 1993. Skills, rules and knowledge; signals, signs, and symbols, and other distinctions in human performance models. *IEEE Trans Syst Man Cybern* 13(3):257–266.

Rosse, C., and Mejino, J.L.V. 2003. A reference ontology for bioinformatics: The foundational model of anatomy. *Journal of Biomedical Informatics* 36:478–500.

9 Augmented Reality in Aging and Medical Education

Pascal Fallavollita and Nassir Navab

CONTENTS

9.1 INTRODUCTION

The aging population poses a significant burden on healthcare systems internationally. The substantial population disparity between older adults who require care and the younger population who must provide it will place an overwhelming economic burden on long-term care facilities in the future, thus making it necessary to identify economical at-home care alternatives. Augmented reality (AR) has proven to be a versatile and applicable technology in the medical field, as it has been utilized in dealing with illnesses such as phobias, muscular dystrophy, and cognitive impairments. However, its adoption for use in elderly care has been minimal due to the lack of progressive technologies that are user-friendly for older adults.

In contrast to the area of aging, gross anatomy is an essential component of medical education for the general population. The methods used to teach this element have changed dramatically over the last few decades. Traditionally, gross anatomy has been taught through cadaver dissection and textbooks. However, the use of these resources has declined due to financial considerations, time constraints, and ethical issues. Together, these limitations and the expansion of medical imaging have led to the development of a variety of technological resources for medical education.

In recent years, AR systems have developed to the extent that they can not only address the limitations of traditional teaching methods but may also increase the rate at which people understand gross anatomy.

This chapter presents a survey of existing AR solutions that aid the aging population and contribute to enhancing medical education.

9.2 AGEING

The baby boomer cohort includes all those born from 1946 to 1964. This represents the largest generational cohort in history with a population of almost one billion individuals. Now, in the twenty-first century, this generational cohort has begun entering late adulthood. This is placing enormous pressure on modern healthcare systems to support this substantial population and their increasing healthcare needs. By 2030, there is expected to be a 135% increase in the elderly population as the baby boomer cohort continues to age (Knickman and Snell 2002). The resultant disparity between the elderly who require care and the younger generation who are required to provide it will be an escalating problem for the medical community. A global issue of this magnitude requires an interdisciplinary and multidimensional investigation that initiates global health interventions and health policy reform.

AR is growing rapidly and becoming more mature and robust by combining virtual information with the real environment during real-time performance. There is some evidence that specially designed AR systems can support older adults in terms of mobility and independence. However, there is a lack of technological solutions that use AR to address the requirements of the older population. We have conducted a short investigation using three major databases—*PubMed*, *Medline*, and *Google Scholar*—to review existing AR solutions in the area of aging. The following combinations of keyword searches were utilized to produce the results shown below:

- *'augmented reality'* & *'therapy'*
- *'augmented reality'* & *'elderly'*
- *'augmented reality'* & *'aging'*
- *'augmented reality'* & *'dementia'*
- *'augmented reality'* & *'Alzheimer's'*

This investigation identified 49 relevant publications, 15 of which were deemed to be significant. For the purpose of this book chapter, we condensed the results to eight papers focused on two categories of elderly care. Table 9.1 lists these categories.

TABLE 9.1

Results of Survey Analysis for AR Solutions in Aging

AR Category of Use	Number of Publications
Elderly care—cognitive improvement	3
Elderly care—at-home living	5

9.2.1 ELDERLY CARE—COGNITIVE IMPROVEMENT

Gamberini et al. (2009) describes the nature and evaluation of *Eldergames*—a prototype offering older adults several games to train their cognitive functions, especially those that deteriorate with aging (memory, reasoning, etc.). *Eldergames* can be used either individually or in groups of up to three people. The platform is a tabletop device where real objects are used to interact with digital objects on the screen. The system exploits the potentialities provided by recent technological advances by utilizing an intuitive interface (Gamberini et al. 2009). It resembles a normal table around which people gather to play cards or other social games but embeds many more functions, including monitoring of performance, specific programs suiting the registered users' abilities, and connection with remote players (Gamberini et al. 2009).

Francisco et al. (2013) published a study that promotes *Visualax*, a visually relaxing AR application that uses music and visual therapy to help older adults manage their mental stress. The developed system enables the users to relax and unwind anytime, anywhere. The goal of the software is to reduce the stress level of the user through audio and visual presentation, by integrating augmentation of the original setting with the application of appropriate concepts from music and visual therapy using a web camera (Francisco et al. 2013).

McCallum and Boletsis (2013) proposed an architecture consisting of AR technology (as an output mechanism) combined with gesture-based devices (as an input method). Their work is intended to provide a theoretical justification for the use of such technologies that are integrated into an architecture that forms a basis for creating more effective games for older adults.

9.2.2 ELDERLY CARE—AT-HOME LIVING

The field of assistive technology has focused on developing systems and techniques to improve the problems caused by the declining physical capabilities of older adults. As information systems increase in daily importance, the possibilities of their use in caring for the elderly population expand and the problems older people experience in interacting with such systems become more pressing. With this motivation, Lawson et al. (2007) conducted a Wizard of Oz evaluation of novel interfaces to an online reminder system to support the daily activities of older people with non-intrusive and persuasive reminders.

Kamieth et al. (2010) aimed at providing answers to a number of issues, such as (a) the adequacy of virtual reality for enhancing user experience for the elderly and disabled and (b) the convenience of virtual reality for a daily handling of smart home environments. To this extent, the authors concluded that the addition of other modalities, such as natural language voice recognition or AR, was primordial in fostering the acceptance of innovative solutions to improve accessibility for people with special needs.

Hsiao and Rashvand (2015) demonstrated that the lack of physical and mental fitness of older adults threatens their effectiveness in contributing positively to society. In order to solve this problem, they propose a low-cost and innovative adoption of AR functions through an agile deployment of mobile-based augmented reality embedded in massively available intelligent smartphones (Hsiao and Rashvand 2015). A set of downloadable, AR-enabled, embedded learning and exercising programs, designed upon users' historical and habitual improvement data, would enable a collective sequence of required activities optimized for individual users.

Schall et al. (2013) assessed the utility of AR cues in alerting elderly drivers with age-related cognitive impairments of potential roadside hazards, such as pedestrians. The question was whether cognitively impaired elderly drivers benefited from, or were distracted by, the additional information intended to alert or warn them. The results of the study were promising, as AR cues improved driver response rates and response times to potential hazards.

Lastly, Saracchini et al. (2015) aimed to offer a technological solution that could improve elderly people's everyday autonomy and life quality through the integration of information and communication technologies. In order to achieve this goal, a new AR technology was developed along with carefully designed internet services and interfaces for mobile devices. Such technology only requires the infrastructure that already exists in most residences and healthcare centers.

9.2.3 CONCLUSION

The growth and development in terms of both the number and complexity of AR research targeting elderly care clearly shows the efficacy of its use for this population group. Improvements in mobility, transportation, medication schedules, socialization, and cognition in the elderly are all plausible benefits of AR applications today. Yet, the real benefits lie in the combination of all these applications into an interdisciplinary and multidimensional application.

This chapter identifies a significant gap in the dissemination of modern AR. The applications of this technology in elderly care have the potential to drastically change the landscape of elderly care in the future. Our investigation first calls for the research community to quantitatively analyze and quantify the benefits of certain AR applications for elderly populations. Then, through analysis of previous literature, this investigation would recommend the development of an all-inclusive, interdisciplinary AR application that fully replaces the need for a primary caregiver for elderly patients. This application would ideally draw on all domains of AR applications to optimize the technologies' efficacy and provide alternative, at-home care for the growing elderly population.

9.3 MEDICAL EDUCATION

In most institutions, cadaver dissection and textbooks are the two major resources for anatomical education. Cadaver dissection allows students to understand the size, shape, and positioning of the body's structures. It also offers trainees an opportunity to gain knowledge of the textures, material properties, and other physical characteristics of these structures. Additionally, the dissection process may expose students to pathological conditions or anatomical abnormalities (Codd and Choudhury 2011). Despite these benefits, the use of cadaver dissection as a teaching method has diminished due to high maintenance costs and limited laboratory time (Thomas et al. 2010; Fang et al. 2014). Furthermore, cadavers are difficult to obtain in countries where cultural practices or legal restrictions oppose cadaver dissection. To mitigate this limitation, textbooks are often used in conjunction with cadaver dissection to help students identify the body's structures and their functions. As an easily transportable teaching method, textbooks are useful for private study. However, their evident disadvantage is that all visual information is presented to the student through two-dimensional diagrams and photographs (Codd and Choudhury 2011).

The limitations of cadaver dissection and textbooks as traditional teaching methods have led to the development of other resources for learning gross anatomy (Thomas et al. 2010). Over the last few decades, the expansion of medical imaging has permitted the creation of advanced technological systems for this module of medical education (Codd and Choudhury 2011). Most recently, three-dimensional anatomy visualization applications have emerged, including virtual reality (VR) and AR systems (Thomas et al. 2010). VR systems completely immerse the student into an artificial environment, which they experience through computer-based sensory stimuli. With AR systems, the student is not immersed into a virtual environment, but rather an enhanced version of reality (See Figure 9.1). Such systems overlay digital information on a structure viewed by the student through a device. The following sections provide a classification of articles in the areas of learning, usability, and curriculum integration of various AR and VR technologies.

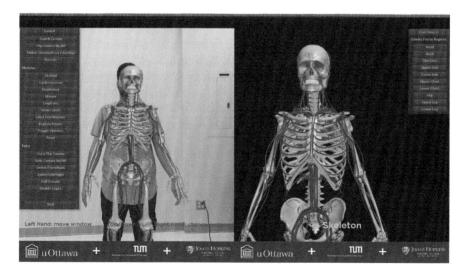

FIGURE 9.1   (Left) AR view of the circulation system. (Right) Corresponding virtual view.

9.3.1 LEARNING IMPACTS

Few studies directly compared AR/VR learning systems to traditional cadaver and atlas-based anatomy education. Instead, AR/VR systems were measured against other distance learning tools (Curnier 2010; Seixas-Mikelus et al. 2010; Thomas et al. 2010; Khot et al. 2013; Stefan et al. 2014; de Faria et al. 2016; Ferrer-Torregrosa et al. 2016; Huang et al. 2016; Küçük et al. 2016; Messier et al. 2016; Peterson and Mlynarczyk 2016; Moro et al. 2017; Ramlogan et al. 2017). In these studies, participants were randomly divided into model and control groups. The model group was equipped with an AR/VR system to supplement anatomy learning, while the control group relied on notes, images, and/or videos. The participants of each group were asked to complete a written examination in order to assess their anatomy learning. Overall, the model group showed superior spatial comprehension of anatomical structures and perceived a lower cognitive load than the control group. The results also indicated that AR/VR systems were significantly better at promoting motivation and autonomy than the other distance learning tools used by the participants in the control group. In another study (Codd and Choudhury 2011), the authors concluded that there was no statistical significance when comparing VR models to traditional dissections and that the VR model could not replace dissection (as it cannot convey the tactile information that a cadaver can).

9.3.2 USABILITY STUDIES

Most studies equated the AR/VR system's usability to user comprehension, which was evaluated through Likert scale questionnaires (Thomas et al. 2010; Fang et al. 2014; Stefan et al. 2014; Huang et al. 2016; Ma et al. 2016; Krueger et al. 2017). The results generally suggest that participants found AR/VR systems easy to understand. Some studies presented an in-depth assessment of usability by evaluating specific tools within the AR/VR system, as well as comparing the chosen interface to traditional interfaces like the keyboard and mouse. Participants typically preferred the AR/VR system's interface. A number of studies also listed general features that increase usability, such as system mobility and adaptability, within the learning environment. Lastly, the usability of AR/VR systems in anatomy learning largely depended on their capacity to support a smooth transition between reality and the augmented or virtual environment.

9.3.3 CURRICULUM INTEGRATION

The literature pertaining to the incorporation of AR/VR systems into the anatomical curriculum was limited (Curnier 2010; Thomas et al. 2010; Kockro et al. 2015; Ferrer-Torregrosa et al. 2016; Peterson and Mlynarczyk 2016). Most studies focused on the usability, development, and initial implementation of these technologies. Generally, an increase in student dependence on AR/VR systems was predicted, as the curriculum is trending towards more independent and distance learning activities. Some studies also suggested that the incorporation of AR/VR systems into the curriculum would help manage growing class sizes, in which demonstration becomes less feasible.

9.4 CONCLUSION

Anatomy learning supported by AR and VR systems enables meaningful and situated learning. Moreover, the immersive learning environment created by these technologies facilitates the transfer of knowledge into professional practice. The empirical research currently published on AR/VR systems in anatomy learning mainly focuses on usability and distance learning comparisons. In order to determine the true educational value of AR/VR systems, future studies should directly compare these technologies to traditional cadaver and atlas-based anatomy learning.

Although studies show that AR/VR systems are effective in conveying anatomy information, they cannot completely replace cadaveric dissection. While many systems incorporate both visual and tactile representations of anatomical structures, cadaveric dissection offers certain sensations that have yet to be reproduced by these technologies. Furthermore, most AR/VR systems cannot simulate the deformation and motion of anatomical structures. The development of these functionalities in future AR/VR systems will increase their usability and acceptance in the classroom.

ACKNOWLEDGMENTS

We would like to thank Arsani Yousef and Madelon Clifford for the work they conducted during their undergraduate studies project, which involved the gathering of survey articles.

REFERENCES

Codd, A.M. and Choudhury, B. 2011. Virtual reality anatomy: Is it comparable with traditional methods in the teaching of human forearm musculoskeletal anatomy? *Anatomical Sciences Education* 4, no. 3: 119–125.

Curnier, F. 2010. Teaching dentistry by means of virtual reality-the Geneva project. *International Journal of Computerized Dentistry* 13, no. 3: 251–263.

de Faria, J.W.V., Teixeira, M.J., de Moura Sousa Júnior, L., Otoch, J.P. and Figueiredo, E.G. 2016. Virtual and stereoscopic anatomy: When virtual reality meets medical education. *Journal of Neurosurgery* 125, no. 5: 1105–1111.

Fang, T.Y., Wang, P.C., Liu, C.H., Su, M.C. and Yeh, S.C. 2014. Evaluation of a haptics-based virtual reality temporal bone simulator for anatomy and surgery training. *Computer Methods and Programs in Biomedicine* 113, no. 2: 674–681.

Ferrer-Torregrosa, J., Jiménez-Rodríguez, M.Á., Torralba-Estelles, J., Garzón-Farinós, F., Pérez-Bermejo, M. and Fernández-Ehrling, N. 2016. Distance learning ects and flipped classroom in the anatomy learning: Comparative study of the use of augmented reality, video and notes. *BMC Medical Education* 16, no. 1: 230.

Francisco, J., Comendador, B.E., Concepcion Jr., A., Tapao, R. and Dalluay, V.L. 2013. VisuaLax: Visually Relaxing augmented reality application using music and visual therapy. *International Proceedings of Economics Development and Research* 63: 21.

Gamberini, L., Martino, F., Seraglia, B. et al. 2009. Eldergames project: An innovative mixed reality table-top solution to preserve cognitive functions in elderly people. *IEEE Human System Interactions, 2009. 2nd Conference on Human System Interactions*, pp. 164–169.

Hsiao, K.F. and Rashvand, H.F. 2015. Data modeling mobile augmented reality: Integrated mind and body rehabilitation. *Multimedia Tools and Applications* 74, no. 10: 3543–3560.

Huang, H.M., Liaw, S.S. and Lai, C.M. 2016. Exploring learner acceptance of the use of virtual reality in medical education: A case study of desktop and projection-based display systems. *Interactive Learning Environments* 24, no. 1: 3–19.

Kamieth, F., Dähne, P., Wichert, R. et al. 2010. Exploring the potential of virtual reality for the elderly and people with disabilities. In *Virtual Reality*, Jae-Jin Kim (Ed.). Rijeka, Croatia: InTech. DOI: 10.5772/13591.

Khot, Z., Quinlan, K., Norman, G.R. and Wainman, B. 2013. The relative effectiveness of computer-based and traditional resources for education in anatomy. *Anatomical Sciences Education* 6, no. 4: 211–215.

Knickman, J.R. and Snell, E.K. 2002. The 2030 problem: Caring for aging baby boomers. *Health Services Research* 37, no. 4: 849–884.

Kockro, R.A., Amaxopoulou, C., Killeen, T. et al. 2015. Stereoscopic neuroanatomy lectures using a three-dimensional virtual reality environment. *Annals of Anatomy-Anatomischer Anzeiger* 201: 91–98.

Krueger, E., Messier, E., Linte, C.A. and Diaz, G. 2017. An interactive, stereoscopic virtual environment for medical imaging visualization, simulation and training. *Proceedings of the SPIE Medical Imaging*. Denver, CO, 10136: 101361H.

Küçük, S., Kapakin, S. and Göktaş, Y. 2016. Learning anatomy via mobile augmented reality: Effects on achievement and cognitive load. *Anatomical Sciences Education* 9, no. 5: 411–421.

Lawson, S.W., Nutter, D. and Wilson, P. 2007. Design of interactive technology for ageing-in-place. In *International Conference on Universal Access in Human-Computer Interaction*, pp. 960–967. Springer, Berlin, Heidelberg.

Ma, M., Fallavollita, P., Seelbach, I. et al. 2016. Personalized augmented reality for anatomy education. *Clinical Anatomy* 29, no. 4: 446–453.

McCallum, S. and Boletsis, C. 2013. Augmented reality & gesture-based architecture in games for the elderly. *Studies in Health Technology and Informatics* 189: 139–144.

Messier, E., Wilcox, J., Dawson-Elli, A., Diaz, G. and Linte, C.A. 2016. An interactive 3D virtual anatomy puzzle for learning and simulation-initial demonstration and evaluation. *Studies in Health Technology and Informatics* 220: 233–240.

Moro, C., Štromberga, Z., Raikos, A. and Stirling, A. 2017. The effectiveness of virtual and augmented reality in health sciences and medical anatomy. *Anatomical Sciences Education* 10, no. 6: 549–559.

Peterson, D.C. and Mlynarczyk, G.S. 2016. Analysis of traditional versus three-dimensional augmented curriculum on anatomical learning outcome measures. *Anatomical Sciences Education* 9, no. 6: 529–536.

Ramlogan, R., Niazi, A.U., Jin, R., Johnson, J., Chan, V.W. and Perlas, A. 2017. A virtual reality simulation model of spinal ultrasound: Role in teaching spinal sonoanatomy. *Regional Anesthesia and Pain Medicine* 42, no. 2: 217–222.

Saracchini, R., Catalina-Ortega, C. and Bordoni, L. 2015. A mobile augmented reality assistive technology for the elderly. *Comunicar* 23, no. 45: 65–74.

Schall Jr, M.C., Rusch, M.L., Lee, J.D. et al. 2013. Augmented reality cues and elderly driver hazard perception. *Human Factors* 55, no. 3: 643–658.

Seixas-Mikelus, S.A., Adal, A., Kesavadas, T. et al. 2010. Can image-based virtual reality help teach anatomy? *Journal of Endourology* 24, no. 4: 629–634.

Stefan, P., Wucherer, P., Oyamada, Y. et al. 2014. An AR edutainment system supporting bone anatomy learning. *IEEE Virtual Reality*, pp. 113–114.

Thomas, R.G., William, J.N. and Delieu, J.M. 2010. Augmented reality for anatomical education. *Journal of Visual Communication in Medicine* 33, no. 1: 6–15.

10 Cost Effective Simulation
A Mixed Reality Approach

Ziv Yaniv, Özgür Güler, and Ren Hui Gong

CONTENTS

10.1 INTRODUCTION

Clinical training is still primarily based on the apprenticeship model. Training starts with acquisition of the procedure-specific knowledge and continues with knowledge acquisition by observing the procedure and then practicing while providing patient care (Aggarwal et al. 2007). This training model is at odds with a key ethical principal: "primum non nocere"—first, do no harm. In addition, this approach limits the trainee's experience to the clinical cases encountered during the training period. Rarer, more complicated cases may not be observed, and potential errors and strategies for their mitigation may not be experienced. These observations have led multiple clinical disciplines to identify simulation as a promising approach towards increasing competency prior to providing patient care and reducing the length of the learning curve during which patient care is provided (Ziv et al. 2003; Aggarwal et al. 2010; Lateef 2010).

Simulation is applicable as a training tool for the acquisition and improvement of several skill types (Aggarwal et al. 2010; Lateef 2010), which we broadly categorize as:

1. *Cognitive skills*: the knowledge associated with a procedure.
2. *Motor skills*: the manual dexterity required to perform a procedure.
3. *Teamwork skills*: the leadership and communication required for working as a team.

Currently, most simulation-based training is performed at dedicated centers due to the infrastructure requirements and the financial costs associated with many simulators. A key factor correlated with simulation cost is the desire for high fidelity, with increased realism and model complexity leading to increased costs. While intuitively we expect that greater fidelity will lead to better skill acquisition, this is not a simple linear relationship.

The relevance of increased fidelity for skill acquisition has been shown to be dependent on factors such as the trainee's skill level and the relevance of physical resemblance for acquisition of a specific skill (Aggarwal et al. 2010; Norman et al. 2012; Hamstra et al. 2014). For some skills, low-cost, low-fidelity simulators may be sufficiently effective. For example, Brewer et al. (2016) and Clarke et al. (2016) show effective cognitive skill acquisition for cardiac and neurosurgery using a mobile device and a game-based approach to teach the stages of cardiac surgery and to identify burr hole surgery instruments. Another example is presented in Matsumoto et al. (2002), who describe the effective acquisition of motor skills in endourological procedures using a simulator constructed from a Styrofoam cup, drinking straws, and molded latex. While these examples illustrate that low-fidelity simulators can be effective tools, the ideal would be to use high-fidelity, low-cost simulators.

In this chapter, we describe two high-fidelity, low-cost, mixed reality simulators. The first is a simulator to improve the acquisition of the cognitive skills associated with the use of image-guided intervention (IGI) systems, originally described in Güler and Yaniv (2012). The second is a simulator aimed at improving the acquisition of the basic motor skills associated with x-ray fluoroscopy performed during the voiding cystourethrography (VCUG) examination, originally described in Gong et al. (2014). In both cases, cost containment is achieved using open source software and consumer grade hardware.

10.2   TABLETOP IMAGE-GUIDED NAVIGATION SIMULATOR

Improved clinical outcomes and lower overall costs have resulted in a growing transition from open to minimally invasive interventions. A hallmark of this trend is the use of advanced intraoperative imaging devices, which can replace the traditional direct line-of-sight to the surgical target. However, understanding the underlying surgical scene from intraoperative imaging is a much harder task, so the clinical outcome highly depends on the physician's ability to interpret the images and infer the spatial relationships between anatomical structures and tools using the limited information provided by the imaging apparatus.

IGI systems aim to augment the physician's ability to perceive the underlying spatial relationships between anatomical structures and tools. This is achieved by integrating multiple sources of information, including preoperative and intraoperative medical images, with data from tracking and robotic devices (Yaniv and Cleary 2006b; Peters and Cleary 2008). IGI systems were initially introduced in neurosurgery (Maciunas 2006), orthopedics (Mavrogenis et al. 2013), and ENT (Caversaccio and Freysinger 2003), where the surgical targets are rigid or semirigid. Since then, their use has spread to clinical areas that deal with soft tissue. Among others, these include interventional radiology (Maybody et al. 2013) and cardiology (Rickers et al. 2003).

The majority of physicians learn the principles and operation of these advanced systems during residency, fellowship, or at a later stage in their careers. At these different stages, physicians become siloed in their specialties (Hanauer 2010), and knowledge is generally not shared between disciplines. For example, a fundamental principle of tool tracking in IGI systems is that the relationship between the tracked sensor and the tool is assumed to be rigid. As a consequence, tools that can exhibit some bending will produce larger tracking errors. This information appeared in the orthopedics literature in 2004, with the tracked tool being a K-wire or thin drill bit (Langlotz 2004). In the interventional radiology literature, this principle was "rediscovered" in 2013 (Appelbaum et al. 2013; Maybody et al. 2013), and the tracked tool was a needle exhibiting improved accuracy with the sensor at the needle tip, as compared to the needle hub. Avoiding rediscovery of fundamental principles allows for more efficient adoption and usage of technologies across clinical specialties.

As clinicians often first encounter IGI systems at an advanced stage in their training, they do not learn the principles underlying these systems in a classroom setting. Physicians learn how to use a specific IGI system either at a training facility or more often in a clinical setting while providing patient care. The issues involved using this training model were described earlier in this chapter and were also highlighted in Tjardes et al. (2010), who identified the need for "systematic development of education and training modules using navigation technology."

The fundamental principles underlying the majority of IGI systems are similar, irrespective of the clinical specialty and IGI system in use. While in theory teaching these principles using an IGI system in a simulation setting is straightforward, in practice IGI systems are costly and therefore not readily available for use as simulators for educational purposes. This is particularly a challenge if one wants to reach a large number of trainees across multiple clinical disciplines. Additionally, there is a need to educate operating room staff in the use of IGI systems in a realistic manner outside of the actual operating room. To illustrate this, most IGI systems use a tracked reference frame that is assumed to be securely attached to the patient. However, accidental bumps of the reference frame by the operating room staff have been cited as a reason for reduced guidance accuracy, which has motivated the development of a novel attachment mechanism (Wellborn et al. 2017). Without a proper understanding of this issue, it is likely that the support staff are not as careful as they need to be to ensure accurate guidance. Our aim is to provide effective training by using a cost-effective, high-fidelity, mixed reality simulator as an educational tool for illustrating the fundamental concepts underlying IGI systems.

10.2.1 HARDWARE AND SOFTWARE

Based on the observations listed above, we have developed a low-cost, high-fidelity, mixed reality simulator to improve the learning outcomes of trainees introduced to the fundamental principles underlying IGI systems. Furthermore, we have developed presentations and short instructional videos to illustrate simulator usage and several fundamental principles underlying IGI. Figure 10.1 shows

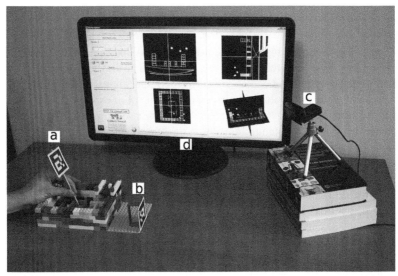

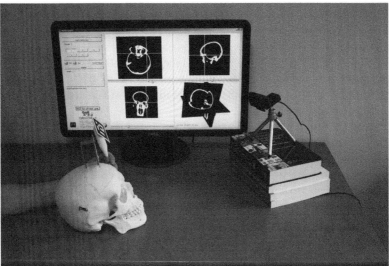

FIGURE 10.1   Tabletop simulator setups, generic configuration using LEGO phantom with skewer pointer and "neuro" configuration using skull phantom with 3D printed pointer: (a) tracked pointer tool; (b) dynamic reference frame; (c) webcam tracker; (d) multi-planar visualization.

two simulator configurations corresponding to different levels of physical resemblance to a clinical IGI system.

10.2.1.1 Overview

The simulator provides functionality similar to that of a basic commercial navigation system and is all but free. It is comprised of four programs that include (1) camera calibration, (2) pointer tool calibration, (3) preoperative planning, and (4) intraoperative registration and navigation. The camera calibration program estimates the extrinsic and intrinsic camera parameters, enabling us to use a webcam as a tracking device. It assumes that the camera has a fixed focal length and requires that the autofocus be disabled if it supports this function. The pointer tool calibration program estimates the translation between the tracked marker attached to the pointer tool and its tip via pivot calibration (Yaniv 2015).

The planning, registration, and guidance programs are the most relevant for training. The planning program allows the operator to localize target and fiducial points on the preoperative CT that are later used for paired-point rigid registration. The operator begins by loading the CT and linearly modifying the displayed intensities for optimal viewing (in the nomenclature, this operation is referred to as setting the window and level). Point localization is performed on reformatted slices of the CT volume displaying the standard radiological views: axial, sagittal, and coronal. The operator scrolls through any of the reformatted stacks, possibly zooming or panning the image, and selects a point using the mouse. Using a linked cursor approach, all other views are updated to display the slice that corresponds to the cursor location. Once all points are localized, the operator saves the settings, which are then used by the guidance program. The registration and guidance program allows the operator to use the tracked and calibrated pointer tool for digitizing the fiducial points on the physical phantom, perform registration, navigate, and then digitize the target points and evaluate the target registration error. The display employs the standard radiological views and a three-dimensional (3D) view, continuously updated based on the location of the tracked tool's tip. The tool mesh representation is overlaid onto the reformatted views in the virtual world so that the representation corresponds to its position in physical space. Similar to commercial IGI systems, we utilize a dynamic reference frame (DRF) that is rigidly attached to the "patient" so that the registration is maintained when the "patient" is moved. During navigation, if either the DRF or tracked tool are not visible, then the display is cleared to preclude navigation.

10.2.1.2 Accessibility

To make the simulator accessible to the broadest possible audience, we utilized two open source toolkits, OpenCV (Bradski 2000) and IGSTK (Enquobahrie et al. 2007), whose licenses allowed us to distribute our software freely, and as open source, under a Berkeley Software Distribution (BSD) license. The instructional material describing simulator usage and IGI concepts, which is included as part of the simulator distribution, is provided under a creative-commons by attribution license. The goal of accessibility also influenced our choice to mimic interventions in which a simple pointer tool is the only requirement. In its most basic form, the pointer tool can be represented by a pencil or skewer. For those who prefer an experience that is physically more similar to commercial navigation systems, we provide a stereolithography model file derived from a clinically used pointer tool that is easily printed using a 3D printer.

The two primary challenges we faced when creating an accessible and cost effective IGI simulator were eliminating the need for acquiring a CT scan of the "patient" at every location where the simulator is used and reducing the cost associated with tool tracking while still providing sufficient accuracy.

The first challenge was addressed by using standardized phantoms and providing their CT scans. We provide CT scans of a generic LEGO phantom and several anatomical phantoms from two commercial vendors: SOMSO Modelle GmbH (Coburg, Germany) and CIRS Inc (Norfolk, VA, USA). These include models of the skull, scapula, humerus, vertebra, pelvis, and abdomen. These models are relevant to three clinical specialties that currently employ IGI systems: orthopedics, neurosurgery, and interventional radiology. The rigid anatomical phantoms from SOMSO Modelle have a fixed physical structure. The abdominal phantom from CIRS has an internal structure that varies slightly from phantom to phantom and may change over time. Currently, the vendor provides an option to purchase the phantom as part of a kit that includes both the phantom and its CT scan. The use of a generic phantom constructed from LEGO blocks was motivated by their widespread availability and the accurate reproducibility of phantom construction, given the instructions included in the distributed material. The geometric accuracy of the LEGO phantom relies on the tolerance of block manufacturing. With LEGO knob tolerance listed as 0.02mm, which is sufficiently accurate for our purposes.

The second challenge, cost-effective tool tracking, was addressed by replacing the expensive, specialized hardware used to perform tracking with a monocular webcam-based approach. This is a compromise whereby we are willing to tolerate a measurable reduction in accuracy to gain a significant reduction in cost. By accepting tracking errors of several millimeters instead of the submillimetric accuracy of commercial tracking systems, we are able to reduce costs from several thousand dollars to less than one hundred dollars.

To transform a user's webcam into a tracking device, we calibrate it using the OpenCV implementation of Zhang's camera calibration algorithm (Zhang 2000), which requires the acquisition of multiple images of a planar checkerboard pattern. As part of the simulator package, we provide two pdf files that the user prints for use with our camera calibration software. The first is a checkerboard pattern used for calibration; the second is a different checkerboard pattern with a known physical size that the operator uses to evaluate the accuracy of the camera calibration. If the calibration accuracy is not sufficient, then it can be improved by acquiring additional images in poses not represented by the initial set of images. To perform tracking, we attach unique square binary markers to all the tools. As part of the simulator package, we provide a pdf file containing five unique markers that the user prints and attaches to the tracked tools and phantom. Marker, creation, and tracking are facilitated using the ArUco library (Garrido-Jurado et al. 2014). This library allows one to define unique, binary-encoded markers, detect them in the images, and estimate their pose by minimizing the marker corner reprojection error via the Levenberg-Marquardt algorithm. When incorporating this functionality into the Image-Guided Surgery Toolkit (IGSTK), we followed the IGSTK interface conventions for tracking devices, making it a trivial task to replace the webcam-based tracker with a commercial tracker. This approach facilitates modification of the simulator programs for use in relevant clinical interventions, as described by (Wu et al. 2017), who modified the intraoperative registration and guidance program for use with electromagnetic tracking in robotic nasopharyngeal biopsies.

10.2.1.3 Instructional Material

The instructional material describing simulator usage and IGI concepts covers multiple subjects, which are not procedure-specific, including:

- The mixed-reality concept underlying IGIs. This uses a tracked pointer tool to reformat the volumetric image, and the tool representation is overlaid onto the image, corresponding to its location in the physical world.
- The workflow of a typical IGI system, which is comprised of preoperative planning, tool calibration, and intraoperative registration and navigation.
- The use of a dynamic reference frame that is rigidly attached to the patient to allow the physician to move the patient while maintaining the registration between the image-space and physical space.
- The concept of registration; aligning the virtual image-space with the physical space.
- The nomenclature associated with paired-point rigid registration: fiducial localization error (FLE), fiducial registration error (FRE), and target registration error (TRE) as introduced in Maurer et al. (1997).
- The effect of fiducial configuration on TRE, avoiding near-collinear configurations, and the fact that FRE and TRE are uncorrelated (Fitzpatrick 2009).

10.2.2 EVALUATION

To evaluate the effectiveness of the IGI simulator as a training tool, we conducted a study at the Medical University of Innsbruck, Austria (Özbek et al. 2014). Thirty medical students were taught the general concepts underlying IGI systems using one of three approaches: a standard lecture, simulator use alone, and a combination of lecture and simulator use. The participants were randomly assigned to one of three groups of ten. All groups met on the same day for a one-hour session and five days later for a written exam. Additionally, students completed a Likert scale questionnaire that assessed whether they had prior knowledge with respect to the subject matter, whether they invested time in preparing for the exam, and their level of engagement. The distribution of grades showed no statistically significant difference between the three teaching approaches with low grades across the board. Figure 10.2 shows a box and whisker plot of the grade distribution per teaching approach. Based on the responses to the Likert questionnaire, we observed that (a) the majority of participants (83%) were previously unfamiliar with the subject matter taught in this study; (b) all students except one invested less than thirty minutes preparing for the exam; (c) simulator usage inspired confidence, with 70% of the participants in the two groups that used the simulator being confident about their subject knowledge as compared to 40% in the lecture-based approach; and (d) simulator usage was more

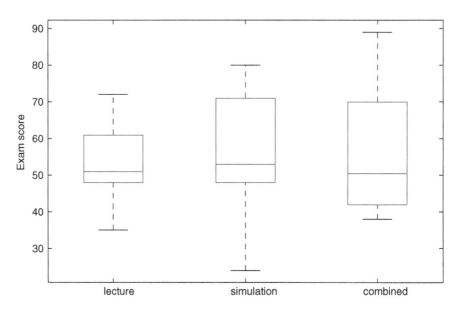

FIGURE 10.2 Grade distributions for the three teaching approaches. The median grades were 51.0 (lecture), 53.0 (simulator), and 50.5 (combined lecture and simulator).

engaging, with 90% of the participants in the combined approach and 100% of the simulator-based group expressing interest in the material as compared to 60% in the lecture-based approach. These results are in line with other simulation-based studies that have shown that there is no relationship between the subjective measure of confidence and the objective measure of competence (Hishikawa et al. 2010; Cordero et al. 2013). In our case, simulator usage was found to be more engaging and instilled confidence in the trainees, but it did not offer improved cognitive benefits as compared to a standard lecture-based approach. It should be noted that limitations of the study were that the training was given outside of the standard curriculum, the exam grade had no effect on the students' transcript, and no additional incentives were given to succeed; this possibly accounts for the low grade distribution.

10.3   X-RAY FLUOROSCOPY SIMULATOR FOR VOIDING CYSTOURETHROGRAPHY

The voiding cystourethrography (VCUG) examination is a radiological procedure for detecting and grading vesicoureteral reflux, a condition in which urine flows back from the bladder towards the kidneys (Agrawalla et al. 2004). This condition can lead to kidney infection, resulting in scarring and potentially long-term kidney damage. VCUG is commonly performed in children who experience recurring urinary tract infections, have voiding abnormalities, or have been prenatally diagnosed with hydronephrosis. It is the most common x-ray fluoroscopy imaging procedure in pediatric radiology departments (Schneider et al. 2001).

The procedure involves the insertion of a catheter into the bladder, filling the bladder with contrast material, and finally having the patient void (urinate). Detection and grading are based on x-ray fluoroscopy images acquired throughout the procedure. Using intermittent imaging, the following images are acquired: early bladder filling view, full bladder view, voiding urethra view, renal view after voiding, and bladder view after voiding (Agrawalla et al. 2004). As reflux may be intermittent, better detection can be achieved if the examination is repeated in a cyclic fashion (Gelfand et al. 1999).

Exposure of pediatric patients to ionizing radiation associated with x-ray imaging is of particular concern given the long period of time during which they can develop complications associated with this exposure. Given the currently accepted linear-no-threshold risk model (Royal 2008), this remains a concern even for low dose exposure. As a consequence, the reduction of radiation exposure and the concept of "as low as reasonably achievable" (ALARA) patient doses are applied in all pediatric fluoroscopy imaging (Strauss and Kaste 2006).

In the context of VCUG, it has been shown that the amount of radiation associated with the procedure is not negligible (Lee et al. 2009), with guidance on how to achieve an ALARA dose described in (Ward 2006). It also has been shown that trainees performing VCUG expose the patient to higher radiation doses than experienced radiologists (Lim et al. 2013).

A recent study illustrated that using standardized training can significantly reduce radiation exposure during VCUG (Shah et al. 2015). In this study, a competency check-off form was introduced, with residents allowed to perform VCUG alone only after an attending clinician had consistently observed and certified that they performed the procedure in a correct and safe manner. Techniques for limiting radiation exposure were explicitly listed as part of the form. Comparing the median cumulative dose observed in procedures performed by residents six months prior to the introduction of the standardized training to the six months following showed a 36% dose decrease. While the check-off process standardized the residents' fluoroscopy training, it did not change the fact that they were learning to perform the procedure while providing patient care. Simulation can potentially address this concern.

Virtual reality-based fluoroscopy simulators have been previously described in the context of cardiology (Dawson et al. 2000) and orthopedics (Jaramaz and Eckman 2006). These simulators primarily aim to enhance cognitive skills. A mixed reality simulator that aims to enhance both cognitive and motor skills in the context of orthopedics was described in (Bott et al. 2011). This high-fidelity simulator uses a standard C-arm fluoroscope to control image acquisition, a mannequin, and a costly commercial electromagnetic tracking system to obtain the spatial relationship between the two. The simulated x-rays, also known as digitally reconstructed radiographs (DRRs), are created using the known spatial relationship between the C-arm and mannequin in combination with a 3D CT. Similar to the goals of this simulator, our aim is to reduce radiation exposure to patients undergoing the VCUG procedure by enhancing the trainees' cognitive and motor skills prior to providing patient care.

10.3.1 Hardware and Software

We developed a low-cost, high-fidelity, mixed reality VCUG imaging simulator. The simulator allows the trainees to practice image acquisition using the same equipment as in clinical use with a minor modification to fluoroscopy control. As the focus is on reducing radiation exposure, the simulator does not include the procedure's catheter insertion phase. The goal of using the simulator is that the trainee acquires the cognitive and motor skills required for VCUG imaging. In this context, this means that they are able to position the machine relative to the patient to acquire the desired images at the desired time (e.g., beginning of voiding) with relevant collimation and zoom. As VCUG imaging has a spatiotemporal aspect, four-dimensional (4D) (3D+time) CT is used to generate DRRs, thus enabling the trainee to practice timed image acquisition. The functionality provided by the simulator mimics that of the fluoroscopy machine in clinical use and includes the following capabilities: collimation, zoom, intensity inversion, image save, and an audible alarm indicating that a total fluoroscopy time of five minutes has elapsed. As our intent was to provide a high-fidelity simulator, yet at the same time contain costs, we used the same webcam-based tracking approach as in the IGI simulator described previously and employed a simple box phantom to mimic the patient. Figure 10.3 shows the simulator in use.

The key simulator elements include (1) a patient model consisting of a 4D CT and a physical phantom; (2) webcam-based tracking; (3) DRR generation; and (4) operation and control of the simulator.

10.3.1.1 Patient Model

The patient model consists of a virtual component defined by a 4D CT and a physical component represented by a box-shaped phantom. The virtual component comprises

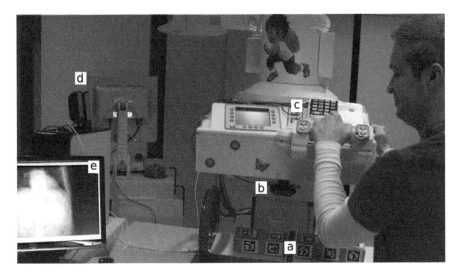

FIGURE 10.3 VCUG simulator in use: (a) box phantom representing patient; (b) webcam tracker; (c) keypad controlling simulated imaging; (d) speakers for audible alarm indicating total fluoroscopy time of five minutes; (e) simulated fluoroscopy.

a set of volumetric images to which we associate timestamps, which indicate when the volume represents the patient using the elapsed time since the beginning of the simulation. We support cyclic processes such as breathing by specifying the last timestamp, without specifying a corresponding volume, and this indicates that the simulation time should be reset. The physical component is a simple box phantom with multiple tracked binary markers attached at arbitrary locations.

This enables us to track the phantom across a wide range of poses, including significant rotations corresponding to positioning the patient on their back or on either side as required during VCUG imaging. The use of a simplistic physical model is possible because we do not simulate the catheter insertion phase of the procedure and because of the imaging technique used in pediatric VCUG. The patient is strapped to a rotating bed, and different views are acquired by translating the fluoroscope and rotating the bed. As a consequence, there is no advantage to using a more elaborate physical phantom, as the physician does not directly touch the patient. The last piece of information that completes the patient model is the rigid transformation that maps between the virtual coordinate system of the 4D CT and the physical coordinate system of one of the markers attached to the phantom. We designate this as the *root* marker. This is an arbitrary user-specified transformation that depends on the contents of the CT and the choice of *root* marker and is denoted $_{CT}T^{root}$. The only constraint is that it be consistent with the physical world so that the head-foot direction is aligned with the long axis of the box. Once this connection between the virtual and physical coordinate systems is defined, the pose of the CT volume in physical space is determined using the tracked pose of the physical phantom.

10.3.1.2 Webcam Tracking

Webcam-based tracking is performed in a manner similar to that employed for the IGI simulator. After camera calibration, a standard webcam is used to track the pose of binary markers. Unlike the previous simulator, we need to track the phantom while it is undergoing significant translations and rotations of up to 180°, so using a single planar marker is not sufficient. Instead, we place markers on the three visible sides of the box phantom, with the constraint that the camera is always able to see at least two markers, creating a composite marker. To use this composite marker, we need to estimate the spatial transformations between all the individual markers and the *root*, as this is the marker that represents the patient's pose. This is done via a one-time calibration.

We use a graph theoretic approach to formulate the calibration process. We define a graph whose vertices are the markers and whose edges are the transformations between them. The edges are weighted based on the quality of the transformation; the more accurate the transformation, the lower the weight. The calibration process starts with a graph without edges and is optionally terminated when we have a connected graph (there is a path between every pair of vertices). This connected graph allows us to compute the transformations between all the markers and the *root* marker. In practice, calibration is performed by repeatedly changing the pose of the phantom in front of the camera and updating the transformations between the visible markers. The poses of markers a and b relative to the camera are estimated as $_bT^{cam}$ and $_aT^{cam}$, thus creating the transformation between them as $_aT^b = (_bT^{cam})^{-1}{_aT^{cam}}$.

The quality of this $_a T^b$ is taken to be the maximum between the quality of $_b T^{cam}$ and $_a T^{cam}$, which is a conservative estimate. We use the angle between the ray originating at the camera and passing through the center of the marker and the marker's normal direction as the quality measure for the pose estimate, so the smaller the angle, the higher the pose quality. If there is no edge between these markers, it is created using the estimated transformation and associated weight, but if there is an edge it is updated only if the current transformation has a lower weight and higher quality. Once the graph becomes connected, there is a path from each marker to the *root*. We then compute the best transformation between every marker and the root using Dijkstra's shortest path algorithm (Dijkstra 1959).

During tracking, when marker a is visible, the pose of the root marker is given by

$$_{root} T^{cam} = {_a T^{cam}}\, _{root} T^a .$$

$_{root} T^a$ is known from calibration, and $_a T^{cam}$ is the current estimate from the webcam tracker. When multiple markers are visible, we select the one that has the minimal angle between the ray originating at the camera and passing through its center and its normal direction in the camera coordinate system.

10.3.1.3 DRR Generation

DRR generation is performed in a customizable manner so that the images created by the simulator are visually similar to those created by the specific fluoroscopy machine in use. This requires that we estimate the fluoroscopy machine's imaging parameters, obtain the transformation between the x-ray and webcam coordinate systems, and generate the DRRs with an acceptable refresh rate.

The fluoroscopy machine is modelled using the standard pinhole camera model (Yaniv and Cleary 2006a) with the following set of parameters: focal length, location of the principle point in the x-ray image, distortion coefficients, and the rigid transformation between the camera and world coordinate systems. In our case, the world coordinate system coincides with the phantom model, and the transformation is denoted as $_{model} T^{x\text{-}ray}$. To estimate these parameters, we acquire a single x-ray image of a 3D, tracked calibration phantom. which consists of two planes embedded with 36 metal spheres arranged in a regular grid. The sphere configuration defines seven line segments: four on the top plane with 3-mm spheres and three on the bottom plane with 2-mm spheres. The sphere projections are first localized in the x-ray image using a multiscale blob detection algorithm (Lindeberg 1998). They are then classified into two groups based on their size. The lines in each group are detected using the RANSAC algorithm (Fischler and Bolles 1981), and the correspondence between the two-dimensional projections and 3D spheres is established. The camera parameters are then estimated using a least squares formulation that minimizes the reprojection error via the Levenberg-Marquardt algorithm (Hartley and Zisserman 2003).

To obtain the transformation between the webcam and x-ray coordinate systems, we place a marker that is visible to the webcam on the 3D phantom. The marker is attached in a known position, $_{marker} T^{model}$, and we acquire its pose, $_{cam} T^{marker}$, while acquiring the x-ray image used for calibration. Once the fluoroscopy machine is calibrated, the transformation between the x-ray and webcam coordinate systems is readily computed using the available transformations:

$$_{cam}T^{x\text{-}ray} = {}_{model}T^{x\text{-}ray}{}_{marker}T^{model}{}_{cam}T^{marker}$$

Finally, to generate a DRR, we need to position the CT in the appropriate pose in the x-ray coordinate system. This is readily achieved with the known transformations:

$$_{CT}T^{x\text{-}ray} = {}_{cam}T^{x\text{-}ray}{}_{root}T^{cam}{}_{CT}T^{root}$$

The DRR is then generated using a regular sampling-based ray-casting approach. To achieve near real-time performance, the DRR is generated using the Graphics Processing Unit. With an NVIDIA GeForce GTX 560 Ti card and a DRR size of 512×512, the DRRs are generated at a rate of 11 Hz. As we are dealing with a 4D CT, two concurrent threads are used. The first queries the box phantom's pose and generates DRRs from the active volume. The second monitors the time and loads the relevant volume based on the time stamps.

10.3.1.4   Simulator Operation and Control

To acquire images during the VCUG examination, the operator activates x-ray acquisition while interactively translating the fluoroscopy device relative to the patient and possibly rotating them. Our simulator employs the clinical setup, inherently supporting the physical manipulation of the fluoroscopy unit and patient bed. Additional functionality that is often used during image acquisition is magnification of regions of interest and the use of collimation to reduce radiation exposure. Other key functions include image saving, inversion of grayscale intensities, and an audible alarm indicating that five minutes of fluoroscopy time have elapsed, with the option to reset it. All these functions are activated from the fluoroscope's control panel, and all these capabilities are supported using a standard keypad. While the use of a keypad differs from the clinical system's controls, the functional keypad layout mimics that of the clinical system. More importantly, to provide a similar ergonomic experience as when operating the clinical system, we mounted the keypad over the clinical machine's controls.

10.3.2   EVALUATION

To evaluate the realism of the simulator as a training tool, we conducted a survey-based study at the Department of Radiology in Children's National Medical Center, Washington DC, USA. As our virtual patient, we used a 4D CT dataset comprised of ten volumes obtained throughout the respiratory cycle. The image size was $512 \times 512 \times 512$ with a voxel size of $0.98 \times 0.98 \times 2.5$ mm.

Six attending radiologists, three fellows, and two resident radiologists participated in the study. All participants were familiar with the operation of the clinical fluoroscopy system and the VCUG procedure. A five-minute instructional session demonstrating simulator usage was given to all participants. Each clinician was then asked

TABLE 10.1

Evaluation Results for Simulator Realism Using Likert Scale (1- strongly disagree, 2- disagree, 3- no opinion, 4- agree, 5- strongly agree)

Question	Score ($\mu \pm \sigma$)
Collimation is realistic.	3.8 ± 1.3
4-level zooming is realistic.	3.8 ± 1.0
Fluoroscopic images are realistic.	4.4 ± 0.5
Imaging responsiveness is realistic.	4.1 ± 0.8
Dose alarm is realistic.	4.2 ± 1.0
Image save is realistic.	4.1 ± 1.1
Control pad closely mimics the clinical hardware.	3.5 ± 1.2
4D CT to model a dynamic physiologic process is realistic.	4.1 ± 0.6
Use of a patient phantom is sufficiently realistic.	4.0 ± 0.8
The range of motion the system provides is realistic (positioning of virtual patient and motion of imager).	4.5 ± 0.5
Hardware setup, wire connections, and computer placement detracts from the system's realism.	4.1 ± 0.8
Overall	4.0 ± 0.9

to operate the simulator, utilizing all of the functions that were described above, and to complete a questionnaire evaluating the simulator's realism with respect to the supported functionality. The questionnaire was comprised of two sections, free-form comments, and a set of statements evaluated using a five-point Likert scale, with a score of one being "strongly disagree," and a score of five being "strongly agree." Table 10.1 provides a detailed summary of this evaluation. The main issues with the simulator realism had to do with collimation, zoom, and the control pad.

The first issue raised by the evaluators was that collimation changes are immediately visible on the display without the need for acquiring an x-ray. This is different from the clinical system in which collimation changes are only visible after a new x-ray is acquired. This is readily addressed by updating the displayed image only when a new simulated x-ray is acquired. It should be noted that the newer generation of fluoroscopy machines support "virtual" collimation by visually displaying changes in the collimation without the need for active x-ray acquisition, similar to the simulator's functionality. The second issue identified by the participants was that the zoom functionality of our simulator exhibited pixilation at high magnification. This is due to two factors: the sampling rate we used to speed up the DRR generation and the spatial resolution of the CT from which the images were derived. The latter is the primary reason for the reduced quality, as aliasing artifacts are visible in the head-foot direction even without magnification. This behavior is expected, as the CT's sampling resolution in the cranial caudal direction is much lower than in the axial direction (2.5 vs 0.98 mm). The final issue was that the button locations on the control pad were different from those on the clinical machine controls. Given that the control locations are machine- and vendor-specific, we decided to continue using the keypad as our control mechanism, as it is cost-effective and generic.

Although the participants identified the issues above, overall the simulator was found to provide a realistic imaging experience with an average score on the Likert scale of 4.0 ± 0.9.

10.4   DISCUSSION AND CONCLUSIONS

Simulation technology has made inroads into training in multiple clinical disciplines and has proven to be beneficial for the acquisition of cognitive, motor, and teamwork skills. While this is clearly a benefit, there are financial costs associated with simulator-based training. An existing concern with respect to medical education in general are its high and rising costs (Walsh and Jaye 2013). This is also a concern with respect to simulator-based medical education (Walsh 2015). Cost-effective simulation solutions are clearly one approach to addressing this concern.

The two simulators described in this chapter address the need for cost-effective simulation in the context of teaching the fundamental concepts of IGI systems and the techniques used for VCUG imaging. The tabletop IGI simulator is essentially free and can be set up in any classroom or office space. In its generic configuration, the simulator only requires a computer, a webcam. and LEGO blocks, with all the software, CT scans, and instructional material provided at no cost. The x-ray fluoroscopy simulator is more specialized and requires access to the clinical equipment, as it can be viewed as an add-on to the equipment, which allows the trainee to practice image acquisition without exposing themselves or patients to unnecessary x-rays.

Evaluation of the IGI simulator as a teaching tool showed it was equivalent to a standard lecture-based teaching approach, although it was found to be a much more engaging tool. Additionally, while the use of the simulator inspired confidence, this was not reflected by improved knowledge retention. It is clear that measuring the subjective confidence of individuals is not sufficient to determine whether the use of a simulator is beneficial, as the only relevant quantity is competence.

Interesting anecdotal experiences gained when presenting the IGI simulator demonstrated the need for physical similarity to increase clinical acceptance. Initially, we presented the simulator using the generic configuration, LEGO "patient," and skewer-based pointer. While the clinicians understood that these represented a generic scenario, their response was not as enthusiastic as we expected. When we presented the same simulator but with physically realistic phantoms based on the appropriate clinical discipline, such as skull for neurosurgery, pelvis for orthopedics, and abdomen for interventional radiology, the responses were considerably more positive. We believe this experience is related to fundamental differences in training between engineers and clinicians. The former are taught to think abstractly by solving a generic problem naturally using a single phantom to represent all anatomical structures, while the latter are taught to think concretely by treating a specific condition with specialization in a specific anatomical structure.

This experience motivated the evaluation of the x-ray fluoroscopy simulator with respect to its realism and potential acceptance as an educational tool, primarily the usage of a box phantom and not an anthropomorphic phantom. That evaluation study showed that in the specific context of VCUG imaging, the use of an anthropomorphic phantom was not necessary. We believe the enthusiasm for this simulator is because it deals with a specific clinical procedure, as compared to the IGI simulator, whose goal was to teach fundamental principles of navigation outside the context of a specific navigation system and clinical procedure.

Based on our experience developing the two simulators described in this chapter, we believe cost-effective, mixed reality simulators have the potential to improve clinical training, while containing costs and making high-quality, affordable health care more widely accessible. Finally, in the spirit of open science, it should be noted that all the material associated with the IGI tabletop simulator, including the software in binary and source code form, the CT scans, and all additional material are freely available online from: http://yanivresearch.info/igiTutorial/igiTutorial.html.

REFERENCES

Aggarwal, R., O.T. Mytton, M. Derbrew, D. Hananel, M. Heydenburg, B. Issenberg, C. MacAulay et al. 2010. Training and simulation for patient safety. *Quality & Safety in Health Care* 19, no. 2 (August): i34–i43.

Aggarwal, R., T.P. Grantcharov, and A. Darzi. 2007. Framework for systematic training and assessment of technical skills. *Journal of the American College of Surgeons* 204, no. 4 (April): 697–705.

Agrawalla, S., R. Pearce, and T.R. Goodman. 2004. How to perform the perfect voiding cysto-urethrogram. *Pediatric Radiology* 34, no. 2 (February): 114–119.

Appelbaum, L., L. Solbiati, J. Sosna, Y. Nissenbaum, N. Greenbaum, and S.N. Goldberg. 2013. Evaluation of an electromagnetic image-fusion navigation system for biopsy of small lesions: Assessment of accuracy in an *in vivo* swine model. *Academic Radiology* 20, no. 2: 209–217.

Bott, O.J., K. Dresing, M. Wagner, B.-W. Raab, and M. Teistler. 2011. Informatics in radiology: Use of a C-arm fluoroscopy simulator to support training in intraoperative radiography. *Radiographics* 31, no. 3 (June): E65–E75.

Bradski, G. 2000. The openCV library. *Dr. Dobb's Journal* 25, no. 11: 120–126.

Brewer, Z.E., W.D. Ogden, J.I. Fann, T.A. Burdon, and A.Y. Sheikh. 2016. Creation and global deployment of a mobile, application-based cognitive simulator for cardiac surgical procedures. *Seminars in Thoracic and Cardiovascular Surgery* 28, no. 1 (March 1): 1–9.

Caversaccio, M., and W. Freysinger. 2003. Computer assistance for intraoperative navigation in ENT surgery. *Minimally Invasive Therapy and Allied Technologies* 12, no. 1 (March): 36–51.

Clarke, D.B., N. Kureshi, M. Hong, M. Sadeghi, and R.C.N. D'Arcy. 2016. Simulation-based training for burr hole surgery instrument recognition. *BMC Medical Education* 16: 153.

Cordero, L., B.J. Hart, R. Hardin, J.D. Mahan, P.J. Giannone, and C.A. Nankervis. 2013. Pediatrics residents' preparedness for neonatal resuscitation assessed using high-Fidelity Simulation. *Journal of Graduate Medical Education* 5, no. 3: 399–404.

Dawson, S.L., S. Cotin, D. Meglan, D.W. Shaffer, and M.A. Ferrell. 2000. Designing a computer-based simulator for interventional cardiology training. *Catheterization and Cardiovascular Interventions: Official Journal of the Society for Cardiac Angiography & Interventions* 51, no. 4 (December): 522–527.

Dijkstra, E.W. 1959. A note on two problems in connexion with graphs. *Numerische Mathematik* 1, no. 1 (December): 269–271.

Enquobahrie, A., P. Cheng, K. Gary, L. Ibanez, D. Gobbi, F. Lindseth, Z. Yaniv, S. Aylward, J. Jomier, and K. Cleary. 2007. The image-guided surgery toolkit IGSTK: An open source C++ software toolkit. *Journal of Digital Imaging* 20, no. 1 (November): 21–33.

Fischler, M.A., and R.C. Bolles. 1981. Random sample consensus: A paradigm for model fit-ting with applications to image analysis and automated cartography. *Communications of the ACM* 24, no. 6 (June): 381–395.

Fitzpatrick, J.M. 2009. Fiducial registration error and target registration error are uncorrelated. *SPIE Medical Imaging: Visualization, Image-Guided Procedures, and Modeling*, 7261: 726102-726102–12.

Garrido-Jurado, S., R. Muñoz-Salinas, F.J. Madrid-Cuevas, and M.J. Marín-Jiménez. 2014. Automatic generation and detection of highly reliable fiducial markers under occlusion. *Pattern Recognition* 47, no. 6 (June 1): 2280–2292.

Gelfand, M.J., B.L. Koch, A.H. Elgazzar, V.M. Gylys-Morin, P.S. Gartside, and C.L. Torgerson. 1999. Cyclic cystography: Diagnostic yield in selected pediatric populations. *Radiology* 213, no. 1 (October): 118–120.

Gong, R.H., B. Jenkins, R.W. Sze, and Z. Yaniv. 2014. A cost effective and high fidelity fluo-roscopy simulator using the image-guided surgery toolkit (IGSTK). *SPIE Medical Imaging: Image-Guided Procedures, Robotic Interventions, and Modeling*, 9036: 903618-903618–11.

Güler, Ö., and Z. Yaniv. 2012. Image-guided navigation: A cost effective practical introduction using the image-guided surgery toolkit (IGSTK). In *Annual International Conference of the IEEE Engineering in Medicine and Biology Society*, 6056–6059.

Hamstra, S.J., R. Brydges, R. Hatala, B. Zendejas, and D.A. Cook. 2014. Reconsidering fidel-ity in simulation-based training. *Academic Medicine: Journal of the Association of American Medical Colleges* 89, no. 3 (March): 387–392.

Hanauer, S.B. 2010. A poor view from specialty silos. *Nature Reviews. Gastroenterology & Hepatology* 7, no. 1: 1–2.

Hartley, R., and A. Zisserman. 2003. *Multiple View Geometry in Computer Vision*. Cambridge, UK: Cambridge University Press.

Hishikawa, S., M. Kawano, H. Tanaka, K. Konno, Y. Yasuda, R. Kawano, E. Kobayashi, and A.T. Lefor. 2010. Mannequin simulation improves the confidence of medical students performing tube thoracostomy: A prospective, controlled trial. *The American Surgeon* 76, no. 1: 73–78.

Jaramaz, B., and K. Eckman. 2006. Virtual reality simulation of fluoroscopic navigation. *Clinical Orthopaedics and Related Research* 442 (January): 30–34.

Langlotz, F. 2004. Potential pitfalls of computer aided orthopedic surgery. *Injury* 35, no. 1: S-A17-23.

Lateef, F. 2010. Simulation-based learning: Just like the real thing. *Journal of Emergencies, Trauma and Shock* 3, no. 4: 348–352.

Lee, R., K.E. Thomas, B.L. Connolly, M. Falkiner, and C.L. Gordon. 2009. Effective dose esti-mation for pediatric voiding cystourethrography using an anthropomorphic phantom set and metal oxide semiconductor field-effect transistor (MOSFET) technology. *Pediatric Radiology* 39, no. 6 (June): 608–615.

Lim, R., R.D.A. Khawaja, K. Nimkin, P. Sagar, R. Shailam, M.S. Gee, and S.J. Westra. 2013. Relationship between radiologist training level and fluoroscopy time for voiding cysto-urethrography. *AJR. American Journal of Roentgenology* 200, no. 3 (March): 645–651.

Lindeberg, T. 1998. Feature detection with automatic scale selection. *International Journal of Computer Vision* 30, no. 2 (November 1): 79–116.

Maciunas, R.J. 2006. Computer-assisted neurosurgery. *Clinical Neurosurgery* 53: 267–271.

Matsumoto, E.D., S.J. Hamstra, S.B. Radomski, and M.D. Cusimano. 2002. The effect of bench model fidelity on endourological skills: A randomized controlled study. *The Journal of Urology* 167, no. 3 (March): 1243–1247.

Maurer, C.R., J.M. Fitzpatrick, M.Y. Wang, R.L. Galloway, R.J. Maciunas, and G.S. Allen. 1997. Registration of head volume images using implantable fiducial markers. *IEEE Transactions on Medical Imaging* 16, no. 4 (August): 447–462.

Mavrogenis, A.F., O.D. Savvidou, G. Mimidis, J. Papanastasiou, D. Koulalis, N. Demertzis, and P.J. Papagelopoulos. 2013. Computer-assisted navigation in orthopedic surgery. *Orthopedics* 36, no. 8: 631–642.

Maybody, M., C. Stevenson, and S.B. Solomon. 2013. Overview of navigation systems in image-guided interventions. *Techniques in Vascular and Interventional Radiology* 16, no. 3: 136–143.

Norman, G., K. Dore, and L. Grierson. 2012. The minimal relationship between simulation fidelity and transfer of learning. *Medical Education* 46, no. 7 (July): 636–647.

Özbek, Y., Ö. Güler, A. Ertugrul, G. Göbel, Z. Yaniv, and W. Freysinger. 2014. Teacher-centred vs. practical learning in image-guided surgery—A study. In *Conference on Medical Informatics in Europe*. Istanbul, Turkey.

Peters, T., and K. Cleary. 2008. *Image-Guided Interventions: Technology and Applications.* 2008 ed. New York: Springer.

Rickers, C., M. Jerosch-Herold, X. Hu, N. Murthy, X. Wang, H. Kong, R.T. Seethamraju, J. Weil, and N.M. Wilke. 2003. Magnetic resonance image-guided transcatheter closure of atrial septal defects. *Circulation* 107, no. 1: 132–138.

Royal, H.D. 2008. Effects of low level radiation-What's new? *Seminars in Nuclear Medicine* 38, no. 5 (September): 392–402.

Schneider, K., I. Krüger-Stollfuss, G. Ernst, and M.M. Kohn. 2001. Paediatric fluoroscopy—A survey of children's hospitals in Europe. I. Staffing, frequency of fluoroscopic procedures and investigation technique. *Pediatric Radiology* 31, no. 4 (April): 238–246.

Shah, S., S.L. Desouches, L.H. Lowe, N. Kasraie, and B. Reading. 2015. Implementation of a competency check-off in diagnostic fluoroscopy for radiology trainees: Impact on reducing radiation for three common fluoroscopic exams in children. *Pediatric Radiology* 45, no. 2 (February): 228–234.

Strauss, K.J., and S.C. Kaste. 2006. The ALARA (as Low as Reasonably Achievable) concept in pediatric interventional and fluoroscopic imaging: Striving to keep radiation doses as low as possible during fluoroscopy of pediatric patients—A white paper executive summary. *Pediatric Radiology* 36, no. 2 (September): 110–112.

Tjardes, T., S. Shafizadeh, D. Rixen, T. Paffrath, B. Bouillon, E.S. Steinhausen, and H. Baethis. 2010. Image-guided spine surgery: State of the art and future directions. *European Spine Journal* 19, no. 1: 25–45.

Walsh, K. 2015. The future of simulation in medical education. *Journal of Biomedical Research* 29, no. 3 (May): 259–260.

Walsh, K., and P. Jaye. 2013. Cost and value in medical education. *Education for Primary Care: An Official Publication of the Association of Course Organisers, National Association of GP Tutors, World Organisation of Family Doctors* 24, no. 6 (September): 391–393.

Ward, V.L. 2006. Patient dose reduction during voiding cystourethrography. *Pediatric Radiology* 36, no. Suppl 2 (September): 168–172.

Wellborn, P.S., N.P. Dillon, P.T. Russell, and R.J. Webster. 2017. Coffee: The key to safer image-guided surgery—A granular jamming cap for non-invasive, rigid fixation of fiducial markers to the patient. *International Journal of Computer Assisted Radiology and Surgery* 12, no. 6 (June 1): 1069–1077.

Wu, L., S. Song, K. Wu, C.M. Lim, and H. Ren. 2017. Development of a compact continuum tubular robotic system for nasopharyngeal biopsy. *Medical & Biological Engineering & Computing* 55, no. 3 (March 1): 403–417.

Yaniv, Z. 2015. Which pivot calibration? In *SPIE Medical Imaging: Image-Guided Procedures, Robotic Interventions, and Modeling*, 9415: 941527-941527-9.

Yaniv, Z., and K. Cleary. 2006a. Fluoroscopy based accuracy assessment of electromagnetic tracking. In *SPIE Medical Imaging: Visualization, Image-Guided Procedures, and Modeling*, ed. K.R. Cleary and R.L. Galloway, Jr., San Diego, CA, 61410L.

Yaniv, Z., and K. Cleary. 2006b. *Image-Guided Procedures: A Review*. Image Science and Information Systems Center, Georgetown University, Washington, DC.

Zhang, Z. 2000. A flexible new technique for camera calibration. *IEEE Transactions on Pattern Analysis and Machine Intelligence* 22, no. 11 (November): 1330–1334.

Ziv, A., P.R. Wolpe, S.D. Small, and S. Glick. 2003. Simulation-based medical education: An ethical imperative. *Academic Medicine: Journal of the Association of American Medical Colleges* 78, no. 8 (August): 783–788.

11 Augmented Reality-Based Visualization for Echocardiographic Applications

Gabriel Hanssen Kiss, Cameron Lowell Palmer,
Ole Christian Mjølstad, Håvard Dalen,
Bjørn Olav Haugen, and Hans Torp

CONTENTS

11.1 INTRODUCTION

Echocardiography has become a routine test for diagnosing, managing, and following up on heart disease. Echocardiography provides information related to both the anatomy of the heart and its global or local functions (Sutherland et al. 2006; Armstrong and Ryan 2009). To derive this information, several standard sectional views of the heart need to be found and imaged by the cardiologist. These views, which typically include apical two-, three-, and four-chamber views, as well as subcostal and parasternal views, are cut planes through the heart that go through anatomic landmarks. Traditionally, echocardiography is performed by a cardiologist or a cardiac sonographer who has undergone an extensive training program. The last decade marked the beginning of a new trend with the introduction of several handheld ultrasound devices, mainly aimed at nonexpert users who have minimal knowledge or ultrasound-related training. Despite recent advancements related to device miniaturization, the acquisition and interpretation of ultrasound images remains challenging and is highly operator dependent when compared to other imaging modalities such as x-ray computerized tomography and magnetic resonance imaging. Early research has shown that handheld ultrasound units have great potential in acute situations (Andersen et al. 2011) and in the general practitioner's office (Mjølstad et al. 2012), both for visualizing anatomy and evaluating function, assuming that the clinical users undergo proper training. Furthermore, it was shown that medical students who were given minimal ultrasound training (nine hours of combined theoretical and practical training) could acquire clinically relevant ultrasound images and interpret them with great accuracy (Andersen et al. 2014). Moreover, adding ultrasound screening (e.g., cardiac and abdominal examination) to all cases admitted to a medical unit leads to a diagnostic change of 18% when examined by experienced cardiologists (Mjolstad et al. 2012). Adding pocket-size ultrasound to the physical examination performed by trained medical residents corrected, verified, or added important diagnoses to one out of three emergency medical admissions (Andersen et al. 2015). A wide dissemination of the method as an add-on and integrated part of the existing physical examination has been hypothesized by several authors (Dalen, Haugen, and Graven 2013). Thus, there is a need for tools that can help nonexpert ultrasound users improve their skills during tailored training and allow them to acquire high-quality, diagnostically relevant ultrasound images during frontline diagnostics.

Augmented reality (AR) in a medical context is an active field of research, with prototype AR systems being available as early as 1994, when State et al. (1994) proposed a system for visualizing a fetus inside a pregnant woman using an ultrasound. A video mixer was employed for merging video images depicting the scene with a volume rendering of the fetus, and only computational limitations hindered real-time performance. More complex AR setups followed and consisted of head-mounted displays (Bajura et al. 1992; State et al. 1998; Harders et al. 2007) or projector-based setups (Bluteau et al. 2005). An optics-based setup, Sonic Flashlight, was proposed by Stetten et al. (2000) and Stetten and Chib (2001); the system uses a half-silvered mirror to superimpose an ultrasound image on top of the patient's body. As proposed, the setup is portable, aims to enhance needle biopsies, and can place the ultrasound images in the line of sight of the operator, thus avoiding the need to view a separate display, and as such, simplify the hand-eye coordination requirements during ultrasound-guided biopsies. Commercially available medical products based on AR also have been introduced to the market and range from minimally invasive surgery (ProMIS, Haptica, CAE Healthcare) laparoscopic simulators (Lap Sim, Inovus Medical or MiniLap, Teleflex) and needle or screw placement systems (Philips, hybrid OR) to transesophageal (Vimedix, CAE Healthcare) or transthoracic (ECHOCOM GmbH, Leipzig, Germany) ultrasound simulators.

However, many of the previously mentioned alternatives require technically complex setups that interfere with the medical workflow and are not well suited for bedside examinations. Moreover, they are aimed at clinical experts and as such require a priori knowledge and training before their use. To facilitate the adoption of ultrasound by nonexperts, we have started to develop ubiquitous, AR-based visualization tools for echocardiographic purposes that can be used in real time during image acquisition. Furthermore, we aimed to implement most of the augmentation pipeline on a tablet device and as such address challenges such as portability, ease of use, affordability, and maintenance by using off-the-shelf hardware. In the following, the main components of an AR system are discussed, and our approach is explained.

11.2   AR FOR ECHOCARDIOGRAPHIC ACQUISITIONS

To obtain a good ultrasound acquisition, detailed anatomical knowledge of the heart is required. Furthermore, during the acquisition the operator needs to be aware of the relationship between the anatomy of the heart, the current slice plane, and the ultrasound probe movement required to refine it. Our aim is to generate an AR view that contains an image of the scene, including the patient and the ultrasound probe, which will be augmented with the ultrasound image currently acquired and a detailed geometric model of the heart. This heart model will illustrate its anatomy and resemble the depiction of the heart present in most anatomy manuals and with which target users should be familiar. As the operator moves the probe, or the patient changes position, the augmented view is updated and kept consistent. As with any AR system, three problems need to be addressed: calibration, registration, and tracking. Additionally, to increase the realism of the scene, a temporal registration must be solved to allow the virtual heart model to be deformed in sync with the beating heart of the subject imaged with ultrasound.

11.2.1   CALIBRATION

To be able to place virtual objects in the real world, the camera used for imaging the scene needs to be calibrated. As such, correspondence between a three-dimensional (3D) point in world coordinates and a two-dimensional (2D) point in the camera's image space is established. Assuming a standard pinhole camera, the perspective projection matrix (PPM) is computed as follows:

$$PPM = K \times [R \,|\, t] \tag{11.1}$$

The PPM matrix has 3×4 elements, with a rotation, R, of (3×3) and a translation matrix, t, of (3×1) that describe the pose of the camera and hold the transformation from the camera to the origin of the world coordinate system. The internal camera parameters are represented as a 3×3 matrix and for a standard pinhole camera, with no zooming allowed, the K matrix is of the following form:

$$K = \begin{pmatrix} f_u & s & c_u \\ 0 & f_v & c_v \\ 0 & 0 & 1 \end{pmatrix} \tag{11.2}$$

In the matrix, (f_u, f_v) refers to the focal lengths along the $(\vec{u}, \vec{v})$ directions in the camera coordinates, (c_u, c_v), which are the offset to the principal point of the camera. Finally, s is a skew factor, which is 0 for most cameras, as typically the directions $\vec{u}$ and $\vec{v}$ are orthonormal.

Camera calibration is an offline process that needs to be performed only once for a given setup. Most AR toolkits include camera calibration tools, and a PPM matrix describing the camera parameters is given to the user.

11.2.2 TRACKING

The position of the ultrasound probe and the patient with regard to the camera must be tracked to be able to generate a consistent augmented view. There are several possibilities to achieve this, including optical and magnetic tracking systems, localization sensors, and visual marker-based tracking. These systems have varying accuracy and setup complexity, so there is no ideal tracking tool that fits all purposes, and, consequently, the choice is application dependent.

In our case, portability and robustness are more important than a high-level of accuracy; thus, we have chosen a frame marker-based visual tracking approach. This is convenient because all tablets have both front and back facing cameras, and their image quality is sufficient for marker tracking. Both the location and the pose of a frame marker of known shape can be computed given a camera image and a camera calibration matrix.

For the visual marker shown in Figure 11.1a, its corners are identified in the camera image using computer graphics algorithms. Thereafter, it is assumed that the corners are lying on a plane, so the relationship between a 3D point, p, in world coordinates, and a 2D point, q, in the camera image is given by the following homography, H:

$$p(x, y, z) = H \times q(u, v) \tag{11.3}$$

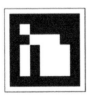

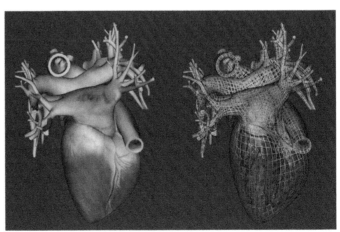

a.   b.

FIGURE 11.1 (a) Typical examples of frame markers used for visual tracking purposes. (b) Anatomical heart model from Zygote, textured, and wireframe rendering.

Equation 11.3 can be solved using a direct linear transformation or more advanced non-linear optimization schemes. There will always be a trade-off between accuracy and computation time. Once H is known, then the position and pose of the frame marker in world coordinates is known, so virtual objects can be placed relative to the frame marker and their position updated when the frame marker is moved in the scene.

Additionally, fusing input from several sensors in the same application can be helpful to improve the robustness of the tracking solution. For cardiac acquisitions, once the position of the probe on the patient's chest is determined, the probe is only tilted and/or rotated to capture the desired plane, and typically no translation occurs. In such a scenario, an orientation sensor can be useful to complement the visual tracker, which may lose track of the frame marker.

11.2.3 ANATOMIC REGISTRATION

Because our intention is to place a geometric heart model in the scene, its position with regards to the ultrasound probe needs to be determined. Furthermore, to give the impression of a beating heart, the model needs to be deformed along the heart cycle. Several heart segmentation algorithms have been proposed in the literature, including Papademetris et al. (2001), Yang et al. (2008), Orderud and Rabben (2008), Leung and Bosch (2010), and Barbosa et al. (2013). Most of them focus on delineating the left ventricle, which is relatively easy to image with ultrasound. Based on a delineation of the left ventricle, the location of given anatomic landmarks (i.e., apex, base, or outflow tract) can be determined, as proposed in Orderud et al. (2009).

Furthermore, based on the size and location of the left ventricle, an anatomic model describing the entire heart can also be deformed and matched with the ultrasound images using a simple deformation model. The chosen method should be fast enough for real-time computation. One alternative for computing the location of the left ventricle in the ultrasound volume is to fit a deformable model to the 3D ultrasound volumes. The left ventricle is modeled as a Doo-Sabin subdivision model, and a Kalman-based, noniterative approach ensuring fast processing times is then used to fit the ventricle to a particular ultrasound volume by adjusting a set of control points that control the shape of the Doo-Sabin model. The measurement vector for the Kalman filter is a set of edge detections that depict the location of the endocardium in the volume of interest and are equally spread on the surface of the left ventricle.

A simple kinematic model simulating the movement of the outer layer of the heart is also implemented. It is known that the position of the apex of the heart is approximately constant throughout the heart cycle, as is the volume of the pericardium. Therefore, the deformation of the outer shell can be represented by a translation of the mitral annular plane along the left ventricle's apex-to-base vector. The magnitude of the excursion can be derived from the apex-to-base distance in the current ultrasound volume, together with the distance of the current voxel from the apex, as detailed in Kiss et al. (2015).

11.3   IMPLEMENTATION DETAILS

The overview of our AR system is presented in Figure 11.2, and this section will describe both the scanner side and tablet components. A continuous stream of 3D ultrasound data is recorded with a high-end ultrasound scanner, and the position of a set of anatomic landmarks is detected and subsequently tracked in each ultrasound frame. The 3D human heart model from Zygote (Zygote, USA) (Figure 11.1b) is deformed and aligned to the ultrasound data. The position of both probe and patient is tracked visually using fiducial markers. Finally, the augmented view is generated on the tablet device using OpenGL ES.

We chose to use a high-end ultrasound scanner because it can record 3D ultrasound volumes of the left ventricle that are directly usable for segmentation and landmark detection purposes. A Vivid E9 ultrasound scanner (GE Vingmed Ultrasound, Norway) was used to acquire 3D apical views of the left ventricle. A custom plugin was implemented on the scanner, and its purpose was to stream ultrasound data together with the position of the anatomic landmarks over a TCP-IP connection. The real-time contour tracking library, a proprietary commercial software solution from GE Vingmed Ultrasound, Norway, was used for left ventricle segmentation and landmark detection purposes. Then, a tracking score that correlated with the quality of the model fit to the ultrasound data as described in Snare et al. (2009) was computed for each volume and sent over the local network.

On the tablet side, we chose the Vuforia SDK (PTC Inc. USA) for camera calibration as well as visual tracking purposes. The Vuforia SDK provides the PPM and is precalibrated for a large set of Android and iOS devices. Because we use the tablet's own camera to capture the scene, the external camera calibration matrix becomes trivial to compute and depends simply on the position of the tablet's camera relative to the display. The relative position of the camera with regards to the display device does not change, so no camera tracking is required.

Vuforia is also employed to track the position and pose of several frame markers and return a model view matrix (MVM) for each of them. The MVM matrix provides the transformation from the camera, which is assumed to be at the origin of the coordinate system and looking down along the z-axis to the frame marker. Two frame markers are used for our application: one to track the position of the ultrasound probe and the other to track the patient. The offset from the center of the marker that is returned by Vuforia to the tip of the ultrasound probe (where the

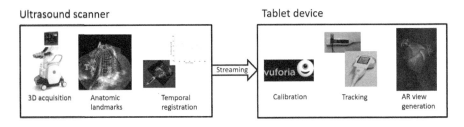

FIGURE 11.2   High-level overview of our AR system, including the components running on the ultrasound scanner and the ones implemented on the tablet device.

virtual image plane will be placed), as well as the position of the heart model with regards to the marker placed on the patient, are represented by two model calibration matrices, and these are determined before the start of the experiments. The frame marker tracking the patient is used for guiding purposes at the beginning to place the heart model at an initial position before the ultrasound data is available. Once an apical view of good image quality is acquired, the heart model is placed in the scene based on that image. By combining the previously computed matrices, the position of the virtual objects in display coordinates can be computed. The final AR view is generated by alpha blending the rendered virtual objects with the camera image. A standard graphics pipeline is implemented that combines the model transformation with the view and the perspective matrices. The position of each vertex $V(x, y, z, 1)$ in the augmented scene is given by the following:

$$\text{gl\_Position} = \text{VAR} \times \text{PPM} \times \text{MVM} \times \text{MCM} \times V \qquad (11.4)$$

The graphics pipeline, illustrated in Figure 11.3, is implemented in a customized version of VES/Kiwi, Kitware Inc., which is a set of libraries that conveniently links The Visualization Toolkit (VTK) and OpenGL ES 2.0 and was available at the start of the development. Currently, VTK has direct support for mobile devices and can be used directly for AR purposes. To improve computational efficiency, the anatomic registration was implemented in the vertex shader, and the deformation applied to each vertex is of the following form:

$$V = \text{MDM} \times \text{MLM} \times V_0 \qquad (11.5)$$

V_0 is the initial position of a vertex on the Zygote mesh, MLD is the local deformation for temporal alignment, and MDM is the mesh deformation matrix to align the Zygote

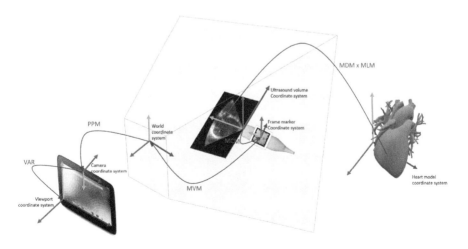

FIGURE 11.3 Illustration of the various coordinate systems and the transformations between them, as described in Equations 11.4 and 11.5. The x-, y-, and z-axes of the coordinate systems are color-coded as red, green, and blue, respectively.

mesh with the segmented left ventricle. Additionally, mesh clipping with a plane representing the ultrasound image plane is implemented to visualize the inner structures of the heart corresponding to the current slice plane. The fragment shader is a standard Gouraud shader, with normal mapping added to improve the appearance of the heart model by displaying fine details without the need for a high-resolution mesh.

11.4   EXPERIMENTAL SETUP

Figure 11.4 shows the lab setup for testing purposes. A Vivid E9 (GE Vingmed Ultrasound, Norway) ultrasound scanner, an ASUS RT- AC66U (AsusTek Computer Inc., Taiwan) wireless router, and an Android tablet Nexus 10 (Samsung, Electronics, Co., Ltd., South Korea) or an iPad Pro (Apple Inc., USA) have been used. Two placements for tablets have been considered, as shown in Figure 11.5. First, we attempted to place the tablet device as close as possible to the patient's chest to achieve a see-through effect. Second, the tablet was placed on a holder near the bed such that it could image the scene using the front-facing camera. After several pilot tests, our expert cardiologists deemed that the second setup was more appropriate, as the tablet was not blocking the ultrasound probe; thus, the patient could be placed in the standard left lateral decubitus position with the device fixed for the duration of the experiment. In this way, the marker tracking was more robust.

To test the usability and the usefulness of our prototype on our target group (i.e., inexperienced ultrasound operators), we invited fourth-year medical students who had received a two-hour introductory ultrasound course as part of their first-year curriculum to test our system. The first twelve students to respond were asked

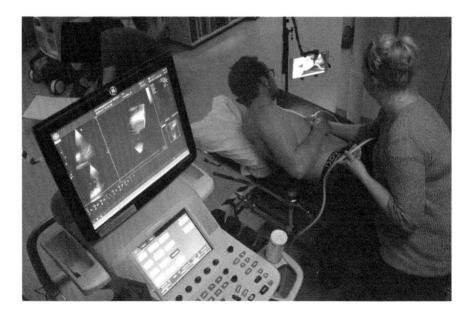

FIGURE 11.4 Setup for the experiments with medical students; all settings on the ultrasound device are predefined such that the student can focus only on the AR view.

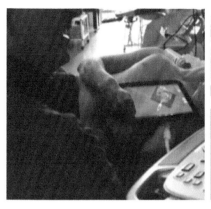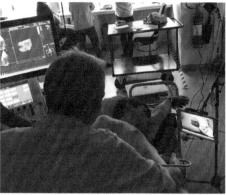

FIGURE 11.5   Two different placements of the tablet device. On the left, the tablet is placed as close as possible to the patient for *in situ* visualization. On the right, the tablet is mounted on a stand with the clinician seeing a mirrored view of the scene.

to perform the test. The Regional Committee for Medical and Health Research Ethics approved the study's conduction. Figure 11.5 illustrates the typical setup and interaction with the AR system. The task the students had to complete was to acquire a standard four-chamber view of the left ventricle, which is the easiest view to image from an apical window relying only on 2D ultrasound images or using the AR-enhanced view. To simplify the test, all the settings of the ultrasound scanner were fixed so that the student could focus on the image itself and not the acquisition parameters. Additionally, all the students did the ultrasound imaging on the same healthy volunteer, which had fair image quality in recordings from an apical view. Prior to scanning, all students received a brief introduction to our system, and a one-minute demonstration on how to acquire a four-chamber view was given by an expert echocardiographer (cardiologist). The medical students were then divided into two equal groups. The first group was shown the AR-enhanced image and asked to find the four-chamber view, and afterwards were asked to complete the same task having access only to the 2D ultrasound image. For the second group, the order was reversed; the students used 2D ultrasound first and then the AR-enhanced image. Figure 11.6 presents the information displayed on the tablet's screen during the two tasks. For the ultrasound-only view, the current 2D slice was shown on the display. In addition to the 2D ultrasound slice, the AR view contained the camera image and the heart model that was anatomically registered to the patient. The yellow mesh represents the segmentation result for the current ultrasound volume. The mesh was color coded either red, yellow, or green depending on the current fitting score. This gave the user a quick feedback sign regarding the quality of the model fit to the data.

All sessions were video recorded, and the time for each task was recorded. When a student was happy with the current image, this was stored as a DICOM loop on the ultrasound scanner. Then, all Digital Imaging and Communications in Medicine (DICOM) images were anonymized, and their quality was scored by two expert echocardiographers independently. Each image was scored on a scale from 1 (worst) to 6 (best), depending on how well the image contained the anatomic landmarks

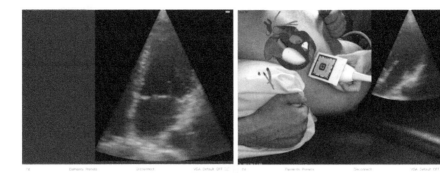

FIGURE 11.6 Screenshots of the AR system for the two different modes used for testing. Left: 2D ultrasound-only mode, showing an ultrasound slice as it would appear on a scanner. Right: AR-enhanced view, with the heart model cut along the acquisition plane in order to present the anatomic location. Note that the image is mirrored because the front camera is used. The mirrored view was considered more natural with regards to hand movements by the experts.

required for a four-chamber image, if the apex was centered, if the image was suitable for mitral annulus evaluation, and the degree of misalignment at the apex. The average of these values yielded the final image score. Additionally, all students were asked to fill out a standard system usability scale (SUS) form (Brooke 1996), which is designed to measure the user acceptance of a given system. Furthermore, based on the SUS form, both the usability and learnability of the system could be measured.

11.5   RESULTS

First, to validate the feasibility of Vuforia for frame marker tracking, an *in vitro* study was carried out. The depth and rotational accuracy of visual tracking were tested by placing a frame marker at 15, 20, 30, 60, and 100 cm along the z-axis of the camera and at three different angles ($-30°$, $0°$, and $30°$) along the y-axis under ambient lighting, making sure that strong reflections on the marker surface were avoided. The value ranges for depth and elevation angle were chosen to match the ones encountered in practice, with the measurements repeated five times for each setup. Figure 11.7 presents all the measurements for the various depths and axis angles. Overall, the mean error ± standard deviation when estimating the position of the frame marker with regards to the camera across all depths was -0.31 ± 0.38 cm. The mean angle errors ± standard deviations when estimating the angle of the frame marker with regards to a given axis angle are $-0.05° \pm 1.77°$, $2.91° \pm 0.29°$, and $-3.39° \pm 0.15°$ for $0°$, $-30°$, and $30°$ respectively.

Figures 11.8 and 11.9 present the results obtained during the experiments involving the medical students. First, the time spent to obtain an ultrasound image with and without the use of AR tools is given in Figure 11.8a; the average time to acquire the ultrasound images was 84 seconds when only the 2D image was shown, whereas for the AR view it was 128 seconds. The overall SUS score given as a percentage as well as the usability and learnability scores for each participant are given in Figure 11.8b, while the scores from the two experts, as well as their average scores are plotted in Figure 11.9.

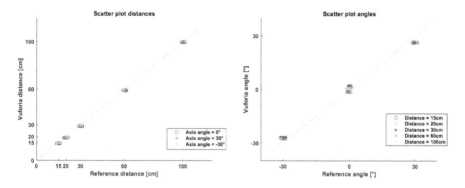

FIGURE 11.7 *In vitro* testing of Vuforia for visual tracking purposes. Both distance and angular errors are plotted.

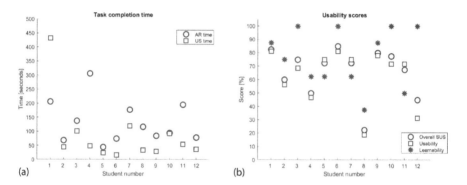

FIGURE 11.8 On the left (a), task completion times for the AR- and ultrasound-only modes. On the right (b), the overall SUS, usability, and learnability scores are presented. Red denotes students that used the AR view first, while blue represents students who were presented the 2D ultrasound image first.

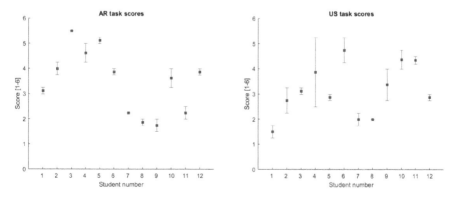

FIGURE 11.9 Image score for the four-chamber-view ultrasound images acquired in the AR mode and 2D ultrasound-only mode. The first six students acquired the AR-guided image first, while the second group was presented with the ultrasound view first.

11.6   DISCUSSION

We have developed an AR prototype system that gives instantaneous feedback regarding the current anatomical location, as well as the quality of the acquired image during the ultrasound acquisition process. It is particularly well suited for ultrasound acquisitions because they are operator dependent, and their clinical usefulness is directly linked to their quality. Implementing the system on a tablet device with minimal setup required is expected to further lower the adoption threshold of the tool.

The first test involving medical students proved that such an AR system can be used in practice in a standard echocardiographic laboratory. All students managed to obtain a four-chamber image with and without the AR tool, but the students who used AR first had consistently higher scores for the AR-aided acquisition when compared to standard 2D ultrasound imaging. Unfortunately, there was a difference in the ultrasound sector width between the two groups (i.e., students using AR first and students using 2D ultrasound first); this may also explain the score difference, as a wider sector size used during the first setup allows the AR prototype to find the position of the heart for a wider set of probe positions and orientations. Overall, there was no significant difference between AR and the 2D ultrasound-only scores. However, the study size is too small for a proper statistical analysis. Furthermore, the selected task was a simple one, and a more complex testing scenario needs to be devised to highlight the benefits of an AR solution.

Overall, the average time when using AR was 44 seconds more than for the ultrasound-only setup. Showing a color-coded representation of the segmented mesh may explain this result because most of the medical students tried to optimize their view until a green mesh, signaling a very good positioning of the probe, was displayed on the tablet.

The learnability values were higher than the usability scores, which suggests that the medical students considered our system useful for learning purposes. Subsequently, it would be interesting to have students fill out similar forms for AR-only and 2D-only acquisitions so that a direct comparison can be made between the AR setup and 2D standard ultrasound imaging. During the current study, the SUS scores were given after completing both tasks.

The usability score of the system was deemed as average by the students; however, usability was not the main focus of this project, as only a barebones interface with minimal functionality was added. This was a deliberate choice because typical ultrasound devices have a multitude of knobs and buttons that can be adjusted to optimize the quality of the image. This works well for a trained professional but has an intimidating effect on novice users. Exposing only the most important controls is beneficial at an early stage in the training process.

11.7   FUTURE DIRECTIONS

AR systems will mostly benefit novice ultrasound users such as medical students. However, it is unlikely they would have access to high-end ultrasound equipment, so it is highly desirable to have an AR platform that can input images from a portable device. This poses two additional challenges, as typically portable ultrasound devices do not have 3D imaging or ECG functionality. However, early work in our lab has shown that by combining a set of 2D ultrasound images of the left ventricle with their orientation recorded by a clip-on sensor is accurate enough for localizing the heart's orientation in 3D and usable as input for the proposed AR system.

Using just the video stream provided by the tablet's camera severely limits the depth perception of a scene, particularly under real-time computation constraints. The frame marker placed on the patient could be used for advanced occlusion and alpha blending algorithms, but this is not implemented currently, and a semitransparent rendering is adopted instead. Detecting and reconstructing the 3D geometry of the patient profile is desirable to enhance the realism of the augmented view. Project Tango and Microsoft HoloLens are two devices that are designed for high-level depth perception and physical environment reconstruction. Integrating depth information when generating the AR view would further increase the user's feeling of immersion.

In addition to cardiac echocardiography, AR tools are beneficial for other applications, such as fetal or liver scanning. Furthermore, the integration of AR headsets with a surgical navigation system is feasible, and an early prototype for spine surgery has been introduced by Scopis Medical, Germany. Moreover, the collaboration between members of the surgical team can be enhanced as they perceive the same scene from their respective location.

11.8   CONCLUSION

By combining a live stream of ultrasound images with a highly descriptive geometric model of an organ of interest, a better understanding of the anatomy can be achieved. The mental burden of establishing a spatial relationship between the ultrasound slice and the anatomy being imaged is alleviated, which is beneficial for nonexpert users during training. A good correlation between the anatomic model and the ultrasound image is achievable in real time under normal scanning conditions, and both the ultrasound slice and the anatomic model are placed at the correct location in the 3D scene with regards to the patient's position. Finally, a small-scale study has shown that AR-based technology can be used by novice users, who have little to no knowledge of ultrasound in clinical practice.

REFERENCES

Andersen, Garrett Newton, Annja Viset, Ole Christian Mjølstad, Øyvind Salvesen, Håvard Dalen, and Bjørn Olav Haugen. 2014. Feasibility and accuracy of point-of-care pocket-size ultrasonography performed by medical students. *BMC Medical Education* 14 (July): 156. doi:10.1186/1472-6920-14-156.
Andersen, Garrett Newton, Bjørn Olav Haugen, Torbjørn Graven, Oyvind Salvesen, Ole Christian Mjølstad, and Håvard Dalen. 2011. Feasibility and reliability of point-of-care pocket-sized echocardiography. *European Journal of Echocardiography* 12 (9): 665–670. doi:10.1093/ejechocard/jer108.

Andersen, Garrett Newton, Torbjørn Graven, Kyrre Skjetne, Ole Christian Mjølstad, Jens Olaf Kleinau, Øystein Olsen, Bjørn Olav Haugen, and Håvard Dalen. 2015. Diagnostic influence of routine point-of-care pocket-size ultrasound examinations performed by medical residents. *Journal of Ultrasound in Medicine: Official Journal of the American Institute of Ultrasound in Medicine* 34 (4): 627–636. doi:10.7863/ultra.34.4.627.

Armstrong, William, and Thomas Ryan. 2009. *Feigenbaum's Echocardiography*. 7th ed. Philadelphia, PA: LWW.

Bajura, Michael, Henry Fuchs, and Ryutarou Ohbuchi. 1992. Merging virtual objects with the real world: Seeing ultrasound imagery within the patient. In *Proceedings of the 19th Annual Conference on Computer Graphics and Interactive Techniques*, pp. 203–210. SIGGRAPH'92. New York: ACM. doi:10.1145/133994.134061.

Barbosa, Daniel, Thomas Dietenbeck, Brecht Heyde, Helene Houle, Denis Friboulet, Jan D'hooge, and Olivier Bernard. 2013. Fast and fully automatic 3-D echocardiographic segmentation using B-Spline explicit active surfaces: Feasibility study and validation in a clinical setting. *Ultrasound in Medicine & Biology* 39 (1): 89–101. doi:10.1016/j.ultrasmedbio.2012.08.008.

Bluteau, Jeremy, Itaru Kitahara, Yoshinari Kameda, Haruo Noma, Kiyoshi Kogure, and Yuichi Ohta. 2005. Visual support for medical communication by using projector-based augmented reality and thermal markers. In *Proceedings of the 2005 International Conference on Augmented Tele-Existence*, pp. 98–105. ICAT'05. New York: ACM. doi:10.1145/1152399.1152418.

Brooke, John. 1996. *SUS: A Quick and Dirty Usability Scale*.

Dalen, Håvard, Bjørn Olav Haugen, and Torbjørn Graven. 2013. Feasibility and clinical implementation of hand-held echocardiography. *Expert Review of Cardiovascular Therapy* 11 (1): 49–54. doi:10.1586/erc.12.165.

Harders, Matthias, Gerald Bianchi, and Benjamin Knoerlein. 2007. Multimodal augmented reality in medicine. In *Universal Access in Human-Computer Interaction. Ambient Interaction*, pp. 652–658. Lecture Notes in Computer Science. Berlin, Germany: Springer. doi:10.1007/978-3-540-73281-5_70.

In P. W. Jordan, B. Thomas, B. A. Weerdmeester, & A. L. McClelland (Eds.), Usability Evaluation in Industry. London: Taylor and Francis.

Kiss, Gabriel Hanssen, Cameron Lowell Palmer, and Hans Torp. 2015. Patient adapted augmented reality system for real-time echocardiographic applications. In *Proceedings of the Augmented Environments for Computer-Assisted Interventions - 10th International Workshop, AE-CAI 2015 Held in Conjunction with MICCAI 2015*, Munich, Germany, October 9, pp. 145–154. doi:10.1007/978-3-319-24601-7_15.

Leung, K. Y. Esther, and Johan G. Bosch. 2010. Automated border detection in three-dimensional echocardiography: Principles and promises. *European Journal of Echocardiography* 11 (2): 97–108. doi:10.1093/ejechocard/jeq005.

Mjolstad, Ole Christian, Havard Dalen, Torbjorn Graven, Jens Olaf Kleinau, Oyvind Salvesen, and Bjorn Olav Haugen. 2012. Routinely adding ultrasound examinations by pocket-sized ultrasound devices improves inpatient diagnostics in a medical department. *European Journal of Internal Medicine* 23 (2): 185–191. doi:10.1016/j.ejim.2011.10.009.

Mjølstad, Ole Christian, Sten Roar Snare, Lasse Folkvord, Frode Helland, Anders Grimsmo, Hans Torp, Olav Haraldseth, and Bjørn Olav Haugen. 2012. Assessment of left ventricular function by GPs using pocket-sized ultrasound. *Family Practice* 29 (5): 534–540. doi:10.1093/fampra/cms009.

Orderud, Fredrik, and Stein Inge Rabben. 2008. Real-time 3D segmentation of the left ventricle using deformable subdivision surfaces. In *2008 IEEE Conference on Computer Vision and Pattern Recognition*, pp. 1–8. doi:10.1109/CVPR.2008.4587442.

Orderud, Fredrik, Hans Torp, and Stein Inge Rabben. 2009. Automatic alignment of standard views in 3D echocardiograms using real-time tracking. In *Proceedings of the SPIE 7265*, 72650D. SPIE, Washington, DC, USA.

Papademetris, Xenophon, Albert J. Sinusas, Donald P. Dione, and James S. Duncan. 2001. Estimation of 3D left ventricular deformation from echocardiography. *Medical Image Analysis* 5 (1): 17–28. doi:10.1016/S1361-8415(00)00022-0.

Snare, Sten Roar, Svein Arne Aase, Ole Christian Mjølstad, Håvard Dalen, Fredrik Orderud, and Hans Torp. 2009. Automatic real-time view detection. In *2009 IEEE International Ultrasonics Symposium*, pp. 2304–2307. doi:10.1109/ULTSYM.2009.5441530.

State, Andrei, David T. Chen, Chris Tector, Andrew Brandt, Hong Chen, Ryutarou Ohbuchi, Mike Bajura, and Henry Fuchs. 1994. Observing a volume rendered fetus within a pregnant patient. In *IEEE Conference on Visualization, 1994, Visualization'94, Proceedings*, pp. 364–368, CP41. doi:10.1109/VISUAL.1994.346295.

State, Andrei, Mark A. Livingston, William F. Garrett, Gentaro Hirota, Mary C. Whitton, Etta D. Pisano, and Henry Fuchs. 1998. Technologies for augmented reality systems: Realizing ultrasound-guided needle biopsies. In *Proceedings of ACM SIGGRAPH 1998*, pp. 439–446. ACM, New York, NY, USA.

Stetten, George D., and Vikram S. Chib. 2001. Overlaying ultrasonographic images on direct vision. *Journal of Ultrasound in Medicine* 20 (3): 235–240. doi:10.7863/jum.2001.20.3.235.

Stetten, George D., Vikram S. Chib, and Robert J. Tamburo. 2000. Tomographic reflection to merge ultrasound images with direct vision. In *Proceedings of the IEEE Workshop on Applied Imagery Pattern Recognition*, pp. 200–205.

Sutherland, George R., Liv Hatle, Piet Claus, Jan D'Hooge, and Bart H. Bijnens. 2006. *Doppler Myocardial Imaging: A Textbook*. 1st ed. Hasselt, Belgium: BSWK bvba.

Yang, Lin, Bogdan Georgescu, Yefeng Zheng, Peter Meer, and Dorin Comaniciu. 2008. 3D ultrasound tracking of the left ventricle using one-step forward prediction and data fusion of collaborative trackers. In *2008 IEEE Conference on Computer Vision and Pattern Recognition*, pp. 1–8. doi:10.1109/CVPR.2008.4587518.

12 Ultrasound Augmented Laparoscopy
Technology and Human Factors

Uditha L. Jayarathne

CONTENTS

12.1 INTRODUCTION

The advancement of video technology has allowed laparoscopy to become one of the most widely used minimally invasive surgical approaches, in which surgeons attempt surgical procedures through small incisions. While a miniaturized camera inserted through one of these incisions provides real-time visual feedback into the patients' body cavity, long, slender instruments inserted through other small incisions provide means to treat critical surgical targets. However, although a laparoscopic approach is preferred over an open surgical approach in many procedures, due to the significantly lower patient morbidity and improved recovery time (Bonjer et al. 2015), it is very challenging both cognitively and physically even for experienced surgeons. This is partly due to the dislocation of the surgeons' perception from the action site and partly due to limitations in the conventional setup, such as limited dexterity in manipulation and limited depth perception in 2D displays. The invention of robotic surgical systems, such as the *da Vinci*, has solved most of the ergonomic and manipulation issues, while the stereo-display systems have eliminated most of the issues in depth perception.

For many laparoscopic tasks, however, whether it is a resection of a tumor situated deep inside an organ parenchyma (e.g., partial nephrectomy, wedge resection surgeries under video assisted thoracic surgical approach, liver tumor resection) or reconstruction of a bile duct while avoiding critical blood vessels, surgeons need to visualize hidden surgical targets. Because the laparoscopic camera provides visualization of only the organ surface, surgeons often use laparoscopic ultrasound (LUS) to establish a visual channel into the tissue. Conventionally, this LUS video is displayed on a monitor separate to that displaying the laparoscopic video. Therefore, surgeons are required to mentally fuse information from the two displays to guide their surgical actions. It is known that such strategies are challenging (Bonjer et al. 2015), and the mental processes involved require a significant amount of working memory (Prime and Jolicoeur 2010). Given the limited working memory capacity and the time constraints for surgical subtasks (Thompson et al. 2010), these processes may result in incorrect spatial representations (Prime and Jolicoeur 2010), which lead to surgical error.

Spatial representations from perception are much more accurate compared to the cognitively mediated ones (Klatzky et al. 2008), so actions relying on such representations are more likely to be accurate. To reduce surgical error and enable spatial representations from perception, ultrasound (US) information is overlaid in the context of the laparoscopic video. This requires an external means of registration of the images followed by overlay visualization of transformed US information such that the surgeon perceives the geometry of the imaged anatomy accurately. This chapter discusses in detail the technology behind accurate registration between the US imaging system and the laparoscopic camera system, visualization of transformed US information, and the psychophysical aspects of augmented visualization.

12.2   MERGING COORDINATE SYSTEMS

To overlay US data in the context of the laparoscopic video, mapping from the US image coordinate system to that based on the laparoscopic camera needs to be established. This mapping, T_u^{cc}, can conveniently be summarized by the following rigid-transformation chain:

$$T_u^{cc} = T_p^{cc} . T_u^p \qquad (12.1)$$

where T_u^p is the transformation from the US image-based coordinate system to the coordinate system on the US probe, T_p^{cc} is the transformation from the US probe coordinate system to that centered in the camera. T_u^p is a constant transform that can be determined by employing a suitable US calibration procedure (Ameri et al. 2015; Ackerman et al. 2014; Comeau et al. 1998), and T_p^{cc} is the relative pose between the laparoscopic camera and the LUS probe to be updated in real-time. The latter can be estimated either by employing an extrinsic spatial tracking system, such as a magnetic tracking system, or by a completely image-based technique.

12.2.1 EXTRINSIC TRACKING METHODS

A magnetic sensor attached to the laparoscopic camera and to the LUS probe (Cheung et al. 2010), or an optically tracked dynamic reference body (DRB) attached in a similar manner (Leven et al. 2005), provide means of estimation of the transform T_p^{cc} accurately in real time. However, optical tracking alone cannot be used when the US probe has an articulated tip because the variable transformation from the tracking DRB to the transducer cannot be determined easily. A popular solution to this issue is to use a magneto-optic hybrid approach (Feuerstein et al. 2007). In addition to optical and magnetic tracking, in the special case of robot-assisted laparoscopy, robot kinematics can be used to estimate T_p^{cc}, even though the accuracy and precision may not be sufficient for clinical use (Leven et al. 2005).

When extrinsic tracking systems are employed, several transformations are concatenated to estimate T_p^{cc}. Typically, this concatenated chain consists of the transformation from the sensor attached to the LUS probe to the tracking system T_p^t, the transformation from the sensor attached to the laparoscopic camera body to the tracking system T_c^t, and the constant transformation from the sensor attached to the camera body to the coordinate system centered on the camera T_c^{cc}. The transformation chain can thus be written as follows:

$$T_p^{cc} = T_c^{cc} \cdot \left[T_p^t \right]^{-1} \qquad (12.2)$$

The transformation T_c^{cc} is commonly known as the hand-eye transformation, a term borrowed from the robotics community. Estimation of this transformation can be done using any of the algorithms proposed in the literature (Feuerstein et al. 2007; Heller et al. 2012; Thompson et al. 2016; Morgan et al. 2017). The accuracy of estimation of this transformation is of paramount importance in an US overlay system, as it plays a critical role in image alignment. It is also crucial that these calibration steps are not overly time consuming and do not add significant overhead to the existing operating room (OR) workflow.

Extrinsic tracking methods have several limitations despite their convenience of use. The majority of ORs are not magnetically clean, meaning that the magnetic field generated by magnetic tracking systems may be distorted by the presence of ferro-magnetic materials. Distorted fields result in reduced accuracy and precision in tracking. Optical tracking systems, on the other hand, require line-of-sight, which may be difficult to maintain in practice. Moreover, the placement of the DRB on the handle of the laparoscope to provide line-of-sight may contribute to magnification of error at the tip of the probe by the lever-arm effect. Typically, the long transformation chains associated with systems employing extrinsic spatial tracking methods result in error accumulation, while the equipment cost and work-flow overhead due to sensor attachment and calibration are other factors limiting their use in the clinic.

12.2.2 INTRINSIC TRACKING METHODS

The transformation T_p^{cc} can be estimated based on purely image-based techniques without employing extrinsic tracking systems. Image-based techniques can estimate this transformation directly and thus avoid error accumulation from multiple sources.

While intrinsic tracking methods eliminate additional costs associated with tracking hardware, they add minimal overhead to the existing OR work flow. However, several challenges exist in estimating this rigid transformation based purely on image information.

Most of the clinically used LUS probes have a semicylindrical shape so that any image-based pose estimation technique that relies on the probe shape fails to resolve ambiguities in the probe roll direction. Moreover, these probes do not contain adequate texture on their surface to be used by a salient-feature-based approach. To remedy this issue, a fiducial marker pattern is often attached to the back surface of the probe (Leven et al. 2005; Pratt et al. 2012; Jayarathne et al. 2013) (see Figure 12.1a and b). These markers can be printed on materials that can be sterilized and are biocompatible for use in the clinic (Pratt et al. 2015). The fiducial points in the image space can be localized by employing specialized salient-point detection algorithms (Pratt et al. 2012; Bennett and Lasenby 2014) in real time and passed to a pose estimation algorithm. Theoretically, one could print any textured pattern and employ Scale-invariant Feature Transform (SIFT) (Lowe 2004) or any other

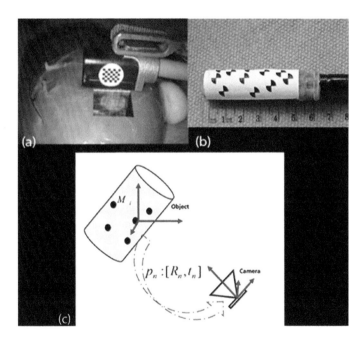

FIGURE 12.1 (a) US image information visualized in the context of a monocular laparoscopic image. To improve depth perception, the image is rendered in a cut-away. (Courtesy of Dr. Philip Pratt, Imperial College, London, UK); (b) A fiducial pattern attached to the curved back surface of the clinical LUS probe. (With kind permission from Springer Science+Business Media: *Simultaneous Estimation of Feature Correspondence and Stereo Object Pose with Application to Ultrasound Augmented Robotic Laparoscopy*, 2015, 134–144, Jayarathne, U.L. et al.); (c) Fiducial locations are defined with respect to a local coordinate system of the probe. Given the 3D points and their image space locations, the objective is to estimate the pose P_n that maps the 3D points to a coordinate system centered in the camera.

salient-point-detector to localize an adequate number of feature points in the image space. However, in practice, these methods often fail to robustly detect the interest points due to the high degree of illumination variation in the laparoscopic scene. Moreover, these algorithms detect blobs in the image space, so the features are not well localized (Zeisl et al. 2009). Unless handled properly, these image-space localization uncertainties result in a high degree of uncertainty in the pose estimates. Therefore, fiducial patterns with more localized features (Jayarathne et al. 2013; Pratt et al. 2015; Zhang et al. 2017) are preferred in practice.

Image-based, three-dimensional (3D) pose estimation requires the fiducial locations to be known with respect to a coordinate system defined on the pattern (see Figure 12.1c). The accuracy at which these coordinates is defined affects the accuracy of the pose estimation. For two-dimensional (2D) patterns that are attached to a flat surface of a probe (see Figure 12.1a), the fiducial location can be defined very accurately using a measuring microscope. However, for 3D patterns that are attached to the curved back surface, fiducial localization will require an accurately tracked pointer or a coordinate measuring machine.

Given the local fiducial coordinates and corresponding feature locations in monocular image space, the pose of the pattern with respect to the camera can be computed by solving the perspective-n-point (PnP) problem, which can be solved by many efficient algorithms (Zheng et al. 2013). However, these solutions assume that the correspondence between the 3D points and image space points are determined a priori. For patterns with simple configurations, this correspondence can be determined easily, even with minor feature occlusion and outliers. The planar checkerboard pattern used by (Pratt et al. 2012, 2015) is an example of such an approach (see Figure 12.1a). The simple fiducial configuration of this approach allows the feature detector to interpolate a few undetected features, making it robust to minor feature occlusions. The method, however, may fail under severe occlusion scenarios, which is an unavoidable situation in practical surgery. Moreover, the planar nature of the pattern prevents its use on probes with curved back surfaces that are common in the clinic. If the pattern lies on the curved back surface of the probe in 3D (see Figure 12.1c), some of the features may not be visible, depending on the viewing angle of the camera. In addition, blood or soft tissue may partially occlude the pattern. In addition to partial feature occlusions, the imperfections of the feature detectors result in outliers to be detected. The algorithm that solves for the feature correspondence should be robust to these conditions and provide accurate matching. Erroneous feature correspondences result in incorrect estimates to be computed by the pose estimation algorithm. For highly localized features such as checkerboard features, the appearance-based feature descriptor such as that computed for SIFT cannot easily be computed. Therefore, matching of such features may have to rely on entirely geometric approaches (Meer and Link 1998) that are sensitive to feature occlusion and clutter.

12.2.2.1 Simultaneous Estimation of Feature Correspondence and Object Pose

The correspondence and the pose estimation problem can be solved jointly (Zheng et al. 2013), rather than separately. However, unless a prior on the pose is not assumed, these algorithms may struggle to perform in real-time. The image-based tracking methods proposed by (Jayarathne et al. 2013, 2015) use priors on the pose (Moreno-Noguer et al. 2008) and priors on the motion to reach real-time performance. The algorithm outline is as follows:

Let M_i be the coordinate of the ith point in the local coordinate system and $\text{Proj}(P_n, M_i)$ be the operator that projects M_i with the pose P_n in the camera image. With orientations in Rodrigues representation, P_n is a six-dimensional vector. However, more efficient quaternion representation can be adapted as well. Let us represent the uncertainty in P_n as Σ_n, and let U_j be the 2D coordinates of a feature detected in the image space. We will assume that the camera is monocular first and show that extension to multiview settings are also possible.

Let's assume that we have an initial guess of P_n and Σ_n. The projection of M_i with P_n and associated covariance Σ_n results in a mean projection location m_i and the uncertainty around it Σ_i that are given by Equations 12.3 and 12.4, where $J(.)$ is the Jacobian of the $\text{Proj}(Pn, M_i)$.

$$m_i = \text{Proj}(Pn, M_i) \tag{12.3}$$

$$\Sigma_i = J(M_i)\Sigma_n J(M_i)^T \tag{12.4}$$

Σ_i defines the search region for correspondence (see Figure 12.2a), and one can restrict the search to an elliptical region defined by Equation 12.5, where the value of Ψ is chosen to be 3, thus resulting in 99% confidence in matching.

$$(m_i - u_j)^T \Sigma_i (m_i - u_j)^T \leq \Psi \tag{12.5}$$

Each point lying inside the search region is a putative match. A Euclidean distance-based heuristic is used to determine the probability that each of the features match with m_i, with higher probability assigned to features lying closer to m_i. If no feature is found within the search region, then the fiducial point is considered to be not detected.

For each feature match, the pose P_n and its covariance is updated using Kalman filter state update equations.

$$P_{n+1} = P_n + K(u_j - \text{Proj}(P_n, M_i)) \tag{12.6}$$

$$\Sigma_{n+1} = (I - KJ(M_i))\Sigma_n \tag{12.7}$$

where K is the Kalman gain.

Fiducial points are then projected back into image space by using the updated pose and the updated covariance. Note that for the matched fiducial point, the updated image space covariance shrinks down to noise variance in the image space, while the covariance for others generally reduces as a result of the established correspondence (see Figure 12.2b). A match for another fiducial is determined as described above, followed by a pose and covariance update (see Figure 12.2c). After three such updates, the change in the covariance in the image space becomes insignificant.

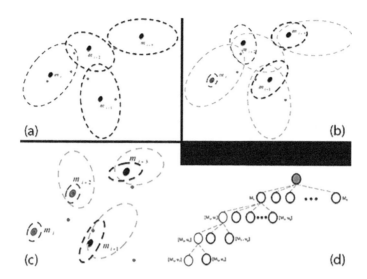

FIGURE 12.2 (a) Given the prior on the pose, the image space locations of the model points (in black) are determined with their image space covariance (dashed ellipses). The output of the feature detector is depicted by red dots. A putative match is sought in the search region in blue, and the pose and its covariance is updated; (b) Due to the established correspondence hypothesis, the image space covariance shrinks. Note the reduction in the size of elliptical regions compared to their previous size (in gray). The image space covariance for the matched model point has now shrunk to measurement noise (in blue); (c) The image space covariance is further reduced after two correspondence hypotheses. One last correspondence hypothesis is made at this stage before the correctness of the hypotheses is evaluated using the Equation 12.8; (d) the correspondence hypotheses are managed in a tree-data structure traversed in depth-first order. Each child node contains a correspondence pair, the current pose, and its covariance. Indicated in blue are the nodes that have been visited in the discussed scenario.

At this point, all the fiducials are projected in the image with the current pose and paired with the closest feature. The fiducials that do not have a feature within a pre-defined distance range are considered undetected. The error in Equation 12.8 is then computed to evaluate the fitness of the computed pose to the data:

$$E(P) = \sum_{(M,U)\in\text{Matches}} \left\| U - \text{Proj}(P,M) \right\| + \lambda \left| \text{NotDetected} \right| \qquad (12.8)$$

where $\left| \text{NotDetected} \right|$ represents the cardinality of the not detected point set, and λ is a tunable parameter. If the error in Equation 12.8 drops below a predefined threshold, then the updated pose is accepted as the pose of the probe and refined to yield a more accurate estimation. Otherwise, the algorithm repeats with the next probable correspondence candidate.

The search space for six-dimensional pose is traversed in depth-first order in a tree data-structure (see Figure 12.2d). For example, assume that during the first projection, k number of features lie in the search ellipse for fiducial $M1$. All the k possible fiducial-feature combinations are ordered by the distance to $M1$ from left to right. After the first projection, the pose will be updated assuming that *M1-U1* is a correct correspondence, and the rest of the fiducials are projected back. Assume that this time, three fiducials came inside the search region for a different fiducial *M3*. The pose is updated again assuming that *M3-U5* is a correct correspondence. Let's assume that after the second pose update, two features lie in the search region for fiducial *M5*. Now if we assume that *U7* is much closer to *M5* than *U9*, then the pose is updated assuming *M5-U9* is a correct correspondence. At this level, the fitness of the computed pose to data is assessed by computing the error in Equation 12.8. If the error drops below a predefined threshold value, then the assumed correspondences are correct. If not, the depth-first search backtracks and assumes *M5-U9* is a correct correspondence and evaluates the error. This continues until a solution that minimizes the error in Equation 12.8 is found.

The algorithm allows a significant amount of clutter and partial occlusion of the fiducial pattern to be present. Once three correspondences are identified and the fiducials are projected to the image space, the fiducials without any features inside their search region are considered to be undetected. However, the fiducials associated with the three correspondences themselves could have been undetected in the first place. This issue can be solved by modeling the probability of not detecting a fiducial as a process of sampling without replacement (Moreno-Noguer et al. 2008). Given an estimate of the fiducial occlusion probability, this probability can be pre-computed to reduce run-time computational overhead.

12.2.2.2 Priors

The simultaneous pose and correspondence estimation framework described above starts with an initial guess of the pose and its covariance and converges to a solution that is consistent with the data. This initialization can be provided by a Gaussian Mixture distribution (Moreno-Noguer et al. 2008) that models the entire search space for pose as a linear combination of weighted Gaussians. Such distributions can be machine-learned by samples acquired either by simulation (Jayarathne et al. 2013) or by employing an extrinsic tracking system (Jayarathne et al. 2015). During initialization, starting from the Gaussian component with the highest weighting, each Gaussian component is sequentially selected to provide the mean pose and the covariance for algorithm initialization. If a pose is not found for a Gaussian component, then the component with the next highest weight is selected. If the algorithm converges to a solution, then the initial pose and covariance for the next frame can be predicted based on Kalman filter state prediction step, assuming a suitable model for probe motion between frames (Jayarathne et al. 2013, 2015). These motion-based priors are typically much stronger than pose priors. Therefore, the algorithm converges rapidly, thus enabling real-time performance.

12.2.2.3 Extension to Multiple Views

The monocular pose estimation scheme described above relies on Extended Kalman Filter (EKF) equations to update the pose and its covariance from measurements and for pose prediction for the next frame. However, EKF is unstable with stereo and multicamera systems, where the pose is updated from two or more measurements that are highly correlated. The solution is to use a different flavor of Kalman filter called the Unscented Kalman filter (UKF) (Wan et al. 2000) that can handle higher degrees of non-linearity. For better numerical stability, the Square-Root Kalman filter (Jayarathne et al. 2015), whose practical run-time complexity is better than that of UKF, can be used.

The stereo/multicamera-based method results in slightly more accurate estimates compared to the monocular image-based method. Figure 12.3 illustrates the results of an experiment conducted with an optical tracking system providing the reference. A stereo-endoscopic camera was used for the experiments so that the monocular image-based method could be compared to the binocular image-based method. Note that the optical tracking-based reference is computed with respect to the camera center. Therefore, the reference may contain errors propagated from the hand-eye calibration and pattern-to-tracker registration procedure. Figure 12.3a and b show results for two estimates, namely the rotation about the y-axis and the translation along the z-axis respectively, which highlight the superiority of the stereoscopic image-based method compared to its monocular image-based counterpart. According to the

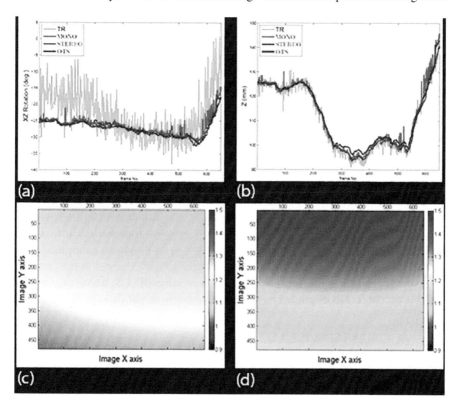

FIGURE 12.3 Rotation estimates about the y-axis (a) and the translation estimates along the z-axis (b) computed by the image-based methods. Mean TRE maps computed by the monocular image-based method (c) and the stereoscopic image-based method (d). (With kind permission from Springer Science+Business Media: *Simultaneous Estimation of Feature Correspondence and Stereo Object Pose with Application to Ultrasound Augmented Robotic Laparoscopy*, 2015, 134–144, Jayarathne, U.L. et al.)

Figure 12.3a and b, monocular image-based estimates (in red) deviate significantly from the reference (in black), particularly when the probe moves further away from the camera while the stereoscopic image-based method (in blue) closely follows the reference. The conventional stereoscopic triangulation-based method (in green) suffers from instability, while the rotational estimates about the y-axis deviate significantly from the reference. Figure 12.3c and d show the mean target registration error (TRE) maps generated by the monocular and stereo image-based methods, considering each US pixel as a target. These maps further illustrate the superior performance of the stereoscopic image-based method over its monoscopic counterpart.

12.2.2.4   Alternative Intrinsic Tracking: Registration through Photoacoustic Effect and Air-Tissue Interface

When the US probe is not visible in the camera image, the image-based methods described above cannot be applied. Particularly in prostatectomy procedures using transrectal ultrasound (TRUS) image guidance, the probe is not directly visible to the camera. In such a situation, a registration method that relies on features visible in both modalities needs to be employed. Cheng and colleagues (Cheng et al. 2012) proposed registering the 3D TRUS probe to the stereo laparoscopic camera using the photoacoustic effect. A pulsed laser light is projected on to the tissue, which results in a wideband acoustic signal due to *thermoelastic* expansion. This signal is picked up by an US probe with a 2D transducer array. Finally, the registration is performed through the laser spots segmented in both the video image and in US space. Even though clinically acceptable registration accuracies can be obtained using this approach, the added instrumentation to deliver laser light into the surgical site adds significant overhead. As a remedy, (Adebar et al. 2012) proposed registering 3D US using a registration tool featuring fiducials visible both in the endoscopic video and 3D US. The tool is pressed against the air-tissue interface until its fiducials are seen in the US, which are localized in the coordinate system of the US probe. Special fiducials visible in the camera allow estimation of the pose of the tool with respect to the camera-based coordinate system. With the constant transformation from the US-visible fiducial to the camera-visible fiducials known through a calibration process, one can register the 3D US coordinate system to that centered in the camera. One major limitation of this technology is that it requires 3D US, which may not be available except in TRUS-guided radical prostatectomy surgeries.

12.3   AUGMENTED VISUALIZATION

Registration of the US coordinate system with that centered in the camera allows US information to be rendered in the context of the laparoscopic video. Traditionally, this information is rendered on a virtual plane placed at the correct pose in front of a virtual camera, whose intrinsic parameters match that of the laparoscopic camera. Laparoscopic video is typically set as the background texture providing context for the US information, with the transparency of the US image being adjusted to blend it with the background (Leven et al. 2005; Feuerstein et al. 2007; Cheung et al. 2010; Pratt et al. 2012). As seen in Figure 12.4a, in this naïve approach the virtual US image is often perceived to be floating above the rest of the scene despite its correct

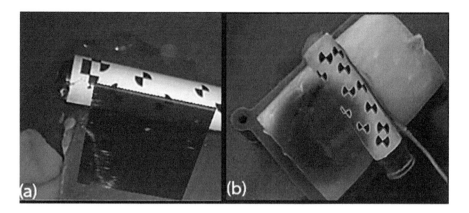

FIGURE 12.4 (a) A 2D US image overlaid in the laparoscopic image using the computed pose estimates. Note that this naïve rendering method results in the perception that the image is floating above the rest of the scene. (With kind permissions from Springer Science+Business Media: *Simultaneous Estimation of Feature Correspondence and Stereo Object Pose with Application to Ultrasound Augmented Robotic Laparoscopy*, 2015, 134–144, Jayarathne, U.L. et al.), (b) A US volume reconstructed in real time, visualized in the context of the laparoscopic image through a circular opacity window. Note that the surface features provide strong occlusion cues that result in improved depth perception. (With kind permissions from Springer Science+Business Media: *Simultaneous Estimation of Feature Correspondence and Stereo Object Pose with Application to Ultrasound Augmented Robotic Laparoscopy*, 2015, 134–144, Jayarathne, U.L. et al.)

spatial location. Having such inaccurate cues may cause erroneous actions to occur, with undesirable clinical consequences. To remedy this, (Hughes-Hallett et al. 2014) proposed superimposing US data in a cutaway that provides an improved perception of depth (see Figure 12.1a).

In many conventional laparoscopic procedures, the camera is located directly above the probe due to constraints in the port placement. In this configuration, the oblique angle between the camera imaging plane and the registered US image plane makes the interpretation of US information from the overlaid image very difficult. This issue easily could be solved if a synthetic image can be generated to represent the surgical scene viewed at an appropriate vantage point. Even though synthesizing such a view from images captured from a monocular camera is a technically challenging problem, it could be a possibility using a stereoscopic laparoscope (Scharstein 1996). Interestingly, a visualization scheme enabling this functionality has not been introduced for laparoscopic applications at this time.

Another solution to the issue of the location of the camera is to reconstruct a 3D US volume as the surgeon scans the organ surface and visualizes it in the context of the LUS image using a ray casting technique (Jayarathne et al. 2017). This technique allows direct visualization of 3D features of hidden anatomy, in contrast to the cognitively demanding 3D structure inference from 2D images. In addition, the reconstructed 3D volume could be helpful in registering preoperative images to the patient anatomy, allowing the preoperative plan to be brought into the surgical scene.

Because a 3D volume is visualized, users can perceive geometry and the location of the hidden structures irrespective of the camera vantage point.

In the approach described in (Jayarathne et al. 2017), a 3D voxel grid is filled in real time from each US image captured with its corresponding pose. The extent of the rectangular volume is determined a priori using a scout scan. To achieve a high-quality reconstruction, a hybrid reconstruction scheme is adapted and implemented in the Graphics Processing Unit (GPU) (Ludvigsen 2010). After the voxel grid is updated, it is rendered at the correct spatial location determined by pose data using a ray casting method that employs a one-dimensional transfer function. The rendering pipeline is implemented entirely in the GPU to enable real-time performance. The rendered volume is blended with the surface view provided by the camera image through a circular opacity window termed *keyhole*, whose transparency varies as a function of the Euclidean distance from its center (see Figure 12.4b). To improve depth perception, inside the keyhole the opacity function is modulated by image gradients to approximate the *pq*-space-based rendering scheme (Lerotic et al. 2007) without a dense surface reconstruction. This method works equally well on monocular and stereo laparoscopy; however, it relies heavily on a properly designed transfer function to highlight target structures from the less interesting background. Designing such a transfer function that works well for real anatomy and pathology may be challenging and is a topic for future research.

12.4   PERCEPTION AND HUMAN FACTORS

Even though many methods have been proposed to solve the tracking problem and the visualization problem in US-augmented laparoscopy, very few studies have been conducted on the associated human factors. In a recent study, (Jayarathne et al. 2017) studied the perceptual factors associated with 3D US visualization in the context of monocular laparoscopy. This psychophysical experiment involved experienced US users, surgical residents, and one experienced surgeon. The subjects localized hidden spherical targets placed at different depth levels (5, 15, and 25 mm from the surface) inside a block of PVA-C (Poly-vinyl Alcohol-Cryogel) using US in a laparoscopic environment. An optical tracking system was employed to track the laparoscopic camera, US probe, and the PVA-C phantom to provide registration between the US and video. Once the target was localized, the subjects were asked to point to its centroid using an optically tracked pointing tool at three different poses to compute the perceived location by triangulation. The time required to complete the task also was measured. Four modes of visualization were tested: conventional visualization where the US image and the laparoscopic image were displayed on separate monitors; real-time 3D US reconstruction and visualization with alpha-blending; 3D US visualization *in situ* through a circular opacity window (*keyhole*); and the hybrid visualization approach, where the subjects had access to the original 2D US image together with the keyhole visualization approach. At the end of the localization task in the PVA-C phantom, subjects were given a set of phantoms with spherical targets placed at the same depth levels as in the PVA-C filled phantoms but clearly visible in the laparoscopic image. The perceived location was computed using the same triangulation method, providing the baseline localization performance for an individual subject.

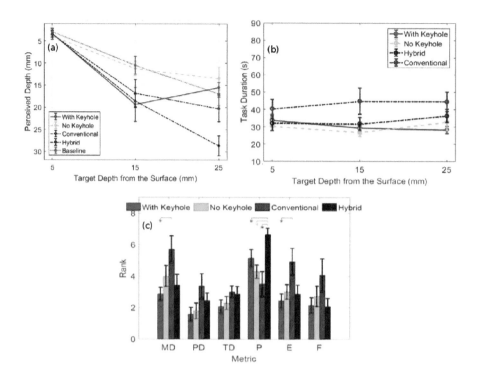

FIGURE 12.5 Results of the perceptual study reported. (Jayarathne, U.L. et al., *Simultaneous Estimation of Feature Correspondence and Stereo Object Pose with Application to Ultrasound Augmented Robotic Laparoscopy*, Springer International Publishing, 134–144, 2015.): (a) Depth perception, (b) task duration, and (c) subjective ranking based on NASA TLX. (With kind permissions from Springer Science+Business Media: *Simultaneous Estimation of Feature Correspondence and Stereo Object Pose with Application to Ultrasound Augmented Robotic Laparoscopy*, 2015, 134–144, Jayarathne, U.L. et al.)

To avoid any bias, the order of the visualization modes was counter-balanced, while the localization in clear phantoms was performed at the end.

The results of the study (see Figure 12.5) revealed that both the target depth and the visualization condition had a significant effect on the depth perception (main effects: Depth: $F(2,40) = 6.354$, $p = 0.006$, Visualization: $F(2.792, 55.837) = 8.793$, $p < 0.001$). Moreover, an interaction between the target depth and the visualization condition was observed (Depth x Visualization: $F(4.601, 92.012) = 3.763$, $p = 0.005$). Post-hoc analysis revealed that, compared to the other visualization approaches, the subjects perceived significantly more depth with the hybrid visualization approach ($p < 0.043$) at more profound depth levels (25 mm from the surface). However, using this approach the depth was slightly overestimated (see Figure 12.5a). The results further revealed that the visualization condition had a significant effect on the target localization time (main effect $F(1.957, 39.134) = 5.031$, $p = 0.012$). No interaction between the visualization condition and the target depth was observed ($F(3.214, 64.270) = 1.243$, $p = 0.058$). Post-hoc analysis further revealed that the subjects required significantly less time with the keyhole visualization method and the hybrid visualization approach compared to the conventional visualization method (see Figure 12.5b). Overall, using the hybrid visualization approach, the subjects demonstrated significantly less cognitive effort, indicated by significantly less time and more accurate depth perception, compared to the conventional US visualization method. This is further verified by the subjects indicating significantly lower mental demand, effort, and frustration and significantly higher performance in the NASA Task Load Index (NASA TLX) compared to the conventional US visualization approach (see Figure 12.5c).

Although it was statistically not significant, an interesting observation from this study is that the subjects tended to perceive more depth from the conventional method of viewing US image in a separate display, compared to the alpha-blending-based and the keyhole-based techniques. Depth cues revealed by the latter approaches were limited by the monocular display, while in the conventional approach the subjects could read the depth of the target from the depth scale associated with the US image. However, building a mental representation of the 3D target location using the conventional method is cognitively demanding, while the depth is underestimated, particularly at more profound levels (Wu et al. 2005). This trend was confirmed by subjects spending significantly more time in the localization task using the conventional technique in contrast to the other techniques, while the target depth was underestimated for deep targets. When US information is overlaid onto the laparoscopic video, cognitive involvement is not required to construct a mental representation of the target location, hence subjects require less time for localization. However, the inadequacy of depth cues in the overlaid information caused subjects to demonstrate a degraded perception of depth. Using the hybrid visualization approach, the subjects combined their percepts with their mental representation of depth acquired by reading the depth scale associated with the US image to demonstrate better localization performance with reduced cognitive demand. Interestingly, using this hybrid approach, the subjects demonstrated a tendency to slightly overestimate depth. Further psychophysical experiments are required to explain this behavior.

12.5 CONCLUDING REMARKS

This chapter discusses the technology behind US augmentation in laparoscopic surgery. State-of-the-art methods of registering the US probe coordinate system with that of the camera are presented in detail, and different means of visualizing US data in the context of the laparoscopic image presented with a discussion on human factors. Initial phantom studies demonstrate that with appropriate visualization schemes, augmenting US information in the laparoscopic video significantly reduces the cognitive demand while helping the operator localize hidden surgical targets more accurately. To prompt wide clinical acceptability, several aspects of the technology need to be further improved.

Image-based intrinsic tracking of the probe seems to have several advantages over its extrinsic tracking counterparts when it comes to clinical translation of the technology.

However, the robustness to occlusion, run-time, and accuracy of the state-of-the-art methods need to be further improved. Tracking by fusing multiple image features such as edges, points, shape, and depth are an interesting avenue of future research. Fusing image-based spatial tracking with other tracking systems, such as robot kinematics, may further improve reliability of the computed estimates. Real-time, freehand, 3D US reconstruction and visualization allow the operators to visualize hidden surgical targets in 3D. However, the state-of-the-art methods assume the organ of interest does not deform significantly during the scan, which is often violated in many soft tissue environments. Therefore, the adaptation of the current methods to highly deformable environments would be another avenue of future research. To reveal the efficacy of these technologies and prompt wide clinical acceptability, it is important to also investigate the human factors of these augmented visualization schemes.

REFERENCES

Ackerman, Martin Kendal, Alexis Cheng, Emad Boctor, and Gregory Chirikjian. 2014. Online ultrasound sensor calibration using gradient descent on the euclidean group. In *2014 IEEE International Conference on Robotics and Automation (ICRA)*, pp. 4900–4905. IEEE. doi:10.1109/ICRA.2014.6907577.

Adebar, Troy K., Michael C. Yip, Septimiu E. Salcudean, Robert N. Rohling, Christopher Y. Nguan, and S. Larry Goldenberg. 2012. Registration of 3D ultrasound through an air-tissue boundary. *IEEE Transactions on Medical Imaging* 31 (11): 2133–2142. doi:10.1109/TMI.2012.2215049.

Ameri, Golafsoun, A. Jonathan McLeod, John S. H. Baxter, Elvis C. S. Chen, and Terry M. Peters. 2015. Line fiducial material and thickness considerations for ultrasound calibration. In edited by Robert J. Webster and Ziv R. Yaniv, 941529. *International Society for Optics and Photonics*. doi:10.1117/12.2081294.

Bennett, Stuart, and Joan Lasenby. 2014. ChESS–Quick and robust detection of chess-board features. *Computer Vision and Image Understanding* 118: 197–210.

Bonjer, H. Jaap, Charlotte L. Deijen, Gabor A. Abis, Miguel A. Cuesta, Martijn H. G. M. Van Der Pas, Elly S. M. De Lange-De Klerk et al. 2015. A randomized trial of laparoscopic versus open surgery for rectal cancer. *The New England Journal of Medicine* 14372 (2): 1324–1332. doi:10.1056/NEJMoa1414882.

Cheng, Alexis, Jin U. Kang, Russell H. Taylor, and Emad M. Boctor. 2012. Direct 3D ultrasound to video registration using photoacoustic effect. *Medical Image Computing and Computer-Assisted Intervention: MICCAI... International Conference on Medical Image Computing and Computer-Assisted Intervention* 15 (Pt 2): 552–559.

Cheung, Carling L., Chris Wedlake, John Moore, Stephen E. Pautler, and Terry M. Peters. 2010. Fused video and ultrasound images for minimally invasive partial nephrectomy: A phantom study. *Medical Image Computing and Computer-Assisted Intervention: MICCAI... International Conference on Medical Image Computing and Computer-Assisted Intervention* 13 (Pt 3): 408–415.

Comeau, Roch M., Aaron Fenster, and Terence M. Peters. 1998. *Integrated MR and Ultrasound Imaging for Improved Image Guidance in Neurosurgery*. In edited by Kenneth M. Hanson, pp. 747–754. International Society for Optics and Photonics. doi:10.1117/12.310954.

Feuerstein, Marco, Tobias Reichl, Jakob Vogel, Armin Schneider, Hubertus Feussner, and Nassir Navabi. 2007. Magneto-optic tracking of a flexible laparoscopic ultrasound transducer for laparoscope augmentation. *Medical Image Computing and Computer-Assisted Intervention: MICCAI... International Conference on Medical Image Computing and Computer-Assisted Intervention* 10 (Pt 1): 458–466.

Heller, J., M. Havlena, and T. Pajdla. 2012. A branch-and-bound algorithm for globally optimal hand-eye calibration. In *2012 IEEE Conference on Computer Vision and Pattern Recognition*, pp. 1608–1615. IEEE. doi:10.1109/CVPR.2012.6247853.

Hughes-Hallett, Archie, Philip Pratt, Erik Mayer, Aimee Di Marco, Guang-Zhong Yang, Justin Vale, and Ara Darzi. 2014. Intraoperative ultrasound overlay in robot-assisted partial nephrectomy: First clinical experience. *European Urology* 65 (3): 671–672. doi:10.1016/j.eururo.2013.11.001.

Jayarathne, Uditha L., A. Jonathan McLeod, Terry M. Peters, and Elvis C. S. Chen. 2013. Robust intraoperative US probe tracking using a monocular endoscopic camera. *Medical Image Computing and Computer-Assisted Intervention: MICCAI... International Conference on Medical Image Computing and Computer-Assisted Intervention* 16 (Pt 3): 363–370.

Jayarathne, Uditha L., Moore John, Elvis C. S. Chen, Stephen E. Pautler, and Terry M. Peters. 2017. Real-time 3D ultrasound reconstruction and visualization in the context of laparoscopy. *Medical Image Computing and Computer-Assisted Intervention: MICCAI... International Conference on Medical Image Computing and Computer-Assisted Intervention*, Quebec City, Canada.

Jayarathne, Uditha L., Xiongbiao Luo, Elvis C. S. Chen, and Terry M. Peters. 2015. *Simultaneous Estimation of Feature Correspondence and Stereo Object Pose with Application to Ultrasound Augmented Robotic Laparoscopy*, pp. 134–44. Springer International Publishing. doi:10.1007/978-3-319-24601-7_14.

Klatzky, Roberta L., Bing Wu, and George Stetten. 2008. Spatial representations from perception and cognitive mediation: The case of ultrasound. *Current Directions in Psychological Science* 17 (6): 359–364. doi:10.1111/j.1467-8721.2008.00606.x.

Lerotic, Mirna, Adrian J. Chung, George Mylonas, and Guang-Zhong Yang. 2007. Pq-space based non-photorealistic rendering for augmented reality. *Medical Image Computing and Computer-Assisted Intervention: MICCAI... International Conference on Medical Image Computing and Computer-Assisted Intervention* 10 (Pt 2): 102–109.

Leven, Joshua, Darius Burschka, Rajesh Kumar, Gary Zhang, Steve Blumenkranz, Xiangtian Donald Dai, Mike Awad et al. 2005. DaVinci Canvas: A telerobotic surgical system with integrated, robot-assisted, laparoscopic ultrasound capability. *Medical Image Computing and Computer-Assisted Intervention: MICCAI... International Conference on Medical Image Computing and Computer-Assisted Intervention* 8 (Pt 1): 811–818.

Lowe, David G. 2004. Distinctive image features from scale-invariant keypoints. *International Journal of Computer Vision* 60 (2): 91–110. doi:10.1023/B:VISI.0000029664.99615.94.

Ludvigsen, H. 2010. Real-time GPU-based 3D ultrasound reconstruction and visualization. Master's thesis, Norwegion University of Science and Technology.

Meer, Peter, and S. Link. 1998. Efficient Invariant Representations. *International Journal of Computer Vision* 26 (2): 137–152.

Moreno-Noguer, Francesc, Vincent Lepetit, and Pascal Fua. 2008. *Pose Priors for Simultaneously Solving Alignment and Correspondence*. European Conference on Computer Vision, Munich, Germany, pp. 404–418.

Morgan, Isabella, Uditha Jayarathne, Adam Rankin, Terry M. Peters, and Elvis C. S. Chen. 2017. Hand-eye calibration for surgical cameras: A procrustean perspective-N-point solution. *International Journal of Computer Assisted Radiology and Surgery*, Springer International Publishing, pp. 1–9. doi:10.1007/s11548-017-1590-9.

Pratt, Philip, Aimee Di Marco, Christopher Payne, Ara Darzi, and Guang-Zhong Yang. 2012. Intraoperative ultrasound guidance for transanal endoscopic microsurgery. *Medical*

Image Computing and Computer-Assisted Intervention: MICCAI... International Conference on Medical Image Computing and Computer-Assisted Intervention 15 (Pt 1): 463–470.

Pratt, Philip, Alexander Jaeger, Archie Hughes-Hallett, Erik Mayer, Justin Vale, Ara Darzi, Terry Peters, and Guang-Zhong Yang. 2015. Robust ultrasound probe tracking: Initial clinical experiences during robot-assisted partial nephrectomy. *International Journal of Computer Assisted Radiology and Surgery* 10 (12): 1905–1913. doi:10.1007/s11548-015-1279-x.

Prime, David J., and Pierre Jolicoeur. 2010. Mental rotation requires visual short-term memory: Evidence from human electric cortical activity. *Journal of Cognitive Neuroscience* 22 (11): 2437–2446. doi:10.1162/jocn.2009.21337.

Scharstein, D. 1996. Stereo vision for view synthesis. In *Proceedings CVPR IEEE Computer Society Conference on Computer Vision and Pattern Recognition*, pp. 852–858. IEEE. doi:10.1109/CVPR.1996.517171.

Thompson, R. Houston, Brian R. Lane, Christine M. Lohse, Bradley C. Leibovich, Amr Fergany, Igor Frank, Inderbir S. Gill, Michael L. Blute, and Steven C. Campbell. 2010. Every minute counts when the renal hilum is clamped during partial nephrectomy. *European Urology* 58 (3): 340–345. doi:10.1016/j.eururo.2010.05.047.

Thompson, Stephen, Danail Stoyanov, Crispin Schneider, Kurinchi Gurusamy, Sébastien Ourselin, Brian Davidson, David Hawkes, and Matthew J. Clarkson. 2016. Hand–eye calibration for rigid laparoscopes using an invariant point. *International Journal of Computer Assisted Radiology and Surgery* 11 (6): 1071–1780. doi:10.1007/s11548-016-1364-9.

Wan, Eric A., and Rudolph Van Der Menve. 2000. The unscented kalman filter for nonlinear estimation. In *Adaptive Systems for Signal Processing, Communications, and Control Symposium*. IEEE, pp. 153–158.

Wu, Bing, Roberta L. Klatzky, Damion Shelton, and George D. Stetten. 2005. Psychophysical evaluation of in-situ ultrasound visualization. *IEEE Transactions on Visualization and Computer Graphics* 11 (6): 684–693. doi:10.1109/TVCG.2005.104.

Zeisl, Bernhard, Pierre Fite Georgel, Florian Schweiger, Eckehard Steinbach, and Nassir Navab. 2009. Estimation of location uncertainty for scale invariant feature points. In *Proceedings of the British Machine Vision Conference 2009*, pp. 57.1–57.12. British Machine Vision Association. doi:10.5244/C.23.57.

Zhang, Lin, Menglong Ye, Po-Ling Chan, and Guang-Zhong Yang. 2017. Real-time surgical tool tracking and pose estimation using a hybrid cylindrical marker. *International Journal of Computer Assisted Radiology and Surgery* 12 (6): 921–930. doi:10.1007/s11548-017-1558-9.

Zheng, Yinqiang, Yubin Kuang, Shigeki Sugimoto, Kalle Astrom, and Masatoshi Okutomi. 2013. Revisiting the PnP problem: A fast, general and optimal solution. In *2013 IEEE International Conference on Computer Vision*, pp. 2344–2351. IEEE. doi:10.1109/ICCV.2013.291.

13 Toward Clinically Viable Ultrasound-Augmented Laparoscopic Visualization

Xinyang Liu and Raj Shekhar

CONTENTS

13.1 INTRODUCTION

Laparoscopic surgery is a preferred alternative to conventional open surgery in many instances, as it is minimally invasive and has many other associated clinical benefits. However, conducting a laparoscopic procedure based solely on intraoperative visualization and without tactile feedback can be challenging. Laparoscopic augmented reality (lap-AR), a method to overlay virtual models or tomographic images on laparoscopic video, has emerged as a promising technology to enhance intraoperative visualization and to compensate for the lack of tactile feedback. In particular, fusing intraoperative data with live laparoscopic video has the advantage of providing real-time updates of an organ's internal anatomy and, thus, enables AR depiction of moving and deformable organs such as those located in the abdomen. Among common intraoperative imaging modalities, laparoscopic ultrasound (LUS) is more amenable to routine use because it is radiation-free, low-cost, and easy to set up and operate in the operating room (OR).

To overlay the LUS image on the camera image, a tracking method is needed to track the pose of the LUS probe relative to the pose of the camera in real time. Common tracking methods are optical tracking, electromagnetic (EM) tracking, computer vision-based tracking, and hybrid tracking (i.e., a combination of the mentioned methods). Each method has its advantages and limitations. Many LUS-based lap-AR (LUS-AR for short) systems have been developed in the past decade. Most of them were validated using phantoms or *ex vivo* tissues in a laboratory or an OR. A few studies were validated using live animals, mostly porcine models, and even fewer studies have presented human data. The reality shows how challenging it would be to translate AR methods to routine clinical use.

In this chapter, clinically promising LUS-AR systems in each tracking category are briefly reviewed. In addition, methods for fast laparoscope calibration that are a prerequisite for extending AR methods to conventional laparoscopes are presented. The chapter concludes with discussing the future directions of a clinical LUS-AR system.

13.2 OPTICAL TRACKING-BASED SYSTEM

13.2.1 BACKGROUND

An established tracking method is optical tracking, which uses an infrared camera to track passive reflective spheres (i.e., optical markers). To track a six degrees-of-freedom (DOF) pose of the imaging tool, it is common to attach four markers on a cross/star-shaped frame (i.e., tracking mount) that is affixed on the imaging tool and maintains a rigid relationship to the imaging tip. Optical tracking is widely used in endoscopic AR applications, such as those based on preoperative images (Shahidi et al. 2002), intraoperative CT (Shekhar et al. 2010; Feuerstein et al. 2008a), and intraoperative LUS (Shekhar et al. 2015; Kang et al. 2014). Although optical tracking can achieve high accuracy, it requires line-of-sight between the optical camera and the markers. In a LUS-AR system, this requires the markers to be affixed on the handles of the laparoscope and the LUS transducer. One advantage of this arrangement is that it keeps the markers away from the patient, thus minimizing safety concerns. However, there are two disadvantages. First, for calibration results to hold, the arrangement does not permit articulation of the imaging tip for those LUS transducers with a flexible imaging tip, whereas flexible-tip transducers are commonly used in laparoscopic procedures for areas that are difficult to reach by a rigid transducer. Second, there is a relatively long distance between the marker and the imaging tip, thus potentially adding to calibration errors due to the lever-arm effect. In the next subsections, an optical tracking-based LUS-AR system that has been evaluated in humans is briefly reviewed (Shekhar et al. 2015; Kang et al. 2014).

13.2.2 System

The system described by Kang et al. includes a stereoscopic vision system (VSII, Visionsense, Philadelphia, PA, USA), an LUS scanner (BK Flex Focus 700, Analogic, Peabody, MA, USA) employing an intraoperative 9-mm rigid transducer, an optical tracking system (Polaris, Northern Digital, Waterloo, ON, Canada), and a desktop computer running image fusion software. The vision system features a stereoscopic, three-dimensional (3D), 5-mm, 0° laparoscope with an integrated light source and fixed focal length, both of which simplify its use in the OR. The 3D laparoscope has been reported to improve depth perception and achieve good clinical outcomes.

The 3D video and LUS images are streamed over high-speed Ethernet from the vision system and the LUS scanner to the computer. Utilizing the tracking data, the LUS images are overlaid on the 3D video in real time, creating two ultrasound-augmented video streams, one for each eye. These two video streams are displayed on a 3D monitor, and users wear passive polarized glasses to experience the 3D effect. OpenCV (Intel, Santa Clara, CA, USA) was used for camera calibration (Heikkilä and Silvén 1997). The Public Software Library for Ultrasound (PLUS) library (Lasso et al. 2014) was used to calibrate the LUS transducer.

To track the two imaging probes, two tracking mounts are attached to their respective handles (Figure 13.1). Because the 3D laparoscope and the LUS transducer must be sterilized before OR use, the tracking mounts must also be disassembled and sterilized separately after calibration. To be able to reuse laboratory calibration results in the OR, the tracking mounts were designed such that they could be easily snapped on the imaging probes in exactly the same position as they were before disassembly. In this manner, the exact optical marker-to-imaging tip geometric relationship is maintained so that a previously performed calibration remains valid.

13.2.3 Clinical Experience

The system described above has been validated using phantoms and through an animal study. Based on these preclinical data and with approval from the Institutional Review Board, clinical evaluation of the system has been performed on 13 patients: 11 (4–18 years old, 4 males, 7 females) undergoing laparoscopic cholecystectomy (one patient also referred for a laparoscopic Puestow procedure) and 2 (14 and 20 years old, both male) undergoing laparoscopic treatment of median arcuate ligament syndrome (MALS). The system calibration, performed a day in advance, preceded each clinical use. After calibration, the laparoscope, the LUS transducer, and the tracking mounts were sent for sterilization. The sterilized items were assembled in the OR at the beginning of the surgery, and four presterilized optical markers were attached on each of the two tracking mounts. The AR visualization was performed for up to 5 minutes prior to starting the actual surgery.

On average, the system took 15 minutes to set up in the OR, with this step taking place in parallel with patient setup in conventional laparoscopic surgery. The AR system was considered easy to use and helpful in the visualization of normally unseen structures, as shown in Figure 13.2.

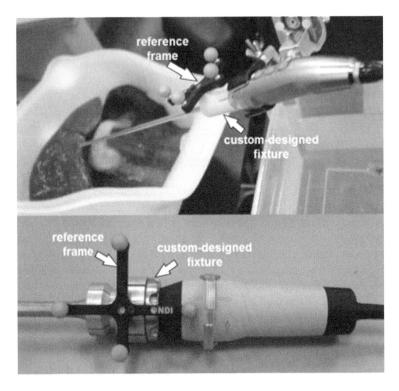

FIGURE 13.1 Tracking mounts for the 3D laparoscope (top) and the LUS transducer (bottom). (Reproduced from Kang, X. et al., *Surg. Endosc.*, 28, 2227–2235, 2014. With permission.)

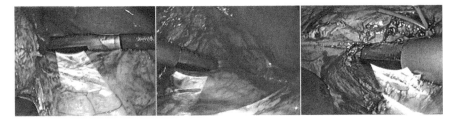

FIGURE 13.2 Snapshots of AR visualization during cholecystectomy (left; showing hepatic artery and cystic duct), Puestow procedure (middle; showing pancreatic duct), and MALS repair (right; showing celiac artery and aorta).

13.3 EM TRACKING-BASED SYSTEM

13.3.1 Background

To address the limitations of optical tracking, as mentioned in Section 13.2.1, one may consider using EM tracking, another commercially available and frequently used real-time tracking method. EM tracking reports the location and orientation of a small (~1-mm diameter) wired sensor inside a 3D working volume with a magnetic field created by a field generator (FG). Compared with optical tracking, EM tracking has the advantages of no line-of-sight requirement as well as its sensor's compact size. In the case of LUS-AR system, these allow the EM sensor to be placed close to the imaging tip of the device. One limitation of EM tracking, however, is the potential distortion of the magnetic field due to ferrous metals and conductive materials inside the working volume. Such materials are commonly found in surgical tools and equipment in a clinical environment. There are extensive studies on EM tracking error and distortion correction, as summarized in a recent review paper (Franz et al. 2014). EM tracking, however, has been used successfully in a few LUS-AR systems (Liu et al. 2016a; Cheung et al. 2010). How and where to affix the EM sensor on the two imaging probes became critical questions for the clinical adoption of these systems. In the next subsections, an EM tracking-based LUS-AR system particularly tailored for clinical use is presented (Liu et al. 2016a).

13.3.2 SYSTEM

The system included the same 3D vision system and the LUS scanner as described in Section 13.2.2. The desktop computer for image fusion was replaced with a laptop computer to improve system portability. An EM tracking system with a tabletop FG (Aurora, Northern Digital, Waterloo, Ontario, Canada) specially designed for OR applications was employed. The FG is designed to be positioned between the surgical table and the patient and incorporates a shield that can suppress distortions caused by the surgical table. EM catheters (1.3-mm diameter) that can stand autoclave sterilization were used; each catheter had a 6 DOF EM sensor at the tip.

To track the laparoscope, it is practical to affix the sensor somewhere near the camera head (i.e., the handle part of the laparoscope) so the sensor is kept outside the patient's body during the surgery. As there are more metal and electronics contained in the camera head than in the telescope (i.e., the long scope cylinder), there is the potential for larger distortion error in EM tracking in the vicinity of the camera head. To reduce this, it is necessary to place the sensor sufficiently away from the camera head. Another consideration to keep the sensor away from the camera head and close to the imaging tip is that during a laparoscopic surgery, the camera head is usually positioned higher than the imaging tip relative to the tabletop FG. Studies have shown that the closer the sensor is to the tabletop FG, the better the EM tracking accuracy (Nijkamp et al. 2016) is. In Liu et al. (2016a), an EM tracking mount was developed based on the above considerations (Figure 13.3a) and would neither interfere with the patient nor block the trocar during the surgery. With this tracking mount, the sensor was positioned approximately 7 cm away (longitudinally) from the camera head and 4 cm away from the outer surface of the telescope. At this location, the measured mean positional and rotational distortion errors (caused by the laparoscope) were 0.31 mm and 0.25°, and the mean positional and rotational jitter errors were 0.10 mm and 0.18°.

To track the LUS transducer with a flexible imaging tip, it is necessary to place the sensor on the movable imaging tip and as close to the outer surface of the LUS transducer as possible to allow insertion through a (12-mm) trocar. As shown in

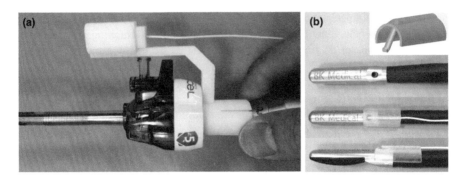

FIGURE 13.3   Snap-on EM tracking mounts for the 3D laparoscope (a) and the LUS transducer (b).

Figure 13.3b, a wedge-like tracking mount was designed to attach to an existing biopsy needle introducer track. With this tracking mount, the sensor was positioned approximately 1.5 mm away from the outer surface of the LUS transducer. At this location, the measured mean positional and rotational distortion errors (caused by the LUS transducer) were 0.13 mm and 0.95°, and the mean positional and rotational jitter errors were 0.02 mm and 0.03°. Both tracking mounts can be snugly and reproducibly snapped on to the two imaging probes and can withstand the commonly used low-temperature sterilization method. The processes of calibration, video processing, and visualization were similar to those for the optical tracking-based LUS-AR system, as described in Section 13.2.2.

13.3.3   LABORATORY VALIDATION

Target registration error (TRE) is a commonly used metric to measure the overall image-to-video registration accuracy. A target point is imaged using the LUS probe, and its pixel location is identified in the LUS image overlaid on the camera image. Aiming the laparoscope at the target point from two different viewpoints, the coordinates of the target point in the tracker coordinate system can be estimated using triangulation (Hartley and Sturm 1997) and compared with the actual location of the target point. In (Liu et al. 2016a), the target point was the intersection of two thin wires. The actual location of the target point was acquired using a tracked stylus. Evaluated over multiple trials, the overall TRE of the system was 2.59 ± 0.58 mm (left-eye channel) and 2.43 ± 0.48 mm (right-eye channel). The ~2.5 mm image-to-video TRE is half the resection margin (5 mm) sought in most tumor ablative procedures (Rutkowski et al. 2012), and therefore is considered clinically acceptable.

The accepted method of imaging a high-speed digital clock with millisecond resolution was used to measure system latency. Any difference in the actual time and the time seen in the AR image is the latency. The AR latency was measured to be 177 ± 12 ms. The latency of the 3D vision system alone was measured to be 119 ± 12 ms. Therefore, the system contributed 58 ms delay to the overall latency. There was no perceptible latency for AR visualization during its practical use.

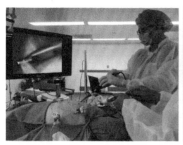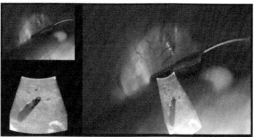

FIGURE 13.4 Left: surgeons, who wore polarized 3D glasses to see stereoscopic video with depth cues using the EM tracking-based LUS-AR system in an animal experiment. Right: snapshot of video showing the original laparoscopic and LUS views, as well as the overlaid AR view. (Reproduced from Liu, X. et al., *J. Med. Imaging (Bellingham)*, 3, 045001, 2016. With permission.)

13.3.4 PRECLINICAL STUDY

An animal procedure, approved by the Institutional Animal Care and Use Committee, was conducted to test the EM tracking-based LUS-AR system. A 40-kg swine was placed in the supine position (face up) on a surgical pad, which was positioned on top of the EM tabletop FG. The swine was positioned such that the EM sensors mounted on the two imaging probes were within the working volume of EM tracking. A 12-mm trocar was placed at the midline mid-abdomen for introducing the LUS transducer, and a 5-mm trocar was placed at the anterior axillary line in the lower abdomen for introducing the 3D laparoscope. The system was successfully used for accurate AR visualization during the experiment. Bending the imaging tip of the LUS transducer did not affect the overlay accuracy. The surgical scene and a representative snapshot of the recorded videos during the experiment are shown in Figure 13.4.

13.4 LUS-AR SYSTEMS BASED ON OTHER TRACKING METHODS

Besides using external tracking hardware, another promising tracking method is the vision-based approach, which uses computer vision techniques to detect intrinsic landmarks and/or user-introduced patterns on the LUS transducer shown in the camera image in real time. The approach has been applied to the LUS probe with a long shaft (Feuerstein et al. 2008b; Leven et al. 2005) as well as the pickup ultrasound probe (Schneider et al. 2016; Pratt et al. 2015), which is usually used in robot-assisted laparoscopic surgery. In (Pratt et al. 2015), KeyDot® markers (Key Surgical Inc., Eden Prairie, MN, USA), made with asymmetrical circular dot patterns, were attached to both (flat) faces of a pickup ultrasound probe. The transformation from the pattern coordinate system to the ultrasound image plane was calibrated (Pratt et al. 2012). OpenCV was used to track the pattern in the camera image, and the pattern's pose relative to the camera was estimated using camera calibration results. The approach has been tested on a human robot-assisted partial nephrectomy case. Immediately prior to resection, the registered ultrasound image was used to confirm

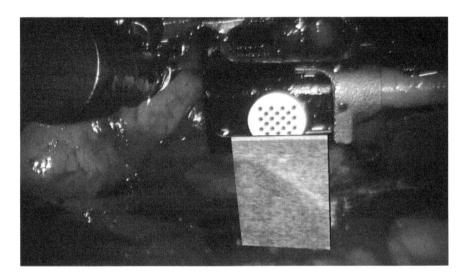

FIGURE 13.5 Still frame illustrating registered ultrasound image of tumor interface. (Reproduced with permission from Pratt, P. et al., *Int. J. Comput. Assist. Radiol. Surg.*, 10, 1905–1913, 2015.)

the location of the tumor. As shown in Figure 13.5, the AR depiction demonstrates the interface between the normal parenchyma and the tumor. Although the AR overlay was proved accurate, the surgeon feedback suggested that the partial occlusion or blending of the surgical scene was a source of distraction from time to time.

To improve tracking accuracy and robustness, and reduce limitations among different tracking methods, the hybrid method emerges as an attractive supplement. A hybrid of optical tracking and EM tracking would effectively remove the line-of-sight requirement of optical tracking and reduce the distortion errors of EM tracking (Nakamoto et al. 2008; Feuerstein et al. 2009). However, this approach requires both optical and EM tracking systems, as well as multiple EM sensors and optical markers. An AR system based on this approach would be more expensive, require more space and time to set up, and be more complicated to use. Another still evolving hybrid method is to combine hardware-based tracking with vision-based tracking, such as the approach of (Plishker et al. 2017), in which LUS image-to-video overlay was initialized by EM tracking and further refined by a vision-based optimization algorithm using intrinsic image features of the LUS probe. Although quite promising, the approach needs further research and development to achieve the accuracy, computational speed, and robustness for clinical use.

13.5   FAST CALIBRATION OF FORWARD-VIEWING LAPAROSCOPES

13.5.1   BACKGROUND

Although a feasible workflow for using the LUS-AR system clinically was introduced in Section 13.2.3, the position of the tracking mount after reassembly in the OR could still change slightly compared to its original position during the calibration. More importantly, other than the highly integrated Visionsense 3D laparoscope, this workflow is not feasible for conventional two-dimensional (2D) laparoscopes, whose optics (e.g., focal length) can be adjusted by the surgeon during the procedure. Therefore, a fast and easy laparoscope calibration method that can be performed in the OR is critical to extend AR methods to conventional laparoscopes. However, the most common camera calibration methods may not address this need because they require a time-consuming process of acquiring multiple images of the calibration pattern. There are two types of commonly used laparoscopes: (1) the forward-viewing laparoscope that has a flat (0°) lens relative to the camera and (2) the oblique-viewing laparoscope that has an angled (e.g., 30°) lens relative to the camera. In the next subsections, a fast calibration method for forward-viewing laparoscopes (Liu et al. 2016b) is briefly reviewed.

13.5.2 METHOD

The system involved a conventional 2D laparoscopic camera with a 0°, 5-mm scope, and an EM tracking system as described in Section 13.3.2. An EM sensor was mounted on the laparoscope similarly to that shown in Figure 13.3. Perceive3D's (Coimbra, Portugal) API based on the single-image calibration (SIC) method (Melo et al. 2012; Barreto et al. 2009) was used. The API features automatic corner detection and calibration of camera intrinsic parameters and lens distortion from a single image of an arbitrary portion of a special calibration pattern. Compared to using the conventional checkerboard pattern, more corners, especially on image periphery, can be detected. This helps better estimate lens distortion. Based on the SIC calibration results, hand-eye calibration was obtained using OpenCV.

The calibration pattern was first printed on paper and clued on a custom-designed calibration plate. An EM sensor and a tubular object for immediate evaluation of calibration accuracy were fixed on the plate and registered with the calibration pattern. A virtual tube model having the same size as the real tube was projected in the camera image using the calibrated camera and hand-eye calibration parameters. There should be a good overlay agreement between the virtual and actual tubes shown in the camera image if the calibration results are accurate. To sterilize and use the calibration plate in the OR, a clinical calibration plate was developed by laser-marking the calibration pattern on Radel polyphenylsulfone, which is a heat- and chemical-resistant polymer.

13.5.3 EXPERIMENTS AND RESULTS

The calibration software incorporating the SIC API and OpenCV functions for hand-eye calibration was implemented using C++ on a laptop computer (4-core 2.9 GHz CPU, 8 GB memory). Calibration time from acquiring a camera image to the generation of results averaged 14.0 seconds (range 3.5–22.7 seconds) based on 20 freehand calibration trials. The time increases as more corners are detected in the image. Calibration accuracy was compared between the common OpenCV method and the fast calibration method. As in Section 13.3.3, TRE was used as the metric, which was obtained by triangulation of the two views of the calibration pattern. With TRE measurements for multiple calibration trails, the TRE for the fast calibration method (1.48 ± 0.31 mm) was comparable to that of the OpenCV method (1.58 ± 0.33 mm).

13.6   FAST CALIBRATION OF OBLIQUE-VIEWING LAPAROSCOPES

13.6.1   BACKGROUND

A second type of commonly used laparoscope is the oblique-viewing laparoscope, which has the advantage of offering a much larger field of view by the rotation of its telescope relative to the camera head. However, this rotation also creates a rotation offset between the actual object shown in the camera image and the projected object obtained using the calibrated parameters before rotation (i.e., initial calibration). A few groups have developed methods to calibrate oblique-viewing rigid endoscopes to correct the rotation offset. One approach was to attach one optical marker on the telescope and another optical marker and a rotary encoder on the camera head to track the rotation (Yamaguchi et al. 2004). The optical marker on the camera head was treated as the reference, and thus the image plane was kept fixed. A later approach improved the Yamaguchi method by removing the rotary encoder and treating the optical marker on the telescope as the reference (Wu et al. 2010). This approach preserves the hand-eye calibration result after the rotation and the camera image rotates about a point in the image (i.e., the rotation center in the image plane O_{IMG}). Other than the methods relying on external trackers, a computer vision-based approach to track the rotation was also reported (Melo et al. 2012).

There are several limitations associated with the aforementioned approaches. First, optical tracking is not ideal for all clinical applications. The optical tracking mount is relatively bulky in size, and maintaining a line-of-sight with the infrared camera for both tracking mounts is challenging and even impossible for certain rotation angles. Second, to obtain the initial calibration, most prior approaches relied on conventional camera calibration methods (Heikkilä and Silvén 1997), which are lengthy procedures to be used in the OR. Third, there is not a universally accepted method to estimate O_{IMG}. The work of (Wu et al. 2010) assumed the principal point resulting from camera calibration to be O_{IMG}. However, this is not generally true, as demonstrated by (Melo et al. 2012), who estimated O_{IMG} using image features such as the circular image boundary contour and the triangular mark on the image boundary of an oblique-viewing arthroscope. However, these image features are not universally available in camera images produced by conventional laparoscopes. In the next subsections, a fast calibration method for oblique-viewing laparoscopes that addresses the above issues is briefly reviewed (Liu et al. 2017a). The method is based on the work of (Wu et al. 2010).

13.6.2   METHOD

In (Wu et al. 2010), two optical markers were fixed on the telescope (OM_1) and the camera head (OM_2), respectively. OM_1 was used as the reference, and therefore the hand-eye calibration result was fixed. An arbitrary point p_{OM_2} in OM_2's space can be transferred to OM_1's space through tracking. During the rotation, p_{OM_2}'s corresponding coordinates in OM_1's space are recorded, forming a set of points, $P_{OM_1} = \left\{ p_{OM_1}^{t_1}, p_{OM_1}^{t_2}, \cdots, p_{OM_1}^{t_n} \right\}$, where t_i is the ith time point. The points in P_{OM_1} should reside on a circle centered at the rotation center in OM_1's space (denoted as O_{OM_1}). For any three points in P_{OM_1}, O_{OM_1} can be estimated based on the geometric formulas provided in (Wu et al. 2010). To improve accuracy and robustness, a RANSAC algorithm was introduced to repetitively select three random points in P_{OM_1} and calculate O_{OM_1}. For each iteration, the distances between the calculated O_{OM_1} and all points (except the three points used to calculate O_{OM_1}) in P_{OM_1} were calculated. Among all iterations, the O_{OM_1} that generates the smallest variance of those distances is chosen as the optimum O_{OM_1}. Once O_{OM_1} is known, it is straightforward to calculate the rotation angle given the tracking data before and after the rotation.

The work of (Liu et al. 2017a) involved a conventional 2D laparoscopic camera with a 30°, 5-mm scope, and an EM tracking system as described in Section 13.3.2. Two EM tracking mounts were attached on the camera head and the telescope, respectively. Compared with optical tracking-based approaches, the EM tracking approach has the advantages of a much more compact configuration, no concerns regarding a loss of line-of-sight, and a greater range of possible rotation.

A universally accepted method to estimate O_{IMG} was developed. Let $C(0°)$ be the principal point calibrated at an initial state. A generic estimation of O_{IMG} would be the midpoint of the line segment connecting $C(0°)$ and $C(180°)$, i.e., $O_{IMG} = \left[C(0°) + C(180°) \right] / 2$, where $C(180°)$ is the principal point estimated after a relative rotation of 180° from the initial state. The calibration steps in Liu et al. (2017a) can be summarized as follows:

1. *Obtain the rotation center in* EMS_1's *(EM sensor on the telescope) space* O_{EMS_1}. This can be achieved using the aforementioned method (Wu et al. 2010).
2. *Obtain the first calibration using the fast calibration method described in Section 13.5.2 and record the current poses of the two sensors (Pose 1).* Root-mean-square (RMS) reprojection error associated with the calibration results was recorded.
3. *Rotate the laparoscope 180° from Pose 1.* Given O_{EMS_1} obtained in Step 1 and Pose 1 obtained in Step 2, any rotation angle θ from Pose 1 can be calculated. Because it is impossible to manually rotate exactly 180° from Pose 1, $\theta \in [175°, 180°]$ is considered to be a good candidate, which can be achieved by one or two adjustments of the rotation.
4. *Obtain the second calibration using the fast calibration method described in Section 13.5.2, record Pose 2, and calculate* O_{IMG}. This completes the calibration. Between the two calibrations, the one with the smaller RMS reprojection error will be set as the Initial Calibration, and its pose will be set as the Initial Pose.

After following the above process, the rotation angle θ can be calculated based on O_{EMS_1}, the Initial Pose, and the current poses of the two EM sensors. The camera matrix can then be updated based on θ, O_{IMG}, and the Initial Calibration. The calibration method was implemented using C++ on a laptop computer with 4-core 2.9 GHz CPU and 8 GB of memory.

13.6.3 EXPERIMENTS AND RESULTS

After attaching the EM tracking mounts, five freehand calibrations were performed repetitively following the above steps. It took an average of 2 minutes and 8 seconds (range 1 minutes and 50 seconds–2 minutes and 25 seconds) to complete the calibration. Because EM tracking accuracy is susceptible to the presence of metallic and conductive materials, experiments were performed in a simulated clinical environment. Setting the tabletop FG on a surgical table, several surgical tools were placed within the working volume of EM tracking. The laparoscope was held in place using a plastic stand to eliminate hand tremor. The clinical calibration plate was fixed on the FG within the field of view of the laparoscope. The calibration results (O_{EMS_1}, O_{IMG}, Initial Calibration, Initial Pose) from one of the five freehand calibration trials were used. The camera head was slightly rotated relative to the telescope, a few angles at a time, both clockwise and counterclockwise. After each rotation, a picture of the calibration pattern was acquired, and corners were automatically detected. The rotation-corrected projections of corners were calculated by applying the updated camera matrix and were compared with the detected corners. The RMS reprojection error averaged 4.9 pixel (range 2.4–8.5 pixel) for rotation angles ranged from –40.3° to 174.7°. For an approximate comparison, the work of (Yamaguchi et al. 2004) achieved a reprojection error of less than five pixels for a rotation in the $\left[0°, 140°\right]$ range. The work of (Wu et al. 2010) achieved a similar accuracy for angles within 75°; however, the reprojection error increased to 13 pixels when the angle increased to 100°. It should be noted that the image resolution in both studies was less than or equal to 320×240, whereas the image resolution in (Liu et al. 2017a) was 1280×720, which was a 12-fold denser pixel matrix.

13.7 FUTURE DIRECTIONS

The long-term goal is to have a practical LUS-AR system for routine clinical use. From the presentation in this chapter, it is apparent that the research community is systematically addressing technical issues and conducting clinical translation. Based on these developments, the clinical adoption of an LUS-AR system in the near future can be anticipated. Among different tracking methods, the hybrid method combining EM tracking and vision-based tracking appears most promising. EM tracking can track the LUS probe with a flexible imaging tip as well as the pickup ultrasound probe. The compact size of EM tracking mounts makes it more suitable to track an oblique-viewing laparoscope. To reduce overlay error caused by inherent imperfections of EM tracking and calibrations, vision-based tracking can be used as a refinement. The approach to attach a dedicated pattern on the LUS probe, similar to that in (Pratt et al. 2012), would greatly improve the robustness of vision-based tracking. After a surgeon attaches the tracking mounts and adjusts the optics of a laparoscope, he/she can perform a fast calibration of the laparoscope based on the methods described in this chapter. As for EM tracking of a flexible LUS probe, although the approach in Figure 13.3b is feasible, a better choice would be to embed the EM sensor inside the probe shaft. The work of (Liu et al. 2017b) demonstrates that it is possible to achieve this, and we are hoping such EM-tracked LUS probes will become commercially available in the near future. The EM-tracked LUS-AR system can be integrated with the routine OR setup. The existing vision system will be used, and the processed AR video, routed through the image management system, can be displayed on all or a subset of OR monitors. The described LUS-AR system has the potential to give surgeons greater confidence, minimize complications, shorten procedure times, reduce blood loss, and expand the range of minimally invasive laparoscopic surgeries.

REFERENCES

Barreto, J.P., J. Roquette, P. Sturm, and F. Fonseca. 2009. Automatic camera calibration applied to medical endoscopy. *Proceedings of British Machine Vision Conference*, London, UK, pp. 1–10.

Cheung, C.L., C. Wedlake, J. Moore, S.E. Pautler, and T.M. Peters. 2010. Fused video and ultrasound images for minimally invasive partial nephrectomy: A phantom study. *Proc MICCAI* 13(Pt 3):408–415.

Feuerstein, M., T. Mussack, S.M. Heining, and N. Navab. 2008a. Intraoperative laparoscope augmentation for port placement and resection planning in minimally invasive liver resection. *IEEE Trans Med Imaging* 27(3):355–369.

Feuerstein, M., T. Reichl, J. Vogel, J. Traub, and N. Navab. 2008b. New approaches to online estimation of electromagnetic tracking errors for laparoscopic ultrasonography. *Comput Aided Surg* 13(5):311–323.

Feuerstein, M., T. Reichl, J. Vogel, J. Traub, and N. Navab. 2009. Magneto-optical tracking of flexible laparoscopic ultrasound: Model-based online detection and correction of magnetic tracking errors. *IEEE Trans Med Imaging* 28(6):951–967.

Franz, A.M., T. Haidegger, W. Birkfellner, K. Cleary, T.M. Peters, and L. Maier-Hein. 2014. Electromagnetic tracking in medicine—A review of technology, validation, and applications. *IEEE Trans Med Imaging* 33(8):1702–1725.

Hartley, R., and P. Sturm. 1997. Triangulation. *Comput Vision Image Understanding* 68(2):146–157.

Heikkilä, J., and O. Silvén. 1997. A four-step camera calibration procedures with implicit image correction. *Proceedings of IEEE Computer Society Conference on Computer Vision and Pattern Recognition*, Washington, DC, pp. 1106–1112.

Kang, X., M. Azizian, E. Wilson, K. Wu, A.D. Martin, T.D. Kane, C.A. Peters, K. Cleary, and R. Shekhar. 2014. Stereoscopic augmented reality for laparoscopic surgery. *Surg Endosc* 28(7):2227–2235.

Lasso, A., T. Heffter, A. Rankin, C. Pinter, T. Ungi, and G. Fichtinger. 2014. PLUS: Open-source toolkit for ultrasound-guided intervention systems. *IEEE Trans Biomed Eng* 61(10):2527–2537.

Leven, J., D. Burschka, R. Kumar, G. Zhang, S. Blumenkranz, X.D. Dai, M. Awad et al. 2005. DaVinci canvas: A telerobotic surgical system with integrated, robot-assisted, laparoscopic ultrasound capability. *Proc MICCAI* 8(Pt 1):811–818.

Liu, X., C.E. Rice, and R. Shekhar. 2017a. Fast calibration of electromagnetically tracked oblique-viewing rigid endoscopes. *Int J Comput Assist Radiol Surg* 12(10): 1685–1695.

Liu, X., S. Kang, W. Plishker, G. Zaki, T.D. Kane, and R. Shekhar. 2016a. Laparoscopic stereoscopic augmented reality: Toward a clinically viable electromagnetic tracking solution. *J Med Imaging (Bellingham)* 3(4):045001.

Liu, X., T.D. Kane, and R. Shekhar. 2017b. GPS lap ultrasound: Embedding electromagnetic sensing to laparoscopic ultrasound. *Proceedings of Annual Meeting of the Society of American Gastrointestinal and Endoscopic Surgeons*. Houston, TX. 31(Suppl 1).

Liu, X., W. Plishker, G. Zaki, S. Kang, T.D. Kane, and R. Shekhar. 2016b. On-demand calibration and evaluation for electromagnetically tracked laparoscope in augmented reality visualization. *Int J Comput Assist Radiol Surg* 11(6):1163–1171.

Melo, R., J.P. Barreto, and G. Falcão. 2012. A new solution for camera calibration and real-time image distortion correction in medical endoscopy-initial technical evaluation. *IEEE Trans Biomed Eng* 59(3):634–644.

Nakamoto, M., K. Nakada, Y. Sato, K. Konishi, M. Hashizume, and S. Tamura. 2008. Intraoperative magnetic tracker calibration using a magneto-optic hybrid tracker for 3-D ultrasound-based navigation in laparoscopic surgery. *IEEE Trans Med Imaging* 27(2):255–270.

Nijkamp, J., B. Schermers, S. Schmitz, S. de Jonge, K. Kuhlmann, F. van der Heijden, J.J. Sonke, and T. Ruers. 2016. Comparing position and orientation accuracy of different electromagnetic sensors for tracking during interventions. *Int J Comput Assist Radiol Surg* 11(8):1487–1498.

Plishker, W., X. Liu, and R. Shekhar. 2017. Hybrid tracking for improved registration of laparoscopic ultrasound and laparoscopic video for augmented reality. *Proceedings of MICCAI Workshop on Clinical Image-Based Procedures: Translational Research in Medical Imaging*, Athens, Greece.

Pratt, P., A. Di Marco, C. Payne, A. Darzi, and G.Z. Yang. 2012. Intraoperative ultrasound guidance for transanal endoscopic microsurgery. *Proceedings of MICCAI* 15(Pt 1):463–4670.

Pratt, P., A. Jaeger, A. Hughes-Hallett, E. Mayer, J. Vale, A. Darzi, T. Peters, and G.Z. Yang. 2015. Robust ultrasound probe tracking: Initial clinical experiences during robot-assisted partial nephrectomy. *Int J Comput Assist Radiol Surg* 10(12):1905–1913.

Rutkowski, A., M.P. Nowacki, M. Chwalinski, J. Oledzki, M. Bednarczyk, P. Liszka-Dalecki, A. Gornicki, and K. Bujko. 2012. Acceptance of a 5-mm distal bowel resection margin for rectal cancer: Is it safe? *Colorectal Dis* 14(1):71–78.

Schneider, C., C. Nguan, R. Rohling, and S. Salcudean. 2016. Tracked "pick-up" ultrasound for robot-assisted minimally invasive surgery. *IEEE Trans Biomed Eng* 63(2):260–268.

Shahidi, R., M.R. Bax, C.R. Maurer Jr, J.A. Johnson, E.P. Wilkinson, B. Wang, J.B. West, M.J. Citardi, K.H. Manwaring, and R. Khadem. 2002. Implementation, calibration and accuracy testing of an image-enhanced endoscopy system. *IEEE Trans Med Imaging* 21(12):1524–1535.

Shekhar, R., O. Dandekar, V. Bhat, M. Philip, P. Lei, C. Godinez, E. Sutton et al. 2010. Live augmented reality: A new visualization method for laparoscopic surgery using continuous volumetric computed tomography. *Surg Endosc* 24(8):1976–1985.

Shekhar, R., X. Liu, E. Wilson, S. Kang, M. Petrosyan, and T.D. Kane. Stereoscopic augmented reality visualization for laparoscopic surgery—Initial clinical experience. 2015. *Proceedings of Annual Meeting of the Society of American Gastrointestinal and Endoscopic Surgeons*. Nashville, TN. Vol. 29(Suppl 1).

Wu, C., B. Jaramaz, and S.G. Narasimhan. 2010. A full geometric and photometric calibration method for oblique-viewing endoscopes. *Comput Aided Surg* 15(1–3):19–31.

Yamaguchi, T., M. Nakamoto, Y. Sato, K. Konishi, M. Hashizume, N. Sugano, H. Yoshikawa, and S. Tamura. 2004. Development of a camera model and calibration procedure for oblique-viewing endoscopes. *Comput Aided Surg* 9(5):203–214.

14 Augmented Reality in Image-Guided Robotic Surgery

Wen Pei Liu and Russell H. Taylor

CONTENTS

14.1 INTRODUCTION

Although minimally invasive surgery provides many advantages, keyhole approaches limit the surgeon's traditional and natural three-dimensional (3D) perception inside the human body. For example, the constrained field-of-view of endoscopes and laparoscopes, plus the lack of haptic feedback can diminish the surgeon's visual and tactile cues. Efforts to improve robotic surgery have looked to augment information visually and through other multisensory feedback and control methods.

This chapter reviews recent approaches in augmented reality (AR) for robotic surgery, including (1) visual AR, (2) visual servo mechanisms, and (3) force servo mechanisms. Sources of information for AR include preoperative and intraoperative medical imaging and sensors. Visual AR is typically video augmentation through which models of critical anatomical structures (e.g., tumors or vessels, see Figure 14.1) (Su et al. 2008; Liu et al. 2013) are overlaid onto the display of the endoscope/laparoscope. The control of the robot, including use of the augmented

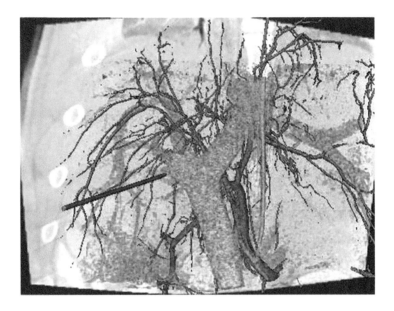

FIGURE 14.1 Artis Zeego CBCT angiography of a porcine liver with arterial (red) and portal venous (blue) phases.

information to affect the robot, remains with the surgeon and so is completely unchanged when compared to a robotic system without visual AR. Conversely, the information integrated with visual and force servo mechanisms assumes some degree of control of an intraoperative device traditionally reserved for the surgeon.

14.2 BACKGROUND

Over the past decade, robotic surgery has become increasingly prevalent for many indications. Current research seeks to increase a surgeon's situational awareness (Simaan et al. 2015) by providing *in situ* guidance and control to help a surgeon carry out surgical plans. Standard-of-care surgical planning typically includes review of preoperative volumetric data (i.e., computed tomography [CT] and magnetic resonance [MR] images [MRI]). During the actual intervention, the surgeon typically must either remember the plan or view the planning information on an external monitor or (in the case of the da Vinci) on a separate display so that images are not aligned with the patient anatomy.

AR methods have the potential to improve a surgeon's situational awareness during robotic surgery by superimposing additional information of the patient's anatomy directly onto the surgeon's view of the anatomy on which he is operating. Augmented information includes visual AR, which combines computer-generated graphical information with the video stream from an endoscopic camera. In more complex systems, augmented information can provide additional sensory feedback and/or control certain aspects of the robotic system.

14.3 MEDICAL IMAGING

Deriving surgical plans from preoperative imaging is a standard-of-care practice for robotic surgery. Objectives include planning traversals for target resection, delineating margins, and forming strategies for reconstruction while controlling critical functional structures. AR has been a popular technique to commute surgical plans into the operating theatre. For example, by segmenting or labeling anatomies in CT or MRI images, methods in computer graphics can generate 3D anatomical models that can be aligned to the operating view. Because these models leverage the ability of varying imaging modalities to visualize subsurface anatomy, the information provided includes structures that are invisible to the human eye.

However, preoperative images may become outdated, as they do not include anatomical changes in the patient that have occurred since the image acquisition. Changes can include deformations due to the positioning of the patient for surgery, changes in stomach and bowel contents, disease progression, and modifications to tissue during surgery. Alternatively, intraoperative imaging visualizes *in situ* anatomic structures in real time, making them arguably a more accurate, safer source of information for AR. A discussion by Hekman et al. (2017) on the value of different intraoperative imaging (ultrasound [US], fluorescence imaging, optical coherence tomography, and MRI) for partial nephrectomy noted an expansion in the use of US and fluorescence. Furthermore, intraoperative imaging has been used in research not only to render subsurfaces of the patient anatomy, but also to provide an anchoring modality for registering higher resolution preoperative images and plans. Current AR research in medical robotics includes examples using preoperative diagnostic imaging, such as CT, intraoperative ultrasound (IOUS), Single-Photon Emission Computed Tomography (SPECT), and other modalities (Liu et al. 2013; Huang et al. 2017). The following reviews some typical clinical uses of these modalities.

14.3.1 CT

Two-dimensional (2D) x-ray imaging has been long established as a cost-effective, real-time modality both preoperatively and intraoperatively. Similarly, the ability of 3D CT images made from multiple x-ray projections to identify abnormalities such as infarctions, tumors, calcifications, hemorrhage, and bone trauma has led to the widespread use of CT in neurology, cardiology, gastroenterology (Saito et al. 2017), urology, and orthopedics (Gibson et al. 2017), among other specialties. Robotic percutaneous biopsies under CT guidance have shown promising results in accuracy and efficacy (Koethe et al. 2014). Hunsche et al. (2017) reported using 2D/3D registration of intraoperative x-ray to preoperative CT during stereotactic robotic-assisted surgery. A study comparing freehand and CT-guided robot percutaneous injections in a phantom showed that the number of required corrections was significantly greater with freehand (Beyer et al. 2016). The emergence of intraoperative Cone-beam Computed Tomography (CBCT) has facilitated the use of CT during surgical interventions (Nithiananthan et al. 2011; Marinetto et al. 2017).

14.3.2   MRI

MRI provides a rich repertoire of means to evaluate physical anatomy and physiological processes of the body in 3D. In interventional radiology, high-resolution MRI viewed through AR has also shown high technical performance for perineural injections (Marker et al. 2017). For intraoperative guidance, the integration of MRI imaging through intraoperative AR has shown effectiveness in neurosurgery (Hirai et al. 2005) and in general surgical applications (Liao et al. 2010). In a urologic clinical study, biopsies guided with preoperative MR fused with IOUS (Hansen et al. 2017) supported high detection rates comparable to clinical standard Gleason scoring. The challenge of using MRI for robotic surgery becomes not only the workspace limitation inside the bore of the MRI scanner, but also the requirement for non-magnetic material during the procedure. For example, material consideration impacts actuation design, in which piezoelectric and pneumatic actuators are the mainstay approaches for robotic manipulation inside MRI.

14.3.3   US IMAGING

2D and 3D US and IOUS imaging provide efficient, low-cost, easily deployed means to image soft tissues. Advanced imaging techniques such as Doppler imaging, US elastography (Salcudean et al. 2009), and photoacoustic US (Rivaz et al. 2010) provide increasingly sophisticated ways to detect tissue properties and to distinguish different anatomic structures.

In diagnostics, for urology and in head and neck patients (Helbig et al. 2008; Pfeiffer et al. 2009), US is often the primary imaging modality, particularly for those with diseases of the prostate and thyroid, respectively. In intervention, these advantages have led to the proliferation of probes being customized for specific clinical applications: transesophageal, intrarectal, endocavity, and the like (Gao et al. 2011). Furthermore, the registration of US images to preoperative CT has demonstrated advantages in staging and surgical planning for papillary thyroid carcinoma as well as nephritic (Leroy et al. 2006) and hepatic (Lange et al. 2003) surgical procedures. In guided surgery, US also can be used as a bridging modality to register other images and plans into the intraoperative scene. For example, Billings et al. (2015) propose a noninvasive improvement to use tracked B-mode US to integrate CT-image-based models for total hip replacement. Similarly, in robotic surgery, Schneider et al. (2016) demonstrate the feasibility of using a tracked, da Vinci-compatible US transducer to register 3D vascular images from a preoperative CT surface model. The latter section on visual servo mechanisms will further explore how US images are being directly used to provide *in situ* guidance and control.

14.3.4   SPECT

SPECT uses gamma cameras to detect radiopharmaceutical tracers, similar to planar scintigraphy. The main difference comes from the ability of SPECT to reconstruct a 3D image using rotating planar images acquired over an arc around the patient, similar to CT. SPECT is often combined with x-ray CT. Together, SPECT/CT provides

3D images representing both the lymphatic system and anatomical structures. This combined imaging method is showing great promise, as sentinel lymph node (SLN) detection rates, as well as indirect metabolic activity, have been reported at 95% incidence and greater (Holman et al. 2014). A robotics SPECT for minimally-invasive SLN mapping was first introduced in 2016 (Fuerst et al. 2015). The authors used a drop-in gamma probe, manipulated with a robotic laparoscopic gripper, for intraoperative abdominal intervention. Evaluation and testing using a phantom for gynecological sentinel lymph node interventions compared to ground-truth data yielded a mean reconstruction accuracy of 0.67 mm.

14.4 VISUAL AR

Robotic surgery requires precise navigation to the clinical target and a 3D understanding of its spatial surroundings. Endoscopic vision is limited to surface features, which are not always sufficient to recognize the location of the organs around the surgical area. Surgical strategy and planning are conducted using preoperative medical images that lend critical insight into the layered, subsurface biological systems. However, the alignment of preoperative plans is often left as a mental exercise. Thus, the emergence of robotic surgery has accentuated a gap that currently exists between preoperative medical imaging and the *in situ* anatomy in surgery. AR in robotic surgery seeks to provide guidance by integrating such information into the endoscopic field of view. The visual AR research approaches reviewed below are categorized into mosaic, subsurface, and depth visualization methods.

14.4.1 Mosaic Visualization

In endoscopic minimally invasive surgery the camera renders the line-of-sight of the work space at a frame rate. What was seen before and after the current camera view is usually discarded. Therefore, inadvertent tissue injury to surface visible structures just outside the current scope of view remains a potential problem. To address this risk, researchers have developed methods to accumulate information between frames by applying mosaicking concepts from computer vision (Richa et al. 2014; Kohler et al. 2016; Dwyer et al. 2017).

Dwyer et al. (2017) described a robotic control interface of an imaging system. Traditionally, for delicate fetoscopic procedures, such as the treatments for twin-twin transfusion, small instrumentation with limited articulation is used to guide the primary interventional tool (e.g., a laser tip). To overcome the narrow field of view, their work proposed to enhance the view at the operating site by assisting operators to scan and create a panoramic scene of the vascular mapping (Figure 14.2). This map is used to guide the laser introducer and instrument to sever the shared blood supply between the fetuses. Their mechatronic design includes a comanipulated instrument that combines concentric tube actuation to a larger manipulator constrained by a remote center of motion. A stereoscopic camera is mounted at the distal tip and used for imaging. They demonstrate that the enhanced dexterity and stability of the tracked imaging device is comparable to electromagnetic-based tracked systems.

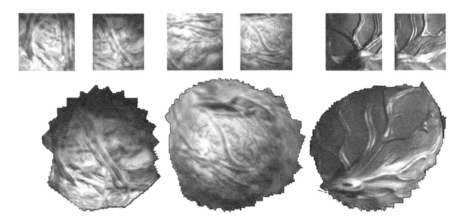

FIGURE 14.2 Mosaics formed from the scanning trajectories; (a) Raster scan of the human *ex vivo* placenta, 30 × 30 mm; (b) Spiral scan of the human *ex vivo* placenta, radius of ≈20 mm; (c) Spiral scan of a model placenta, radius of ≈20 mm. (Reproduced from Dwyer, G. et al., *IEEE Rob. Automat. Lett.*, 2, 1656–1663, 2017. With thanks and kind regards to the authors.)

Similarly, in ophthalmology, researchers created intraoperative mosaics for view expansion. Expanded mosaic views can be used to guide laser photocoagulation, which is currently the standard treatment for sight-threatening diseases worldwide, namely diabetic retinopathy and retinal vein occlusions. For example, Richa et al. (2014) extended the capabilities of a collaborative robot for eye surgery by creating a panoramic view of the retina. Correspondence was established with feature-rich structures, such as vessel branches among images of the fundus through the microscope. The concept of surface reconstruction can extend the application of mosaic views even further. By using a miniature projector for structured light surface reconstruction, Edgcumbe et al. (2015) reported errors less than 2 mm in phantom-based experiments and feasibility in an *in vivo* proof-of-concept porcine trial.

14.4.2 SUBSURFACE VISUALIZATION

Beyond mosaics, to reduce the risk of injury to subsurface critical tissue and improve *in situ* visualization, researchers have explored augmenting the video source with data from medical imaging. Information is often derived from preoperative modalities, as discussed in Section 14.3. Volonte et al. (2013) applied volumes rendered from a standard CT using the OsiriX DICOM workstation. A custom OsiriX plugin was created that permitted the 3D-rendered images to be displayed in the da Vinci surgeon console using the TilePro multi-input display. Displays were controlled by a 3D joystick installed on the console and updated in real time.

Other teams also have reported the successful use of different types of mixed reality and endoscopic video. Previously rendered images were superimposed with transparency on the real scene using a virtual helmet. Su et al. (2008) used AR during robot-assisted partial nephrectomy, in which they overlaid reconstructed 3D computer tomography images onto real-time stereo video footage. Although retrospective, these results showed the possibility of incorporating these images directly in the surgical field during the operation. Pietrabissa et al. (2009) also demonstrated the advantages of AR during the treatment of a splenic artery aneurysm.

Key challenges with *in vivo* adaptation of video AR include subsurface alignment from initial registration to continued updates. In, arguably, more rigid environments, such as neurosurgery and maxillofacial surgery, these challenges are minimized. Wang et al. (2017) reported a streamlined, real-time, markerless image registration method with a shape-based matching algorithm for maxillofacial surgery. Feasibility clinical studies with visual AR have also been explored for craniomaxillofacial surgery. Lin et al. (2016) reported a study on their novel, robot-assisted, AR navigation for mandibular angle split osteotomy with five patients. In comparison to a control group, they achieved a statistically significant average position and angle. Compared to neurosurgery, otolaryngology, orthopedics (Fallavollita et al. 2015), and maxillofacial surgery, the development of AR-based navigation surgery in the abdomen has been much slower. Okamoto et al. (2015) have suggested that the delay can be attributed to more complex intraoperative organ deformations and the existence of established medical imaging intraoperative modalities.

14.4.3 Depth Visualization

For humans, depth is a sensory perception drawn from interpreted cues. Cues stem from texture gradients and lighting as well as from other perceived properties of objects, such as shape, orientation, and dimension. When merging real and virtual images, the relative position in depth may not be perceived correctly even when all alignments are accurate. Thus, the usefulness of an AR image-guidance system is a function of both registration accuracy and techniques in visual perception.

To create compelling depth perception in AR for surgery, Bichlmeier et al. (2007) demonstrated a novel design incorporating context awareness in a series of cadaveric and *in vivo* experiments conducted with a stereoscopic head-mounted display. In their study, they adjusted the transparency of the video images dynamically. Their algorithm was not only based on the position and line-of-sight of the observer, but also the shape of the patient's skin and the location of the instrument. The modified video image of the real scene was then blended with the previously rendered virtual anatomy to create a much more natural blending of augmentation with overlay.

To provide navigational information beyond video augmentation in an otolaryngology application, Liu et al. (2013) used an auxiliary display window to disambiguate relative distances of objects in the viewpoint orthogonal to the camera. Their mixed reality included dynamically updated tracked distances of tool points to targets. Furthermore, a novel, supplemental view of tracked tools within the virtual scene (model meshes of critical information and CBCT slices and volumes) was added as a picture-in-picture. This auxiliary camera perspective was dynamically changed but was set to the lateral, left-to-right sagittal plane, orthogonal to the camera plane after empirical observations (Figure 14.3).

Information about tracked distances is even more compelling when based on intraoperative imaging. In robot-assisted lymphadenectomy, Fuerst et al. (2015) explored the role of depth with a laparoscopic gamma probe (Eurorad, Eckbolsheim,

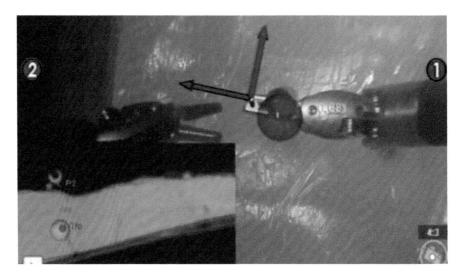

FIGURE 14.3 Screenshot of the enhanced AR scene with a virtual, orthogonal perspective in the lower left corner. As the tracked needle tip approaches the embedded target, enhancements include the change in color (red) of the sphere, a distance label (white, on end effectors), and the virtual perspective (picture-in-picture) showing a red avatar of the tracked point inside the target (yellow).

France; Section II-B) and a SPECT imaging system (SurgicEye GmbH, Munich, Germany). Using an infrared tracking system (Polaris Vicra, Northern Digital Inc, Canada) to maintain patient and endoscope alignment, the live endoscopic video was augmented with a freehand SPECT volume and quantitative distances of radioactive sources. Their hybrid mechanical and image-based in-patient probe reported an accuracy of 0.2 mm.

14.5 VISUAL SERVO MECHANISM

Krupa (2014) presented a method for a three degrees-of-freedom steering of a flexible biopsy needle using two orthogonal cameras. The visual servoing control design tracked a beveled-tip needle in a translucent phantom during experiments that showed a final positioning error of 0.4 mm. Instead of cameras, Chatelain et al. (2015) proposed a US-based biopsy system. A 3D US-based needle tracking algorithm was combined with a duty-cycling visual servoing strategy. Modeled as a polynomial curve, a flexible needle was tracked during automatic insertion using particle filtering on US images.

Percutaneous needle placement is also a critical workflow step for needle ablation procedures in interventional radiology. For example, Won et al. (2017) demonstrated a master-slave robotic system capable of delivering biopsy and radiofrequency ablation. Although it was not the focus of the experimental analysis in their paper, the design accommodated additional manipulation of the robotic arm based on visual feedback, as well as enforcement of critical structure breach. Other applications of active guidance paradigms in medicine include brachytherapy, a type of treatment for prostate cancer, in which needles are used to drop radiotherapy seeds at exact locations that are predetermined from diagnostic imaging. Researchers have looked to MR for synergistic control of real-time needle positioning to help optimize dose deposits (Wartenberg et al. 2016). Further extension of cooperation between a robotic system and a surgeon was demonstrated by de Battisti et al. (2017) with a stochastic criterion through MR-based needle tracking combined with a real-time adaptive plan.

Although often visualized with intraoperative imaging, e.g., CT, MRI, or US, needle placement is inherently challenging due to systemic errors, the dynamics of tissue heterogeneity, the motion of targets within the tissue, and the normal range of organ size/shape fluctuations. Complementary components that constitute a closed-loop needle steering system are further detailed by Rossa and Tavakoli (2017), including modeling needle-tissue interaction, sensing needle deflection, controlling needle trajectory, and hardware implementation. In addition to targeting, visual servo mechanisms in medical imaging can be used for autonomous intraoperative tracking (Degirmenci et al. 2017).

14.6   FORCE SERVO MECHANISM

In contrast to the visual servo mechanisms discussed above, force servo mechanisms share the control of the surgical devices through haptic, human-robot synergy. Gonenc and Iordachita (2016) reported improvements to an established force-sensing system in retinal microsurgery, in which multiple fiber Bragg grating (FBG) sensors were incorporated into sub-mm surgical tools. Because FBG sensors are MR-compatible, many research groups have explored their use in MRI-guided procedures (Monfaredi et al. 2013; de Battisti et al. 2016; Hao et al. 2017; Moreira et al. 2017). An initiative, Project MIRIAM (Minimally Invasive Robotics in an MRI environment), looks to build an MR-compatible robot with FBG-based needle tip tracking (Moreira et al. 2017). Designs that vary the fundamental principles of fiber optics, including light intensity modulation, wavelength modulation, and phase modulation are reviewed by (Su et al. 2017).

Caversaccio et al. (2017) reported the first clinical experience of a robotic, cochlear, surgical workflow incorporating intraoperative force sensing. First, a path to the ear's round window was planned based on preoperative images. Intraoperatively, this path was robotically drilled out with the following safety mechanisms: (1) a force sensor mapping force profile to depth, (2) stereotactic optical tracking of instruments, and (3) multipolar neuromonitoring to confirm the proximity of the facial nerve. Electrode array insertion was manually achieved under microscope visualization with a reported accuracy of 0.2 mm. Postoperative validation used CT to verify electrode array placement, structure preservation, and the accuracy of the drilling and all safety mechanisms.

Force servo mechanisms have also been combined with visual systems and other control paradigms. For example, capabilities from force adaptation with compliant robotic manipulators are capitalized for endomicroscopy in a system proposed by Wisanuvej et al. (2017). Haptic and visual sensing are combined in a stabilizing handheld robot with camera guidance for retinal vein cannulation (Mukherjee et al. 2017). Similarly, Abayazid et al. (2016) used US imaging to control and execute desired needle orientations for a broad application of needle steering workflows. During needle insertion, their design provided intuitive navigation cues about the computed orientation to the human operator through haptic and visual feedback.

14.7 CONCLUSION

While the magnification and stereo capabilities of current minimally invasive surgical systems provide high-resolution views of the workspace surface, navigation through complex critical substructures continues to be a challenge. The ability to continuously maintain correspondence remains a function of experience, and the learning curve is steep. Furthermore, the narrow field of view from minimally invasive surgical (MIS) cameras has increased the need to juggle even more information beyond the current field of view. To address these challenges, researchers have explored AR for image-guided surgery to enrich the surgical scene with virtual content. The results support the efficacy and potential of navigation from applying AR in medical robotics. However, research must be conducted to better understand how to correlate natural and intuitive multisensory manipulation in context with the actual patient. Further integration of AR with active guidance mechanisms will continue to push the boundaries of shared control in robotics towards improved navigation, spatial orientation, and intraoperative confidence. Along with technological difficulties, AR in medicine must meet its challenges to justify utility, portability, and cost.

REFERENCES

Abayazid, M, C Pacchierotti, P Moreira, R Alterovitz, D Prattichizzo, and S Misra. Experimental evaluation of co-manipulated ultrasound-guided flexible needle steering. *International Journal of Medical Robotics and Computer Assisted Surgery*, 12, no. 2 (2016): 219–230.

Beyer, L et al. Evaluation of a robotic assistance-system for percutaneous computed tomography-guided (CT-Guided) facet joint injection: A phantom study. *Medical Science Monitor*, 22 (2016): 3334–3339.

Bichlmeier, C, F Wimmer, S M Heining, and N Navab. Contextual anatomic mimesis hybrid in-situ visualization method for improving multi-sensory depth perception in medical augmented reality. *International Symposium on Mixed and Augmented Reality*, Nara, Japan, 2007, pp. 1–10.

Billings, S, H J Kang, A Cheng, E Boctor, P Kazanzides, and R Taylor. Minimally invasive registration for computer-assisted orthopedic surgery: Combining tracked ultrasound and bone surface points via the P-IMLOP algorithm. *International Journal of Computer Assisted Radiology Surgery*, 10 (2015): 761–771.

Caversaccio, M et al. Robotic cochlear implantation: Surgical procedure and first clinical experience. *Acta Oto-Laryngologica*, 137, no. 4 (2017): 447–454.

Chatelain, P, A Krupa, and N Navab. 3D ultrasound-guided robotic steering of a flexible needle via visual servoing. *IEEE International Conference on Robotics and Automation*. Seattle, WA, 2015, pp. 2250–2255.

de Battisti, M B, B Senneville, M Maenhout, and M Moerland. Fiber Bragg gratings-based sensing for real-time needle tracking during MR-guided brachytherapy. *Medical Physics*, 43 (2016): 5288–5297.

de Battisti, M B et al. A novel adaptive needle insertion sequencing for robotic, single needle MR-guided high-dose-rate prostate brachytherapy. *Physics in Medicine & Biology,* 62, no. 10 (2017): 4031.

Degirmenci, A, P M Loschak, C M Tschabrunn, E Anter, and R D Howe. Enabling autonomous ultrasound-based procedure guidance in cardiac interventions. *ICRA Workshop C4 Surgical Robots: Compliant, Continuum, Cognitive, and Collaborative,* Singapore, 2017.

Dwyer, G et al. A continuum robot and control interface for surgical assist in fetoscopic interventions. *IEEE Robotics and Automation Letters,* 2, no. 3 (2017): 1656–1663.

Edgcumbe, P, P Pratt, G Yang, C Nguan, and R Rohling. Pico lantern: A pick-up projector for augmented reality in laparoscopic surgery. *Medical Image Analysis,* 25 (2015): 95–102.

Fallavollita, P, L Wang, S Weidert, and N Navab. Augmented reality in orthopaedic interventions and education. In *Computational Radiology for Orthopaedic Interventions.* Springer, Cham, Switzerland, 2015, pp. 251–269.

Fuerst, B et al. First robotic SPECT for minimally invasive sentinel lymph node mapping. *IEEE Transactions on Medical Imaging,* 35, no. 3 (2015): 830–838.

Gao, G et al. Rapid image registration of three-dimensional transesophageal echocardiography and X-ray fluoroscopy for the guidance of cardiac interventions. In *International Conference on Information Processing in Computer-Assisted Interventions.* Springer, Berlin, Germany, 2011, pp. 124–134.

Gibson, P et al. The role of computed tomography in surgical planning for trimalleolar fracture. A survey of OTA members. *Orthopaedic Trauma,* 31 (2017): e116–e120.

Gonenc, B, and I Iordachita. FBG-based transverse and axial force-sensing micro-forceps for retinal microsurgery. In *Sensors.* IEEE, Orlando, FL, 2016.

Hansen, N et al. Magnetic resonance and ultrasound image fusion supported transperineal prostate biopsy using the ginsburg protocol: Technique, learning points, and biopsy results. *European Urology,* 70 (2017): 332–340.

Hao, S et al. Fiber optic force sensors for MRI-guided interventions and rehabilitation: A review. *IEEE Sensors Journal,* 17, no. 7 (2017): 1952–1963.

Hekman, M, M Rijpkema, J Langenhuijsen, O Boerman, E Oosterwijk, and P Mulders. Intraoperative imaging techniques to support complete tumor resection in partial nephrectomy. *European Urology Focus,* 17 (2017): 2405–4569.

Helbig, M, K Krysztoforski, P Krowicki, S Helbig, W Gstoettner, and J Kozak. Development of prototype for navigated real-time sonography for the head and neck region. *Head Neck,* 30 (2008): 215–221.

Hirai, N, A Kosaka, T Kawamata, T Hori, and H Iseki. Image-guided neurosurgery system integrating AR-based navigation and open-MRI monitoring. *Computer Aided Surgery,* 10, no. 2 (2005): 59–72.

Holman, L L, C F Levenback, and M Frumovitz. Sentinel lymph node evaluation in women with cervical cancer. *Journal of Minimally Invasive Gynecology,* 21, no. 4 (2014): 540–545.

Huang, B, M Ye, Y Hu, A Vandini, S Lee, and G Yang. A multi-robot cooperation framework for sewing personalized stent grafts. *Arxiv:cs,* 2017: 03195v1.

Hunsche, S et al. Intensity-based 2D 3D registration for lead localization in robot guided deep brain stimulation. *Physics in Medicine & Biology,* 62, no. 6 (2017): 2417–2426.

Koethe, Y, S Xu, and G Velusamy. Accuracy and efficacy of percutaneous biopsy and ablation using robotic assistance under computed tomography guidance: A phantom study. *European Radiology,* 24, no. 3 (2014): 723–730.

Kohler, T, A Heinrich, A Maier, J Hornegger, and R Tornow. Super-resolved retinal image mosaicing. *IEEE 13th International Symposium on Biomedical Imaging,* 2016, pp. 1063–1067.

Krupa, A. 3D steering of a flexible needle by visual servoing. In *Medical Image Computing and Computer-Assisted Intervention*. Springer International Publishing, Basel, Switzerland, 2014, pp. 480–487.

Lange, T, S Eulenstein, M Hunerbein, and P M Schlag. Vessel-based non-rigid registration of MR/CT and 3D ultrasound for navigation in liver surgery. *Computer Aided Surgery*, 8, no. 5 (2003): 228–240.

Leroy, A, P Mozer, Y Payan, and J Troccaz. Rigid registration of freehand 3D ultraound and CT-scan kidney images. *arXiv: Physics /0606216*, 2006.

Liao, H, T Inomata, I Sakuma, and D Takeyoshi. 3-D augmented reality for MRI-guided surgery using integral videography autostereoscopic image overlay. *IEEE Transactions on Biomedical Engineering*, 57, no. 6 (2010): 1476–1486.

Lin, L et al. Mandibular angle split osteotomy based on a novel augmented reality navigation using specialized robot-assisted arms—A feasibility study. *Journal of Craniomaxillofacial Surgery*, 44, no. 2 (2016): 215–223.

Liu, W P et al. A clinical pilot study of a modular video-CT augmentation system for image-guided skull base surgery. *The Society of Photo-Optical Instrumentation Engineers (SPIE) Medical Imaging*, San Diego, CA, 2012.

Liu, W P et al. Toward intraoperative image-guided transoral robotic surgery. *Journal of Robotic Surgery*, 7, no. 2 (2013): 217–225.

Marinetto, E et al. Integration of free-hand 3D ultrasound and mobile C-arm cone-beam CT: Feasibility and characterization for real-time guidance of needle insertion. *Computerized Medical Imaging and Graphics: The Official Journal of the Computerized Medical Imaging Society*, 58 (2017): 13–22.

Marker, D et al. 1.5 T augmented reality navigated interventional MRI: Paravertebral sympathetic plexus injections. *Diagnostic and Interventional Radiology*, 23, no. 3 (2017): 227–232.

Monfaredi, R, R Seifabadi, G Fichtinger, and I Iordachita. Design of a decoupled MRI-compatible force sensor using fiber Bragg grating sensors for robot-assisted prostate interventions. *SPIE*, Orlando, FL, 2013, pp. 8671–8679.

Moreira, P, K Boskma, and S Misra. Towards MRI-guided flexible needle steering using fiber Bragg grating-based tip tracking. *International Conference on Robotics and Automation*, Singapore, 2017, pp. 4849–4854.

Mukherjee, S, S Yang, R A MacLachlan, L A Lobes, Jr, J N Martel, and C N Riviere. Toward monocular camera-guided retinal vein cannulation with an. *International Conference on Robotics and Automation*, Singapore, 2017.

Nithiananthan, S et al. Incorporating tissue excision in deformable image registration: A modified demons algorithm for cone-beam CT-guided surgery. *SPIE Medical Imaging*, Orlando, FL, 2011, pp. 7964–7969.

Okamoto, T, S Onda, K Yanaga, N Suzuki, and A Hattori. Clinical application of navigation surgery using augmented reality in the abdominal field. *Surgery Today*, 45, no. 4 (2015): 397–406.

Pfeiffer, J, G Kayser, and G Ridder. Sonography-assisted cutting needle biopsy in the head and neck for the diagnosis of lymphoma: Can it replace lymph node extirpation? *Laryngoscope*, 119, no. 4 (2009): 689–695.

Pietrabissa, A et al. Mixed reality for robotic treatment of a splenic artery aneurysm. *Surgical Endoscopy*, 24, no. 5 (2009): 1204.

Richa, R et al. Fundus image mosaicking for information augmentation in computer-assisted slit-lamp imaging. *IEEE Transactions on Medical Imaging*, 33, no. 6 (2014): 1304–1312.

Rivaz, H, E Boctor, M Choti, and G Hager. Real-time regularized ultrasound elastography. *IEEE Transactions on Medical Imaging*, 30, no. 4 (2010): 928–945.

Rossa, C, and M Tavakoli. Issues in closed-loop needle steering. *Control Engineering Practice*, 62 (2017): 55–69.

Saito, H et al. Usefulness and limitations of dual-layer spectral detector computed tomography for diagnosing biliary stones not detected by conventional computed tomography: A report of three cases. *Clinical Journal of Gastroenterology,* 11, no. (2) (2017): 1–6.

Salcudean, S E, W Xu, S S Mahdavi, M Moradi, J W Morris, and I Spadinger. Ultrasound elastography—An image guidance tool for prostate brachytherapy. *Brachytherapy,* 8, no. (2) (2009): 125–126.

Schneider, C, C Nguan, R Rohling, and S Salcudean. Tracked "Pick-Up" ultrasound for robot-assisted minimally invasive surgery. *IEEE Transactions on Biomedical Engineering,* 63, no. (2016): 260–268.

Simaan, N, R H Taylor, and H Choset. Intelligent surgical robots with situational awareness: From good to great surgeons. *ASME Dynamic Systems Magazine,* 137, no. 9 (2015): 3–6.

Su, H et al. Fiber optic force sensors for MRI-guided interventions and rehabilitation: A review. *IEEE Sensors Journal,* 17, no. 7 (2017): 1952–1963.

Su, L M, B P Vagvolgyi, R Agarwal, C E Reiley, R H Taylor, and G D Hager. Augmented reality during robot-assisted laparoscopic partial nephrectomy: Toward real-time 3D-CT to stereoscopic video registration. *Journal of Urology,* 73, no. 4 (2008): 896–900.

Volonte, F et al. Stereoscopic augmented reality for da Vincii™ robotic biliary surgery. *International Journal of Surgery Case Reports,* 4, no. 4 (2013): 365–367.

Wang, J, H Suenaga, L Yang, E Kobayashi, and I Sakuma. Video see-through augmented reality for oral and maxillofacial surgery. *International Journal of Medical Robotics,* 13, no. 2 (2017): e1754.

Wartenberg, M, N Patel, G Li, and G S Fischer. Towards synergistic control of hands-on needle insertion with automated needle steering for MRI-guided prostate interventions. *2016 38th Annual International Conference of the IEEE Engineering in Medicine and Biology Society,* Orlando, FL, 2016, pp. 5116–5119.

Wisanuvej, P, P G Giataganas, K L Leibrandt, J L Liu, M H Hughes, and G Z Yang. Three-dimensional robotic-assisted endomicroscopy with a force adaptive robotic arm. *International Conference on Robotics and Automation.* Singapore, 2017, pp. 2379–2384.

Won, H J, N Kim, G B Kim, J B Seo, and H Kim. Validation of a CT-guided intervention robot for biopsy and radiofrequency ablation: Experimental study with an abdominal phantom. *Diagnostic and Interventional Radiology,* 23, no. 3 (2017): 233–237.

15 Augmented Reality for Reducing Intraoperative Radiation Exposure to Patients and Clinicians during X-Ray Guided Procedures

Nicolas Loy Rodas and Nicolas Padoy

CONTENTS

15.1 INTRODUCTION: CLINICAL CONTEXT

Medical augmented reality (AR) technology has the potential to enhance a surgeon's view with information crucial to the current state of the procedure, and it has now been successfully applied in several fields of surgery, such as neurosurgery, orthopedic surgery, and maxillofacial surgery (Chen et al. 2013). Yet, in this chapter, we will discuss recent works that make use of AR for a different kind of medical application besides assisting the surgeon in the immediate execution of a procedure. We refer to the use of AR to reduce the amount of ionizing radiation clinical staff and patients are exposed to during surgical procedures involving x-rays.

15.2 EXPOSURE TO IONIZING RADIATION DURING X-RAY GUIDED PROCEDURES

X-ray-based medical imaging has revolutionized the diagnosis of diseases and the practice of numerous surgical treatments in the past few decades. It also has been a key factor in the paradigm shift from traditional surgery to minimally invasive surgery. X-ray imaging has become fundamental in several fields of medicine, such as interventional radiology/cardiology, orthopedics, urology, neuroradiology, and radiation therapy. However, the use of x-rays for medical purposes carries with it the risk of exposing patients, surgeons, and supporting medical staff members to harmful ionizing radiation. Studies have reaffirmed the hypothesis of a linear no-threshold model of radiation risk, namely that any amount of exposure increases the risk of radiation-induced tissue reactions (epilation, skin necrosis, cataract etc.) and of stochastic effects (cancers) (Roguin et al. 2013). While a patient's exposure can be justified by medical indication and usually occurs in a single episode, medical staff providing patient care may be exposed on a daily basis. The repetitive nature of such an exposure, even when the dose is low, increases the risk of developing negative biological effects, and this risk increases with the dose accumulated over time (Kirkwood et al. 2014). Furthermore, as can be seen in Figure 15.1, when x-ray imaging is used for guidance, such as during interventional procedures, clinicians are obliged to remain next to the patient during the procedure, and their exposure cannot

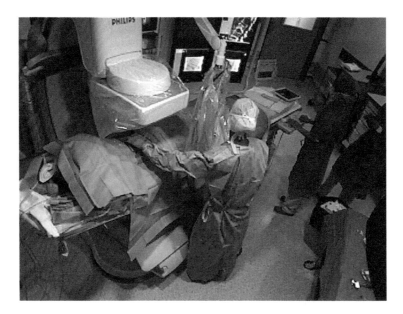

FIGURE 15.1   Fluoroscopy-guided procedure. (Courtesy of Strasbourg's University Hospital, interventional radiology Department, Strasbourg, France.)

be completely avoided (Nikodemová et al. 2011). Indeed, reports have documented the dosage of radiation among interventional physicians as the greatest registered among any medical staff working with x-rays (Roguin et al. 2013).

Despite the use of protective equipment to mitigate the risk of exposure, such as lead aprons, thyroid collars, and shielding screens, several body parts (hands, head, and eyes) remain not fully protected; thus, medical staff's exposure levels can approach the annual limits (Krim et al. 2011). Even though lead screens can provide high protection, often its usage is not practical and can impede the operator's work. A large study across six different EU countries reported that in 23% of the interventional radiology procedures performed in the hospitals under study, no room protective equipment was used (Nikodemová et al. 2011).

15.2.1 Intraoperative Monitoring of Radiation Exposure: Challenges

Large-scale efforts are being made to develop methodologies and tools for better understanding, assessing, and limiting medical radiation exposure. While technical innovation and optimization of the design of medical imaging equipment has enabled the reduction of the patient dose during image acquisition, occupational exposure has proven to be more challenging to address (Sailer et al. 2016). Indeed, staff's exposure results mostly from the x-rays that are not absorbed and are deflected by the patient, which is known as scattered radiation. Its propagation and magnitude are affected by several simultaneously changing factors (Koukorava et al. 2011). Some of them, such as patient characteristics (e.g., obesity) or the complexity of the procedure, are beyond clinicians' control and are risk factors for increased radiation dose (Kirkwood et al. 2014). For instance, complex interventions requiring both longer fluoroscopy times and a large number of x-ray shots, such as complex endovascular procedures, incur a higher dose to the patient and increase the risk of staff's exposure to the generated scatter (Kirkwood et al. 2014). Other factors, such as the personnel's position with respect to the patient, the imaging parameters, or the disposition of protective equipment can be partially controlled. However, these are usually altered during the procedure, thus making highly irradiated areas difficult to predict.

The monitoring of staff's exposure is currently achieved either by means of dosimeters, which provide the effective dose value at the measuring position, or by using estimations provided by the imaging device (e.g., dose area product). Yet, studies have reported large variations in the occupational exposure per procedure and per person's body part (Nikodemová et al. 2011), so the full body exposure of clinicians cannot be assessed solely by dosimeters. Also, correlations between the dose values provided by the imaging device and the exposure of clinicians can hardly be found because such estimations do not consider the parameters affecting scattered radiation propagation, which are external to the device (Carinou et al. 2011). Therefore, operators cannot use such values as an indicator of their likely radiation exposure.

The *invisible* nature of ionizing radiation makes it hard to be aware of radiation exposure and to make optimal use of the radiation protection equipment during a procedure. Proper monitoring of the propagation of scattered radiation and the full-body exposure of staff and patients require to keep track of the three-dimensional (3D) context of the operating room (OR) and imaging parameters, which remains challenging to achieve.

15.3   REDUCING RADIATION EXPOSURE IN THE OR USING AR

Many medical AR systems for enhancing surgical guidance and visualization, and thereby potentially reducing the number of x-ray shots, can be found in the literature. Recently, other works have instead proposed to provide direct visual feedback of radiation's 3D propagation and magnitude using AR to increase radiation awareness. This section reviews recent works on both of these medical applications of AR.

15.3.1   AR TO IMPROVE SURGICAL GUIDANCE AND REDUCE PATIENT/STAFF RADIATION EXPOSURE

Several minimally invasive procedures rely on percutaneous access to inner organs or other tissue, which is generally performed using ultrasound or x-ray imaging for accurately guiding a needle to a target. In the latter case, patient and staff are exposed to a certain amount of radiation depending on the time it takes to reach the target. Such an exposure is higher when fluoroscopy (continuous x-ray imaging) is used to acquire real-time feedback of the needle's trajectory, and, especially in complex procedures, can lead to radiation-induced skin injuries to the patient (Kirkwood et al. 2014). As an alternative, several works have proposed using AR to provide an enhanced visualization of a patient's inner anatomical structures. For instance, Müller et al. (2013) and Seitel et al. (2016) propose to use AR to facilitate the navigation during percutaneous needle insertion and therefore reduce the amount of performed x-ray acquisitions. These approaches rely on the registration of a pre-operative patient's model (CT) to the user's viewpoint, which is achieved either by means of fiducial markers (Müller et al. 2013) or by using the depth data from an Red, Green, Blue-Depth (RGB-D) camera and surface matching algorithms (Seitel et al. 2016). Information such as the insertion trajectory or the target's position can be overlaid onto a video stream serving as guidance visualization during the needle insertion. Similarly, x-ray guidance is crucial during orthopedic and trauma surgery to guide joint replacements, or for the treatment of fractures. To facilitate guidance during such procedures, Navab et al. (2010) propose augmenting a mobile angiographic C-arm with a video camera and mirror construction, as this enables a direct overlay of the x-ray images over the video stream. After a calibration procedure, such a design enables both the camera and the x-ray source centers to be virtually aligned, and therefore to provide an AR visualization of the x-ray images over the video stream. Studies have reported that such an intuitive intraoperative overlay allows surgeons to reduce the number of x-ray acquisitions performed and thereby radiation exposure for several clinical tasks, such as skin incision, entry point localization, and x-ray positioning (Chen et al. 2013).

15.3.2   AR VISUALIZATION OF INTRAOPERATIVE SCATTERED RADIATION

Studies evaluating radiation awareness have reported a considerable proportion of unnecessary exposure and risk underestimation resulting from a lack of awareness and poor knowledge of radiation behavior (Katz et al. 2017). This is partially due to the invisible nature and complex behavior of ionizing radiation. However, appropriate feedback of the current distribution of scattered radiation can increase the awareness of clinical staff and reduce the risk of overexposure. To this end, computer-based systems combining radiation simulation, person tracking, and visualization of radiation in virtual environments have been developed (Bott et al. 2009; Ladikos et al. 2010). Following this line, AR was proposed as a means to render intraoperative ionizing radiation visible (Loy Rodas and Padoy 2015). Through AR, *in situ* visual feedback about the current radiation diffusion can be provided to the user in an intuitive and non-disruptive fashion. As can be seen in Figure 15.2, such a direct visualization enables a clearer understanding of the highly irradiated areas around the operating table and can help optimize the use of protective measures to avoid overexposure. The exposure of the patient or of the clinical staff present in the room can also be visualized in this way (see Figure 15.3).

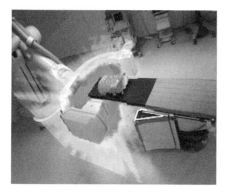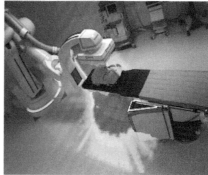

FIGURE 15.2   AR visualization of the 3D diffusion of scattered radiation for two imaging projections: a lateral projection (left) and a posterior-anterior projection (right). Red indicates a higher dose. (From Loy Rodas, N., Context-aware radiation protection for the hybrid operating room. PhD Dissertation, University of Strasbourg, Alsace, France, 2018.)

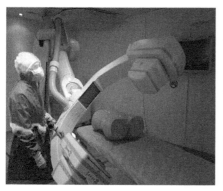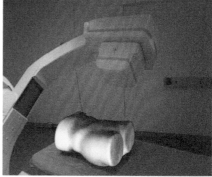

FIGURE 15.3   AR visualization of the body-part dose of clinical staff (left) and of the patient (right) during an Right Anterior Oblique at 135° (RAO135) imaging projection. (From Loy Rodas, N. et al., Pose optimization of a C-arm imaging device to reduce intraoperative radiation exposure of staff and patient during interventional procedures, *IEEE International Conference on Robotics and Automation (ICRA)*, Singapore, 2017.)

The system proposed in Loy Rodas and Padoy (2015) relies on the use of multiple ceiling-mounted RGB-D cameras to perceive and keep track of the current room's layout. A radiation simulation framework applies Monte Carlo methods to compute the propagation of x-rays and the persons' exposure (staff and patient) in the current room conditions. As in Bott et al. (2009), the real imaging parameters (tube kilovoltage, filtration, aperture angle, and beam projection), together with the physics effects modelling the photon interactions that occur at the energy range of x-rays, are considered by the simulation. Additionally, the energy deposited at each voxel of a 3D grid placed around the patient is computed. Then, color and transparency transfer functions are applied to map the energies into RGB/transparency values, enabling to overlay volume rendered radiation isosurfaces on the image. As it can be seen in Figure 15.2, such a visualization provides a clear understanding of the 3D dissemination of scattered radiation and shows intuitively how highly irradiated areas around the patient change according to the device's positioning. Studies have shown that the highest rate of scatter is always produced between the x-ray source and the patient (i.e., backscattering effect) (Carinou et al. 2011). Such a phenomenon can be observed in the visualizations in Figure 15.2. In the left image, which corresponds to a lateral projection, most of the scatter propagates above the table. These visualizations suggest that standing without protection close to the x-ray source should be avoided; this aligns with the radiation safety recommendations from the literature (Koukorava et al. 2011).

Moreover, by applying a background subtraction approach on the depth images, the system can track the position of clinical staff in the room. This is used to compute and display an estimation of the current full-body radiation exposure of each attendee. The points corresponding to the tracked person's shape are colored according to the simulated exposure value at each of its 3D locations. Figure 15.3 shows an example of a person's exposure AR visualization when the x-ray source is positioned over the bed (over-couch). The highest exposure to scattered radiation can be depicted in the person's upper body. Over-couch configurations can generate up to six times more exposure to highly sensitive body parts, such as the thyroid, hands, eyes, and head, and should be avoided (Koukorava et al. 2011). Again, AR provides a clear visualization of an otherwise purely theoretical safety recommendation. Leucht et al. (2015) applied a similar pipeline to provide a visualization of the exposure of the staff's body parts to radiation by means of AR. However, in this case, two RGB-D cameras used for tracking the clinician are physically mounted to a mobile C-arm instead of the ceiling of the room to ensure a more flexible setup.

Figure 15.3 also shows an example of an AR visualization of a patient's exposure obtained with the simulation model from Loy Rodas and Padoy (2015) Red spots can be depicted over an irradiated virtual torso augmented in the image, indicating higher exposure in the areas corresponding to the x-ray beam's entry point. This kind of visualization can be useful to avoid overexposing certain skin areas and/or to sensitize clinicians about the patient's exposure.

15.3.3 Context-aware AR Visualization of Radiation

Facilitating surgical navigation, either by using anatomical landmarks or by AR guidance, can help clinical staff to obtain the required imaging with fewer x-ray shots. In addition to reducing direct radiation exposure and wearing personal protective equipment, knowledge of the direction and magnitude of scatter may help reduce exposure (Katz et al. 2017). Most clinicians working with x-rays have never seen radiation in 3D. Therefore, the use of AR to make ionizing radiation visible and to increase the awareness to radiation exposure is a promising medical application of AR. However, such a novel application has not yet been extensively explored in the literature; hence, we dedicate this section to discussing the challenges and perspectives of an AR system used intraoperatively to provide awareness of radiation exposure.

15.4 MAKING X-RAY RADIATION VISIBLE THROUGH AR: CHALLENGES

A first major challenge for an intraoperative AR radiation safety system is the need to track the many parameters affecting ionizing radiation in real time. Indeed, such a system should be a *context-aware* one. While the current x-ray imaging parameters can be obtained directly from the imaging device's Application Programming Interface (API) (kilovoltage, filtration, collimation, beam projection), a tracking approach is necessary to track the positions of medical equipment and clinicians as well as the disposition of lead protective shields. To this end, vision-based approaches have been applied (Ladikos et al. 2010; Leucht et al. 2015; Loy Rodas and Padoy 2015 but these have not yet proven to be robust enough to overcome the typical challenges encountered in clinical environments (occlusions, illumination, or similarity of colors). However, optical tracking systems could be used to accurately track the positions of lead protective walls, ceiling-suspended shields, and other medical equipment that have a significant impact in the diffusion of ionizing radiation. Such online context tracking should then be considered to simulate radiation. This aspect constitutes a second major challenge, as such a simulation should be performed in real time for a clinical application. While approaches for simulating x-ray propagation using Graphics Processing Unit (GPU)-accelerated methods have been proposed (Badal and Badano 2009; Loy Rodas et al. 2017), the real-time capability of the simulations is dependent on the considered granularity level and the precision required by the application. Indeed, an accurate simulation of the dose to the tissues and/or organs of a patient can take up to a few seconds even on GPU, yet a coarser simulation of the scattered radiation propagation aiming at providing awareness of the highly irradiated areas of the room can be performed in real time (Loy Rodas et al. 2017). Additionally, the simulations need a preoperative model of the patient registered to the same reference frame used in the simulation framework. This would allow showing an intraoperative patient's accumulated dose map through AR similar to that shown in Figure 15.3 but in which all previous irradiations are also considered to avoid overexposing certain skin areas already sensitized due to previous exposure.

Although the use of a patient-specific model would enable the computation of quantitative dose values that would consider the real patient's anatomy, such a model is not always available. However, a generic model may be sufficient to provide qualitative visualizations. In the same way, assessing the exposure of clinicians' body parts to radiation through simulations is challenging. Previous works have modeled clinicians as water boxes to lower computation times (Bott et al. 2009; Loy Rodas and Padoy 2015). However, computing a clinician's accumulated dose per body part requires to estimate and track his/her body pose (Kadkhodamohammadi et al. 2017), register a human model with materials' composition information, and deform that model according to his/her current body pose. Whereas these complex research issues are not within the scope of this book, they remain challenges to consider when bringing this medical AR application to clinical practice.

15.5 VISUALIZATION SOLUTIONS FOR AR-BASED RADIATION SAFETY

As clinicians can already be overwhelmed by the large amount of data and information available during a surgery, key questions to be asked are what would be the best way to present the information for radiation safety while least affecting the clinical workflow and to whom it should be shown (operators, assistant personnel, radiation protection officers etc.). In (Leucht et al. 2015; Loy Rodas and Padoy 2015), the AR visualization is displayed on an external screen. This enables the user to have an overview of the current propagation of radiation and to manually select the viewpoint from where to look at the scene. (Loy Rodas et al. 2016) propose displaying the information related to radiation safety directly in the user's view through a tracked, handheld screen. As shown in Figure 15.4, this gives the impression of seeing radiation "as with one's own eyes," thus enabling a more intuitive visualization.

With the advent of modern optical see-through head-mounted displays (OST-HMD), the typical challenges encountered by mobile AR technologies (indoor mapping, relocalization issues) have now been solved, and commercial devices suitable for medical applications are now available. Indeed, a recent study showed that OST-HMD displays, such as Microsoft's HoloLens, are now suitable enough in terms of contrast perception, task load, and frame rate, for mixed reality surgical interventions (Qian et al. 2017). It is also highlighted that such devices are already used to augment fluoroscopic images directly into the surgeon's view during orthopedics surgery. Indeed, the use of OST-HMDs in surgical scenarios can also reduce the number of performed x-rays and/or fluoroscopy time by facilitating surgical navigation. Furthermore, protective eyewear is commonly used in interventional radiology/cardiology procedures, as the eyes are radiosensitive anatomical structures and even low levels of exposure may induce lens opacities or cataracts (Carinou et al. 2011). An OST-HMD could be designed specifically to simultaneously protect the eyes while also providing an enhanced AR visualization either for radiation awareness (augmenting radiation exposure maps) or for facilitating surgical guidance (augmenting intraoperative images).

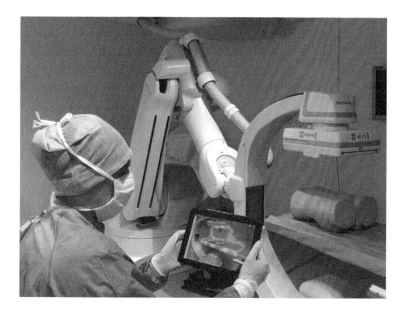

FIGURE 15.4 Mobile AR visualization for radiation awareness using a handheld screen. (From Loy Rodas, N. et al., *IEEE Trans. Biomed. Eng.*, 64, 429–440, 2016.)

Projecting light patterns or holograms on the floor is an alternative to visualizing scattered radiation. The technical feasibility and integration into the clinical workflow will be the criteria to consider for finding an appropriate visualization solution for this application.

15.6 AR AS A TEACHING TOOL FOR RADIATION AWARENESS

Training with real radiation is dangerous and thereby prohibited. Thus, current training is usually based on courses, lectures, and the presentation of theoretical aspects, rather than hands-on training (Katz et al. 2017). Computer-based training and simulation systems have proven to be useful to improve education on C-arm operation and on minimizing radiation exposure (Bott et al. 2009; Katz et al. 2017). Such systems incorporate simulations of scattered radiation computed for a set of user-defined parameters. Visualizations of radiation color maps are then provided over a virtual OR scenario to illustrate the effects that altering parameters such as the imaging device's angulation can have on scatter. Virtual simulators are a good step for moving from theory to practice, yet these are meant to be used outside of the OR. Moreover, it is not possible to simulate every possible scenario that could take place during a real intervention. Teaching about radiation protection with AR would enable to bring the training inside the OR, allowing trainees to learn in real clinical conditions. An AR-based teaching tool could be used in conjunction with interventional surgery training courses or during surgical training involving animals so that trainees can learn *in situ* the effects of the parameters affecting radiation propagation. This also would help with teaching the best radiation safety practices, such as

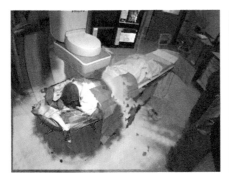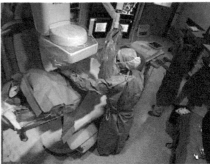

FIGURE 15.5 AR visualization of potential scattered radiation overlaid *a posteriori* for visualization purposes, if the x-ray device was used in such a situation: no lead protective shields (left) and with ceiling/table shields (right) (Loy Rodas 2018) (Strasbourg's University Hospital, Strasbourg, France.)

the proper use of lead protective shields. Studies report that a properly positioned table shield can lead to a reduction of up 99% of the dose to the legs (Koukorava et al. 2011). As shown in Figure 15.5, such knowledge can also be transmitted intuitively by means of AR.

Figure 15.6 shows an example of a radiation awareness prototype system (Loy Rodas 2018) at IHU Strasbourg (France). It is based on Loy Rodas and Padoy (2015), except that the simulations of radiation are performed with GPU-accelerated methods and the system is connected to the angiographic C-arm's API. Therefore, the system has direct access to the device's configuration and can provide an AR visualization of the diffusion of scattered radiation, which is updated in quasi real time as the C-arm parameters change. It can also show a patient's dose map and an AR visualization of the staff's radiation exposure. The system's graphical user interface (depicted in Figure 15.6) is displayed on the surgical screen inside the OR, where users can see the different AR visualizations and interact with the software. Integrating an

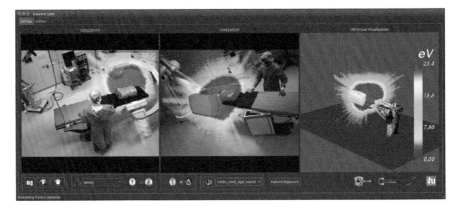

FIGURE 15.6 Radiation awareness demonstrator system (Loy Rodas 2018) at Institut Hospitalo-Universitaire (IHU) Strasbourg, France.

OST-HMD to the system to provide visual feedback directly in the user's view is a feasible and promising step to render such a training tool more intuitive.

15.7 INTEGRATION IN TOMORROW'S FULLY-CONNECTED OR: PERSPECTIVES

Tomorrow's fully context-aware operating and examination rooms will record, process and analyze the large amount of multi-modal surgical data available during a procedure (Maier-Hein et al. 2017). This will enable the development of smart decision-support tools, which will assist healthcare personnel in the performance of routine tasks and permit them to better process and visualize the large amount of information that is generated. Medical AR will be fully integrated into clinical practice and intraoperative images, or other patient data will be augmented directly into the clinicians' view, thus facilitating the performance of image-guided procedures. Radiation awareness systems will also benefit from such knowledge, not only to provide an accurate feedback about the current radiation exposure of staff and patient, but also to correlate such exposure to the underlying activities taking place in the surgical suite. A context-aware radiation safety system will be able to assess the dose generated at each step of the surgery; generate exposure statistics to compare practices among procedures, personnel, and hospitals; and devise safer surgical workflows to enable the minimization of radiation exposure. Such statistics will be computed by considering each person's record of previous exposures to radiation, which will help reduce the risks of the long-term negative effects of exposure.

15.8 CONCLUSION

Recent years have witnessed the appearance of numerous medical AR systems looking to facilitate surgical guidance and data visualization during a surgical procedure. Due to the need to monitor and limit the exposure to ionizing radiation during x-ray guided procedures, a different application for medical AR has recently emerged: the use of AR to reduce the exposure to radiation. Such an application can help to improve the acceptance of x-ray imaging technologies, make the workflow of x-ray guided procedures safer in terms of radiation exposure, and render the benefits of minimally invasive surgery accessible to a wider population. While the development of an intraoperative, context-aware radiation safety system is challenging, the use of AR to facilitate surgical navigation and reduce the number of x-ray shots, or to intuitively teach about radiation diffusion and best protection practices, is feasible today.

REFERENCES

Badal A., Badano A., 2009. Monte Carlo simulation of X-ray imaging using a graphics processing unit. *IEEE Nuclear Science Symposium Conference Record (NSS/MIC)*, IEEE, Orlando, FL, pp. 4081–4084.

Bott O.J., Wagner M., Duwenkamp C., Hellrung N., Dresing K., 2009. Improving education on C-arm operation and radiation protection with a computer-based training and simulation system. *International Journal of Computer Assisted Radiology and Surgery*, 4(4), 399–407.

Carinou E., Brodecki M., Domienik J., Donadille L., Koukorava C., Krim S., Nikodemova D. et al., 2011. Recommendations to reduce extremity and eye lens doses in interventional radiology and cardiology. *Radiation Measurements*, 46(11), 1324–1329.

Chen X., Wang L., Fallavollita P., Navab N., 2013. Precise X-ray and video overlay for augmented reality fluoroscopy. *International Journal of Computer Assisted Radiology and Surgery*, 8(1), 29–38.

Kadkhodamohammadi A., Gangi A., de Mathelin M., Padoy N., 2017. Articulated clinician detection using 3D pictorial structures on RGB-D data. *Medical Image Analysis*, 35, 215–224.

Katz A., Shtub A., Roguin A., 2017. Minimizing ionizing radiation exposure in invasive cardiology safety training for medical doctors. *Journal of Nuclear Engineering and Radiation Science*, 3(3), 030905.

Kirkwood M. L., Arbique G. M., Guild J. B., Timaran C., Valentine R. J., Anderson J. A., 2014. Radiation-induced skin injury after complex endovascular procedures. *Journal of Vascular Surgery*, 60(3), 742–748.

Koukorava C., Carinou E., Ferrari P., Krim S., Struelens L., 2011. Study of the parameters affecting operator doses in interventional radiology using Monte Carlo simulations. *Radiation Measurements*, 46(11), 1216–1222.

Krim S., Brodecki M., Carinou E., Donadille L., Jankowski J., Koukorava C., Dominiek J. et al., 2011. Extremity doses of medical staff involved in interventional radiology and cardiology: Correlations and annual doses (hands and legs). *Radiation Measurements*, 46(11), 1223–1227.

Ladikos A., Cagniart C., Ghotbi R., Reiser M., Navab N., 2010. Estimating radiation exposure in interventional environments. *Medical Image Computing and Computer-Assisted Intervention (MICCAI)*, Springer, Berlin, Germany, 237–244.

Leucht N., Habert S., Wucherer P., Weidert S., Navab N., Fallavollita P., 2015. [POSTER] Augmented reality for radiation awareness. *2015 IEEE International Symposium on Mixed and Augmented Reality*.

Loy Rodas N., 2018. Context-aware radiation protection for the hybrid operating room. PhD Dissertation, University of Strasbourg, Alsace, France.

Loy Rodas N., Barrera F., Padoy N., 2016. See it with your own eyes: Markerless mobile augmented reality for radiation awareness in the hybrid room. *IEEE Transactions on Biomedical Engineering*, 64(2), 429–440.

Loy Rodas N., Bert J., Visvikis D., de Mathelin M., Padoy N., 2017. Pose optimization of a C-arm imaging device to reduce intraoperative radiation exposure of staff and patient during interventional procedures, *IEEE International Conference on Robotics and Automation (ICRA)*, Singapore.

Loy Rodas N., Padoy N., 2015. Seeing is believing: Increasing intraoperative awareness to scattered radiation in interventional procedures by combining augmented reality, Monte Carlo simulations and wireless dosimeters. *International Journal of Computer Assisted Radiology and Surgery*, 10(8), 1181–1191.

Maier-Hein L., Vedula S., Speidel S., Navab N., Kikinis R., Park A., Eisenmann M. et al., 2017. Surgical data science for next-generation interventions. *Nature Biomedical Engineering*, 1(9), 691–696.

Müller M., Rassweiler M., Klein J., Seitel A., Gondan M., Baumhauer M., Teber D., Rassweiler J. J., Meinzer H., Maier-Hein L., 2013. Mobile augmented reality for computer-assisted percutaneous nephrolithotomy. *International Journal of Computer Assisted Radiology and Surgery*, 8(4), 663–675.

Navab N., Heining S. M., Traub J., 2010. Camera augmented mobile C-Arm (CAMC): Calibration, accuracy study, and clinical applications. *IEEE Transactions on Medical Imaging*, 29(7), 1412–1423.

Nikodemová D., Brodecki M., Carinou E., Domienik J., Donadille L., Koukorava C., Krim S. et al., 2011. Staff extremity doses in interventional radiology. Results of the ORAMED measurement campaign. *Radiation Measurements*, 46(11), 1210–1215.

Qian L., Barthel A., Johnson A., Osgood G., Kazanzides P., Navab N., Fuerst B., 2017. Comparison of optical see-through head-mounted displays for surgical interventions with object-anchored 2D-display. *International Journal of Computer Assisted Radiology and Surgery*, 12(6), 901–910.

Roguin A., Goldstein J., Bar O., Goldstein J.A., 2013. Brain and neck tumors among physicians performing interventional procedures. *The American Journal of Cardiology*, 111(9), 1368–1372.

Sailer, A.M., Paulis, L., Vergoossen, L., Kovac A.O., Wijnhoven G., Schurink, G.W.H., Mees B. et al., 2017. Real-time patient and staff radiation dose monitoring in IR practice. *CardioVascular and Interventional Radiology,* 40(3), 421–429.

Seitel A., Bellemann, N., Hafezi, M., Franz A. M., Servatius M., Saffari A., Kilgus T. et al., 2016. Towards markerless navigation for percutaneous needle insertions. *International Journal of Computer Assisted Radiology and Surgery*, 11(1), 107–117.

16 Augmented and Virtual Visualization for Image-Guided Cardiac Therapeutics

Cristian A. Linte, Terry M. Peters,
and Michael S. Sacks

CONTENTS

16.1 INTRODUCTION

The advent of virtual reality and augmented reality (AR) environments in medicine was driven by the need to enhance or enable therapy delivery under limited visualization and restricted access conditions. For most of history, surgery has involved the exposure of the affected organ via typically large incisions, but image guidance has, for the most part, introduced less invasive alternatives for performing traditional interventions. Technological developments and advances in medical therapies have enabled increased use of less invasive treatment approaches for conditions that require treatment via surgical procedures that involve patient trauma and complications.

A cardiac surgeon colleague often says that "surgery is a side-effect of therapy." This statement certainly applies to conventional open-chest, open-heart surgery in which most patient trauma is caused while reaching the target via a median sternotomy, cardio-pulmonary bypass, and cardiac incision. Although this approach affords the surgeon a bloodless environment within which to perform the repair, its efficacy is undetermined until the patient is "closed back up," the cardiopulmonary bypass is disconnected, and heart-lung function is restored.

Concurrent with technological and computational advances, endoscopic imaging (Litynski, 1999) was introduced, which considerably reduced the incision size used for access, and interventional cardiology (Soares and Murphy, 2005) enabled percutaneous treatment under x-ray fluoroscopy or ultrasound (US) image guidance. These developments shifted visual feedback during interventional medicine from direct vision to reliance on medical imaging. Entry into the cardiac chambers is achieved either through the vascular system, with instruments introduced via the femoral artery in the leg, or via the heart wall, typically through the apex, while allowing the heart to remain beating during the procedure and removing the need for major incisions and cardiopulmonary bypass. Cardiac therapy may consist of the replacement or repair of a malfunctioning valve, restoration of myocardial perfusion by inserting a stent or performing a bypass graft, or electrical isolation of tissue regions that cause abnormal heart rhythm by creating scar tissue by heating or freezing.

Cardiac interventions are unique in several perspectives: access, restricted visualization and surgical instrument manipulation, and the dynamic nature of the heart. The invasiveness of the procedure extends beyond the typical measurement of the incision size. Supplying circulatory support via cardiopulmonary bypass (i.e., heart-lung machine) represents a significant source of invasiveness that may lead to severe inflammatory response and neurological damage. Moreover, the delivery of therapy on a soft tissue organ enclosing a blood-filled environment in continuous motion is still a significant challenge. Successful therapy requires versatile instrumentation, robust visualization, and superior surgical skills.

Due to the challenges associated with visualization and access, cardiac interventions have been among the last surgical applications to embrace the movement toward minimal invasiveness (Mack, 2006). This movement originated in the mid-1990s following the introduction of laparoscopic techniques and their use in video-assisted thoracic surgery (Mack et al., 1992).

The adoption of less invasive techniques posed some problems in terms of their workflow integration and yield of clinically acceptable outcomes. However, the morbidity associated with the surgery, together with the success of less invasive approaches in other surgical specialties, have fueled their emergence into cardiac therapy (Linte et al., 2010b). Multiple access routes, including partial sternotomies, limited access thoracotomies, or catheter-based techniques have all been used as an alternative to the traditional full median sternotomy. Initial attempts were aimed at performing coronary artery bypass graft (CABG) surgery via minimally invasive access to the arrested heart without cardiopulmonary bypass. A number of centers reported their experience with robot-assisted atrial septal defect repair, mitral valve (MV) repair and replacement, transluminal or transapical aortic valve implantation or percutaneous pulmonary vein isolation for the treatment of atrial fibrillation. The increasing use of endovascular techniques is one of the most rapid advances in cardiac interventions, rendering vascular-guided interventions as the ultimate, least invasive cardiac therapy approach (Joels et al., 2009).

16.2 IMAGING FOR INTERVENTIONAL CARDIAC GUIDANCE

Medical imaging has provided a means for visualization and guidance during interventions where direct visual feedback cannot be achieved without significant trauma. Similar to traditional image-guided therapeutic systems described by Cleary and Peters (2010), cardiac Image-Guided Interventions (IGI) systems consist of several components: pre- and intraoperative images acquired using different medical imaging modalities; surgical instruments tracked using spatial localization systems; a platform that enables the integration of various images; signals (e.g., electrocardiogram or electrophysiology); and tracking data and their registration to the patient. These systems also incorporate various methods to visualize the multidimensional information and display it to the clinicians to guide the intervention.

In the context of cardiac image guidance, while on-pump, open-chest procedures may benefit from enhanced visualization available through medical imaging, off-pump, beating heart cardiac interventions rely heavily on imaging, thus enabling clinicians to "see" inside the thoracic cavity and heart chambers in the absence of direct visual access.

Preoperative imaging: This procedure is necessary to understand the patient's heart anatomy, identify a suitable treatment approach, and prepare a surgical plan. These data are often in the form of high-quality images that provide sufficient contrast between normal and abnormal tissue (Peters and Cleary, 2008). Three of the most common imaging modalities employed preoperatively are computed tomography (CT), magnetic resonance imaging (MRI), and nuclear medicine.

Intraoperative imaging: Because the surgical sites are inside the closed chest, and often inside the closed, beating heart, they cannot be observed directly. Hence, intraoperative imaging is critical for visualization. While these imaging systems need to operate in real time to provide accurate guidance and be compatible with the standard operating room equipment, they often compromise spatial resolution or image fidelity in favor of real-time operation.

16.3   SURGICAL TRACKING

The tracking technologies most frequently employed in IGI use either optical (Wiles et al., 2004) or electromagnetic (Birkfellner et al., 1998; Frantz et al., 2003; Hummel et al., 2005) approaches. Despite their tracking accuracy on the order of 0.5 mm, the direct line-of-sight requirement associated with optical tracking systems precludes their use for intracardiac interventions. Electromagnetic tracking systems (Franz et al., 2014), on the other hand, do not suffer from such limitations and allow the tracking of flexible instruments inside the body, such as a catheter tip (Linte et al., 2009), endoscope (Frantz et al., 2003; Wood et al., 2005), or a transesophageal echocardiography (TEE) transducer (Wiles et al., 2008). However, their performance may be limited by the presence of ferromagnetic materials in the vicinity of the field generator or inadequate placement of the "surgical field" within the tracking volume. For a more detailed reference to surgical tracking systems and their use in image-guided interventions, we refer the reader to Chapters 2 and 3 of this textbook, which focus on techniques for calibration and registration of tracking systems for intraoperative use.

16.4   NAVIGATION VERSUS POSITIONING IN IMAGE-GUIDED CARDIAC INTERVENTIONS

Linte et al. (2010a) described the concept of the therapy delivery task as a two-stage process: during the initial navigation step, the surgical instrument is brought into the proximity of the target site, while during the subsequent positioning step, the instrument is actually positioned on-target and therapy is delivered. To achieve the desired accuracy and precision, both the navigation and positioning steps are critical, especially when no direct visual guidance is available and the clinician relies on medical imaging and surgical tracking.

16.4.1   TOOL-TO-TARGET NAVIGATION

The preoperative images and anatomical models provide contextual information to identify the region of interest and serve as a road map for instrument navigation. Provided the patient anatomy is registered to the preoperative road map (typically using a tracking system), the surgical instrument representations can be visualized in the same coordinate system as the road map. The navigation step relies implicitly on the preoperative images and models used to provide the surgeon with a "big picture" of the cardiac anatomy, as well as the virtual representations of the surgical instruments whose positions and orientations are encoded by the localization system that is employed.

As most instruments used during cardiac procedures are inserted inside the chest or the heart, electromagnetic rather than optical tracking is typically employed (Linte et al., 2013b, 2010b). Preoperative images are necessary to understand the patient's heart anatomy and navigate the instruments to the region of interest. The most common imaging modalities employed pre-operatively are CT and MRI.

16.4.2 ON-TARGET POSITIONING

The positioning step follows the tool-to-target navigation and entails the accurate and precise manipulation of the target tissue. While the navigation step ensures the surgical instrument is first located in the vicinity of the target to be treated, the positioning step truly ensures accurate targeting and manipulation of the surgical site and is conducted under real-time, intraoperative image guidance. Because the surgical field cannot be observed directly, and the preoperative models and the image/model-to-patient registration are prone to uncertainties, intraoperative imaging such as US, x-ray fluoroscopy, or cone-bean CT are critical for visualization.

The technology must operate in real time to provide accurate guidance and be compatible with the standard OR equipment, but these attributes may only be possible at the expense of spatial resolution or image fidelity. As such, the most common imaging modalities employed intraoperatively are US imaging and x-ray fluoroscopy; the latter is slowly evolving thanks to the recent developments in cone-beam CT technology.

16.5 CLINICAL APPLICATIONS OF IMAGE-GUIDED CARDIAC THERAPEUTICS

16.5.1 VALVULAR INTERVENTIONS

16.5.1.1 Transapical Aortic Valve Replacement (TAVR)

The standard of care for patients with severe aortic valve stenosis is open heart surgery, in which the patient is placed on cardiopulmonary bypass, allowing the surgeon direct tactile and visual access to the surgical target site. However, due to trauma associated with cardiopulmonary bypass and aortic cross clamping, up to one-third of all patients are deemed inoperable due to comorbidities such as pervious cardiac surgeries, chronic lung disease, or renal failure (Iung et al., 2005). In response to this problem, beating heart techniques are being developed. A stent-based, beating-heart aortic valve replacement was first performed in humans in 2002, with over 50,000 cases performed in over 40 countries since then (Haussig et al., 2014). Access to the aortic valve is achieved either transfemorally, via apical entry through the left ventricle (LV) or directly through incision into the descending aorta. The latter two techniques require a mini-thoracotomy for access but provide more direct control of the delivery tool. Stents are either made from a shape-memory alloy or use an inflatable balloon for deployment. Since their inception, a wide variety of devices have come on the market.

Because these procedures are performed while the heart is still beating, surgeons rely on image guidance to safely and effectively perform the therapy. While US (TEE) is ubiquitous in cardiac interventions, it is inadequate as a guidance modality, primarily due to shadow artifacts from the valve stent occluding crucial anatomy (valve nadir and commissures, as well as coronary ostia). Consequently, the TAVR standard of care relies primarily on fluoroscopy, which is the other imaging modality that is ubiquitous in cardiac interventions. Image guidance is crucial to ensure proper stent placement; a stent deployed too far inside the LV may embolize, while

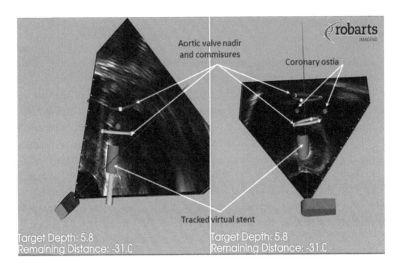

FIGURE 16.1   Mixed reality guidance for transcatheter aortic valve replacement: real-time US image from the TEE probe is integrated with a model of the tracked stent (green) and relevant anatomical landmarks defined using the tracked TEE. Red and green splines defining the valve annulus and commissure regions, and blue and orange spheres mark coronary ostia locations.

a stent deployed too far into the aorta may occlude the coronary ostia. Furthermore, if the stent is not coaxial with the native valve, then there is a significant risk of paravalvular leak.

Commercial systems, such as Siemens DynaCT, use intraoperative C-arm cone beam reconstructions to facilitate optimal valve orientation and positioning during real-time fluoroscopic imaging, while the Philips HeartNavigator system[1] integrates fluoroscopy with echocardiography. Recently, in an attempt to eliminate the need for contrast agents as well as radiation dose to both patient and clinician, researchers have been developing techniques for performing TAVR using echocardiography (TEE) augmented with information from magnetically tracked tools (McLeod et al., 2016). In this technique, magnetic sensors are integrated into or onto both the TEE probe and the catheter delivery tool. The US image data are then augmented with virtual models to indicate the location of relevant tools and patient anatomy (ostia, valve nadir or commissures, Figure 16.1). Segmentations of the aortic root derived from preoperative CT can be registered into the scene if required.

16.5.1.2   MV Applications

MV Modeling for Intraoperative Sizing and Visualization

MV repair has been embraced as the gold standard strategy to treat regurgitation (Braunberger et al., 2001), with the Carpentier's annuloplasty technique

---

[1] https://www.philips.co.uk/healthcare/product/HCOPT20/heartnavigator-planning-and-guidance-software

(David et al., 2013) yielding excellent initial results. The procedure consists of suturing a ring on the MV orifice near the MV annulus hinge region to reduce the orifice size and ensure that the leaflet coaptation completely covers the left atrioventricular cavity (Rausch et al., 2012). Unfortunately, follow-up studies have revealed an undesirable rate of failure and need for repeat MV repair procedures (Acker et al., 2014). This may be attributed to the still existing uncertainty in the optimal shape and size of the annuloplasty rings (Bothe et al., 2013), as well as their peri-operative evaluation prior to insertion during the repair procedure.

Although studies have suggested that patient-specific geometries affect the repair durability and effectiveness (Bouma et al., 2015, 2016), the repair planning process has remained mostly qualitative. It is believed that the complex structure of the MV plays a significant role in the valvular response to the repair (Flameng et al., 2008). Yet isolating the effect of each factor to study the valvular response is feasible neither in *in vitro* nor in *in vivo* animal studies. On the other hand, computational simulations of heart valve behavior have proven to be promising tools to enhance our understanding of the valvular mechanisms and response to pathological alterations (Chandran, 2010; Kheradvar et al., 2015) and their integration into therapy planning or guidance. However, existing computational models have yet to account for all the underlying features that impact MV behavior.

Drach et al. (2018) developed a robust pipeline (Figure 16.2) to build a computational model of MV with a significantly higher level of geometric detail and fidelity. Moreover, the MV model pipeline was extended to enable the building of models with adjustable levels of detail and discretization, thus enabling a framework for multiresolution modeling of MV. This constitutes the first comprehensive study focused on the development of validated, multiresolution, attribute-rich computational models of the MV, while illustrating the benefits of the proposed approach by building a single ovine MV model from *in vitro* data.

Patient-specific virtual models of the MV apparatus generated using this pipeline could be used to plan the repair procedure, as well as augment both the pre- and the intraoperative imaging data with the preprocedural, biomechanical valve repair plan to noninvasively assess and eventually guide the subsequent repair procedure.

Similarly, to support the surgeon during that crucial intraoperative phase, Engelhardt et al. (2016) proposed a computer-based assistance system for exploring and assessing the patient-specific valve geometry (Figure 16.3). The valvular apparatus was assessed by customized instruments located using well-established optical tracking technology (NDI Polaris Spectra®, Northern Digital Inc., Waterloo, Canada). Based on those measurements, morphologic shapes and important distances can be computed for enhancing the surgeon's cognition and three-dimensional (3D) spatial orientation with quantitative information. Moreover, intraoperative support can be provided to assist in surgical decision making, in particular in prosthesis selection and determination of neo-chordae lengths. These digital representations can provide means for documentation of the intraoperative valve geometry and necessary modifications and adjustments that need to be applied to the morphology identified by the surgeon.

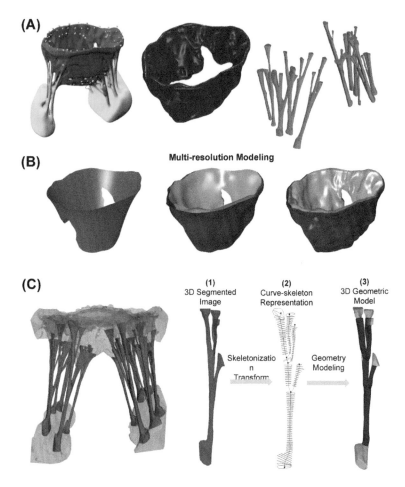

FIGURE 16.2 Data processing steps for constructing multiresolution models of the mitral valve. (A) Model of the mitral valve including leaflets, papillary muscles and chordae tendinae; (B) Multi-scale model of the mitral leaflets; (C) Model of the chordae tendinae obtained by segmenting the chords from 3D images, followed by curve-skeleton representation and refined through geometric modeling. (Courtesy of Michael S. Sacks, PhD, *University of Texas at Austin*.)

MV Repair via Augmented Virtuality Guidance

Just as many patients are judged as high-risk for open-heart aortic valve repair/ replacement, those with functional or degenerative MV disease also may be unable to receive standard of care (on-pump, open-heart surgery) treatment. While MV replacement/implantation devices are widely under development, current options for high-risk patients are limited to MV repair techniques, such as the trans-femoral MitraClip (Abbot Vascular Inc.) and the LV apical access NeoChord (NeoChord Inc.).

Unlike aortic valve replacement, x-ray fluoroscopy is of limited use for guiding MV repairs given the excessive amount of contrast agent required to identify the MV

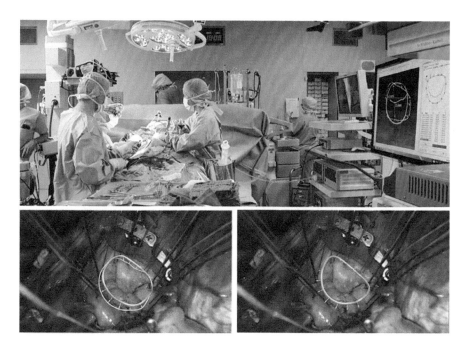

FIGURE 16.3 Proposed assistance system employed in the operating room during a mitral valve repair intervention (*top*). Endoscopic images for annuloplasty ring selection augmented with the patient-specific mitral valve annulus (white) segmented from the transesophageal US images and the virtual ring implant (green) suggested for MV repair (*bottom*). (Courtesy of Sandy Engelhardt, PhD.)

anatomy using this modality. Consequently, beating heart MV repair procedures rely primarily on two-dimensional (2D) and 3D TEE US guidance. In the case of the NeoChord procedure, 2D biplane TEE is used to navigate from the LV apical entry point to the region of the MV. Unfortunately, the limited field-of-view and lower resolution of 3D TEE makes it unsuitable for this stage of the procedure. However, once the device is in the target region, 3D TEE is used to identify the exact target position on the MV leaflet, then the surgeon returns to 2D TEE for the actual grasping of the MV leaflet. In the context of image guidance challenges, the process of final tool positioning and leaflet grasping are well handled by 3D and 2D TEE, respectively.

The NeoNav augmented virtuality guidance platform is an immediate application of the navigation-positioning paradigm, designed to assist with the repair of the MV apparatus by implanting artificial chordae tendinae. The process of safely navigating the tool from its entry site at the LV apex to the mitral apparatus is quite challenging. The NeoNav guidance system uses electromagnetic tracking technology to track and visually integrate real-time US with models of the tool and the anatomy to assist with the navigation and has demonstrated significant improvement in procedure safety and speed (Moore et al., 2013).

Figure 16.4 illustrates the AR view vis-à-vis the traditional, orthogonal, biplane US image guidance display, as well as the total distance traveled by the tool under each user's attempt to navigate the valve repair device from the apex to the mitral

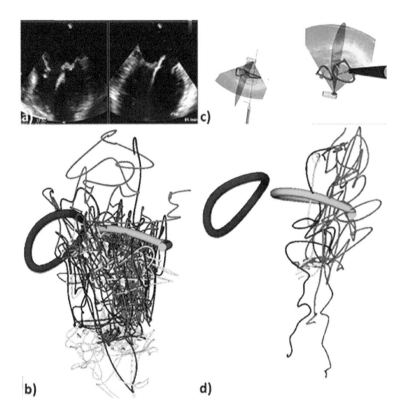

FIGURE 16.4 MV repair navigation assistance via US augmented virtuality. (a) US image guidance alone and (b) tool tip path length during LV apex to mitral apparatus navigation; (c) US-enhanced augmented virtuality platform and (d) corresponding tool tip navigation path, which was accomplished four times faster with many fewer "risky" excursions into the LV outflow tract compared to using US image guidance alone.

apparatus. The traditional biplane US imaging provides minimal intuitive visualization of the anatomy or the interventional instrument, making it difficult to identify the access and target sites and to navigate the instrument from the apex to the mitral apparatus. In contrast, the AR display contains clues such as the mitral and aortic valve annuli locations, which together with the virtual representations of the repair device and US probe, facilitate navigation, as demonstrated by the significantly shorter distance travelled by the repair instrument.

16.5.2 ELECTROPHYSIOLOGY APPLICATIONS: CARDIAC ABLATION PLANNING, VISUALIZATION, GUIDANCE, AND MONITORING

Catheter-based tissue ablation interventions for treatment of arrhythmic conditions still rely heavily on x-ray fluoroscopy guidance despite the limited visualization it provides. The intracardiac ablation path is typically planned prior to the procedure but cannot be faithfully reproduced during the intervention. This difficulty arises because of the lack of sufficient visualization and navigation information for accurate targeting, as well as the lack of information with regards to the geometry and pathophysiology of the ablation lesions. In these cases, despite the complex planning of the planned irreversible isolation of the electrical pathway, patient sequelae are temporary edema and recurring arrhythmia requiring continued treatment and further procedural interventions.

The prototype system for advanced visualization for image-guided left atrial ablation therapy developed at the Biomedical Imaging Resource (Mayo Clinic, Rochester, MN, USA) (Rettmann et al., 2009) uses an architecture that allows the integration of pre- and intraoperative imaging, catheter localization, and electrophysiology information into a single user interface. While sufficiently general to be utilized in various catheter procedures, the system has been primarily tested and evaluated for the treatment of left atrial fibrillation.

The system interfaces to a commercial cardiac mapping system that relays catheter position and orientation information, while the user interface displays a surface-rendered, patient-specific model of the left atrium (LA) and associated pulmonary veins (PV). These are segmented from a preoperative, contrast-enhanced CT scan, along with a point cloud sampled intraoperatively from the endocardial left atrial surface using the tracked catheter. The model-to-patient registration is initialized using a set of anatomical landmarks and continuously updated during the procedure as additional endocardial points are sampled within the left atrium (Rettmann et al., 2011). These data are further augmented with real-time US images acquired using a tracked intracardiac echocardiography (ICE) probe; the images are displayed relative to the left atrial model registered to the patient (Figure 16.5).

In addition, a fast and accurate surrogate thermal model that predicts the lesion geometry and lesion quality (extent of reversible and irreversible thermal damage induced in the tissue) is used to provide a clear visualization of the superimposed lesion on the anatomical model. This surrogate ablation lesion model can display lesion representations in near real time, thus facilitating ablation lesion monitoring and providing cues with regards to the delivery of subsequent ablation lesions to avoid incomplete isolation of the arrhythmic pathway (Linte et al., 2013a). The lesion characterization information can be presented to the clinician in the form of local temperature and exposure maps superimposed onto the patient-specific left atrial model.

16.5.3 ROBOT-ASSISTED INTERVENTIONS

16.5.3.1 Image-Guided Planning Correction for Robot-Assisted Coronary Artery Bypass Graft (CABG)

In current clinical practice, a pre-operative computed tomography (CT) scan of the patient is used to assess candidacy for undergoing a Robot-Assisted Coronary Artery Bypass Graft (RA-CABG) procedure. Based on the preoperative scan, the surgeon identifies the location of the surgical target—the left anterior descending (LAD)—coronary artery, examines whether there is sufficient workspace inside the chest wall for the robot arms, and ultimately estimates the optimal locations of the port

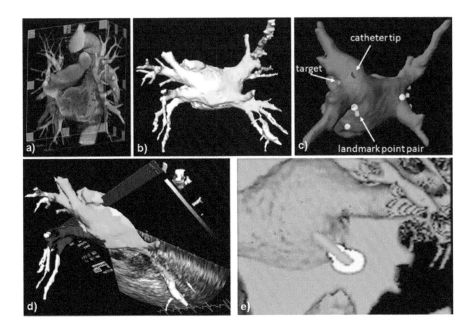

FIGURE 16.5   Prototype image guidance platform for left atrial ablation therapy. (a) volume-rendered CT image; (b) left atrial electro-anatomical (EAM) model; (c) EAM-to-patient registration; (d) integration of real-time ICE images with EAM; (e) superposition of model-predicted ablation lesion characterization onto the EAM used for guidance.

incisions to ensure proper reach of the surgical targets with the robotic instruments. However, it is not unusual that after setting up the patient for the robot-assisted procedure, the surgeon encounters difficulties in reaching the target, and/or robot arm collisions or reduced dexterity (Trejos et al., 2007). In fact, during the procedure, 20%–30% of the RA-CABG interventions require conversion to traditional open-chest surgery (Damiano, 2007), mainly due to the migration of the heart due to lung collapse and chest insufflation; these workflow steps are necessary to create more working volume for the robotic instruments inside the thoracic cavity.

To prevent erroneous planning, it is critical to estimate the global heart displacement during the typical perioperative workflow and use this information to augment or update the original plan based on the original CT image. To address this clinical challenge, Cho et al. (2012) developed a feasible approach to "image" a patient's heart at each perioperative workflow stage using tracked US and to estimate its global displacement. They also developed a technique to register the preoperative instance of the heart (containing the true LAD location identified from the CT dataset [Figure 16.6]) to the perioperatively acquired instances, thus ultimately predicting the intraoperative LAD location.

Cho and colleagues used real-time, 2D TEE to monitor the heart during the interventional workflow. The images were acquired using a spatially tracked TEE probe modified by embedding a 6 DOF NDI Aurora magnetic sensor coil (Northern Digital Inc., Waterloo, Canada) inside the casing of the transducer (Moore et al., 2010).

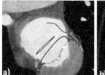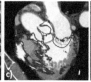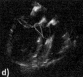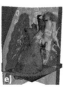

FIGURE 16.6 Preoperative planning stage showing patient's cardiac CT scan with the coronary vessel displayed relative to the valve annuli (a) and the port placement to ensure proper reach of the target vessel with the robotic instruments (b), where the yellow lines represent intercostal spaces; (c) registration of tracked TEE image acquired following intubation (under dual lung ventilation) to preoperative CT image acquired under dual lung ventilation; (d) tracked TEE images acquired following after lung collapse and CO_2 chest insufflation; (e) heart migration during perioperative workflow: dual lung ventilation (red), single lung ventilation (green), and following CO_2 chest insufflation (blue). (Adapted from Cho, D.S. et al., *Med. Phys.*, 39, 1579–1587, 2012.)

These studies suggested that the heart undergoes considerable displacement during the workflow, as shown in Figure 16.6, which must be accounted for during the planning process.

This information is critical for integrating the port placement planning during a robot-assisted intervention using a technique such as that described by Marmurek et al. (2006), which facilitated the use of a laser projection system to augment a direct view of the patient's thorax with the predicted (and in this case updated) port placement configuration to ensure optimal reaching of the desired targets.

16.5.3.2 Augmenting Visualization with Robot Assistance for Cardiac Therapy

While robot-assisted instruments and devices have been developed to reduce incision size, to access hard-to-reach targets, and increase precision and accuracy during target manipulation, they need integrated augmented imaging and visualization as a substitute for direct vision.

Concurrent with developments in augmented and mixed reality visualization for image guidance, catheter-based percutaneous procedures have also advanced, with several cardiac procedures being performed using robot-assisted systems. Hansen Medical Inc. (Mountain View, CA, USA) offers the Sensei X Robotic Navigation System designed for electrophysiology interventions (Antoniou et al., 2011); it features a visualization module that incorporates real-time imaging and 3D electroanatomical mapping, together with a manually controlled input device for catheter motion control. The NIOBE Magnetic Navigation System (Stereotaxis, St Louis, MO, USA) is another remote catheter navigation system operated by a magnetic field created by two computer-controlled 0.08 T permanent magnets (Miyazaki et al., 2010). Lastly, a new magnetically controlled system that utilizes a technology of dynamically shaped magnetic fields was introduced (Catheter Guidance Control and Imaging, Magnetec, Los Angeles, CA, USA) (Gang et al., 2011). The system can be operated in a manual magnetic mode using a joystick-type controller or in automated mode by advancing the catheter along a planned path until firm and continuous tissue contact is achieved.

Most of these interventions entail tissue ablation rather than tissue reconstructive procedures. This trend has primarily been enabled by the limitations of current robotic catheter designs to firmly apply significant force in a lateral direction from the axis of the catheter and to provide sufficiently stable position control to enable tissue manipulation. While there have been significant efforts toward providing minimally invasive visualization for tissue manipulation, the lack of suitable instrumentation impairs the surgeon's ability to manipulate, excise, repair, and remove tissue during complex cardiac procedures. Dupont and his team (Vasilyev et al., 2012) developed and demonstrated concentric tube robot-assisted instruments for tissue approximation, tissue removal, and tissue tracking-based motion compensation.

16.5.4 MR-GUIDED CARDIAC THERAPEUTIC INTERVENTIONS

Although interventional MRI may not be a direct example of augmented or mixed reality, it nevertheless enables guidance of cardiac interventions in a less invasive fashion using patient-specific images acquired in real time and inherently registered to the patient. While the images used for guidance are real and acquired in real time, they are classified as virtual visualization, as no direct view of the interventional site is achieved during MR-guided procedures.

Standard cardiac MR techniques, such as 3D anatomical imaging, cardiac function and flow, parameter mapping, and delayed-enhanced imaging provide valuable clinical data at various procedural stages, especially when augmented with rapid intraprocedural image analysis, thus enabling the extraction and highlighting of critical information about interventional targets and outcomes. Real-time interactive imaging can be used to provide a continuous stream of images displayed to the interventionalist for dynamic device navigation. Interventional devices also can be visualized and tracked throughout a procedure using specialized imaging methods. Operating in such sophisticated environments requires coordination and planning. In their review, Campbell-Washburn et al. (2017) provide an overview of the imaging technology used in MRI-guided cardiac interventions, including clinical targets, image acquisition and analysis tools, and the integration of these tools into clinical workflows.

Setting up an interventional MRI suite or retrofitting an existing suite requires careful planning. Although colocation of interventional MRI facilities with catheterization labs or diagnostic suites facilitates access and streamlines safe bidirectional patient transfer, particularly in the case of combined x-ray/MRI (XMR) procedures, combined suites are designed and equipped with RF-shielded sliding doors to allow direct patient transfer and independent use of facilities.

Wide-bore MRI scanners are ergonomically preferred for interventional applications, enabling interventionists to reach into the scanner bore. To address the ergonomic challenges of patient access in conventional closed-bore scanners, Tavallaei and colleagues (2016) proposed a remote catheter navigation system that allows remote manipulation of the catheter with three degrees of freedom in real time and under MRI guidance.

The capacity to visualize 3D anatomy to facilitate device and catheter navigation and the capacity to assess myocardial tissue as well as local hemodynamics before and immediately after procedures will drive the adoption of interventional MR for congenital, ischemic, and structural heart disease, as well as complex arrhythmias.

16.5.5 IMAGE-GUIDED CARDIAC RESYNCHRONIZATION THERAPY

Coronary artery revascularization (CAR) and cardiac resynchronization therapy (CRT) may improve systolic performance, survival, and quality of life in patients with left ventricular dysfunction. However, the presence and extent of myocardial scar within the relevant vascular targets may reduce clinical response to therapy. 3D vascular imaging techniques, such as coronary CT or MR angiography can be used to characterize vascular targets and to plan both CAR and CRT interventions. Moreover, vascular images can be augmented with spatially matched 3D myocardial scar imaging to provide 3D maps of both relevant vascular structures and related myocardial scar (Figure 16.7).

Revascularization procedures are performed using either percutaneous, fluoroscopically-guided delivery of coronary stents, or surgically through CABG. The preprocedural vascular-scar models have the potential to guide the selection of vascular targets based on the viability of the tissue in the respective territories (White et al., 2006). Therefore, a simultaneous, augmented display of such models during fluoroscopic procedures may be clinically valuable. This information is also relevant to the delivery of the coronary sinus pacemaker leads for resynchronization therapy. These leads are fluoroscopically guided into branches of the coronary venous system to advance the mechanical activation of delayed myocardial segments. To ensure delivery of the coronary sinus lead to the most delayed myocardial segment that does not feature any scar tissue, one potential solution is to augment the intraoperative x-ray fluoroscopy imaging with multicomponent cardiac models featuring myocardial scar maps. However, the future development of lead guidance approaches that integrate vascular models, scar distribution, and activation maps needs more research.

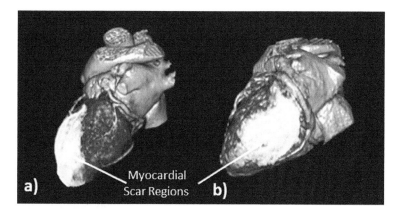

FIGURE 16.7 Volume rendering of fused 3D myocardial scar imaging and coronary Magnetic Resonance Angiography (MRA) datasets featuring prior myocardial infarction referred for CRT. (a) Lateral wall vein without underlying scar despite extensive infarction of the anterior wall; (b) extensive infarction of the lateral wall but a viable anterior wall beneath the anterior interventricular vein.

16.6 SUMMARY AND FUTURE DIRECTIONS

Image-guided cardiac therapeutic technology continues to develop, stimulated both by improvements in computing and image-processing capabilities, hardware to support tracking and visualization, including augmented and mixed reality, as well as an increasing number of clinicians willing to embrace nontraditional technologies. As the push towards less invasive cardiac therapies continues, image-guided intracardiac visualization is experiencing wider adoption and increased clinical exposure, as it has the potential to improve the precision and outcome of surgical procedures. However, wider clinical acceptance of this technology only will occur through close partnerships between scientists, cardiologists, and surgeons, compelling studies that conclusively demonstrate major benefits in terms of patient outcome and cost and a commitment from the manufacturers of therapeutic devices and imaging technology to support these concepts.

REFERENCES

Acker, M.A., Parides, M.K., Perrault, L.P., Moskowitz, A.J., Gelijns, A.C., Voisine, P., Smith, P.K. et al., 2014. Mitral-valve repair versus replacement for severe ischemic mitral regurgitation. *N. Engl. J. Med.* 370, 23–32. doi:10.1056/NEJMoa1312808.

Antoniou, G.A., Riga, C.V., Mayer, E.K., Cheshire, N.J.W., Bicknell, C.D., 2011. Clinical applications of robotic technology in vascular and endovascular surgery. *J. Vasc. Surg.* 53, 493–499. doi:10.1016/j.jvs.2010.06.154.

Birkfellner, W., Watzinger, F., Wanschitz, F., Enislidis, G., Kollmann, C., Rafolt, D., Nowotny, R., Ewers, R., Bergmann, H., 1998. Systematic distortions in magnetic position digitizers. *Med. Phys.* 25, 2242–2248. doi:10.1118/1.598425.

Bothe, W., Miller, D.C., Doenst, T., 2013. Sizing for mitral annuloplasty: Where does science stop and voodoo begin? *Ann. Thorac. Surg.* 95, 1475–1483. doi:10.1016/j.athoracsur.2012.10.023.

Bouma, W., Aoki, C., Vergnat, M., Pouch, A.M., Sprinkle, S.R., Gillespie, M.J., Mariani, M.A., Jackson, B.M., Gorman, R.C., Gorman, J.H., 2015. Saddle-shaped annuloplasty improves leaflet coaptation in repair for ischemic mitral regurgitation. *Ann. Thorac. Surg.* 100, 1360–1366. doi:10.1016/j.athoracsur.2015.03.096.

Bouma, W., Lai, E.K., Levack, M.M., Shang, E.K., Pouch, A.M., Eperjesi, T.J., Plappert, T.J. et al., 2016. Preoperative three-dimensional valve analysis predicts recurrent ischemic mitral regurgitation after mitral annuloplasty. *Ann. Thorac. Surg.* 101, 567–575; discussion 575. doi:10.1016/j.athoracsur.2015.09.076.

Braunberger, E., Deloche, A., Berrebi, A., Abdallah, F., Celestin, J.A., Meimoun, P., Chatellier, G., Chauvaud, S., Fabiani, J.N., Carpentier, A., 2001. Very long-term results (more than 20 years) of valve repair with carpentier's techniques in nonrheumatic mitral valve insufficiency. *Circulation* 104, 8–11.

Campbell-Washburn, A.E., Tavallaei, M.A., Pop, M., Grant, E.K., Chubb, H., Rhode, K., Wright, G.A., 2017. Real-time MRI guidance of cardiac interventions. *J. Magn. Reson. Imaging* 46, 935–950. doi:10.1002/jmri.25749.

Chandran, K.B., 2010. Role of computational simulations in heart valve dynamics and design of valvular prostheses. *Cardiovasc. Eng. Technol.* 1, 18–38. doi:10.1007/s13239-010-0002-x.

Cho, D.S., Linte, C., Chen, E.C.S., Bainbridge, D., Wedlake, C., Moore, J., Barron, J., Patel, R., Peters, T., 2012. Predicting target vessel location on robot-assisted coronary artery bypass graft using CT to ultrasound registration. *Med. Phys.* 39, 1579–1587. doi:10.1118/1.3684958.

Cleary, K., Peters, T.M., 2010. Image-guided interventions: Technology review and clinical applications. *Annu. Rev. Biomed. Eng.* 12, 119–142.

Damiano, R.J., 2007. Robotics in cardiac surgery: The emperor's new clothes. *J. Thorac. Cardiovasc. Surg.* 134, 559–561. doi:10.1016/j.jtcvs.2006.08.026.

David, T.E., Armstrong, S., McCrindle, B.W., Manlhiot, C., 2013. Late outcomes of mitral valve repair for mitral regurgitation due to degenerative disease. *Circulation* 127, 1485–1492. doi:10.1161/CIRCULATIONAHA.112.000699.

Drach, A., Khalighi, A.H., Sacks, M.S., 2018. A comprehensive pipeline for multi-resolution modeling of the mitral valve: Validation, computational efficiency, and predictive capability. *Int. J. Numer. Methods Biomed. Eng.* doi:10.1002/cnm.2921.

Engelhardt, S., Wolf, I., Al-Maisary, S., Schmidt, H., Meinzer, H.-P., Karck, M., De Simone, R., 2016. Intraoperative quantitative mitral valve analysis using optical tracking technology. *Ann. Thorac. Surg.* 101, 1950–1956. doi:10.1016/j.athoracsur.2016.01.018.

Flameng, W., Meuris, B., Herijgers, P., Herregods, M.-C., 2008. Durability of mitral valve repair in Barlow disease versus fibroelastic deficiency. *J. Thorac. Cardiovasc. Surg.* 135, 274–282. doi:10.1016/j.jtcvs.2007.06.040.

Frantz, D.D., Wiles, A.D., Leis, S.E., Kirsch, S.R., 2003. Accuracy assessment protocols for electromagnetic tracking systems. *Phys. Med. Biol.* 48, 2241–2251.

Franz, A.M., Haidegger, T., Birkfellner, W., Cleary, K., Peters, T.M., Maier-Hein, L., 2014. Electromagnetic tracking in medicine—A review of technology, validation, and applications. *IEEE Trans. Med. Imaging* 33, 1702–1725. doi:10.1109/TMI.2014.2321777.

Gang, E.S., Nguyen, B.L., Shachar, Y., Farkas, L., Farkas, L., Marx, B., Johnson, D., Fishbein, M.C., Gaudio, C., Kim, S.J., 2011. Dynamically shaped magnetic fields: Initial animal validation of a new remote electrophysiology catheter guidance and control system. *Circ. Arrhythm. Electrophysiol.* 4, 770–777. doi:10.1161/CIRCEP.110.959692.

Haussig, S., Schuler, G., Linke, A., 2014. Worldwide TAVI registries: What have we learned? *Clin. Res. Cardiol. Off. J. Ger. Card. Soc.* 103, 603–612. doi:10.1007/s00392-014-0698-y.

Hummel, J.B., Bax, M.R., Figl, M.L., Kang, Y., Maurer, C., Birkfellner, W.W., Bergmann, H., Shahidi, R., 2005. Design and application of an assessment protocol for electromagnetic tracking systems. *Med. Phys.* 32, 2371–2379. doi:10.1118/1.1944327.

Iung, B., Cachier, A., Baron, G., Messika-Zeitoun, D., Delahaye, F., Tornos, P., Gohlke-Bärwolf, C., Boersma, E., Ravaud, P., Vahanian, A., 2005. Decision-making in elderly patients with severe aortic stenosis: Why are so many denied surgery? *Eur. Heart J.* 26, 2714–2720. doi:10.1093/eurheartj/ehi471.

Joels, C.S., Langan, E.M., Cull, D.L., Kalbaugh, C.A., Taylor, S.M., 2009. Effects of increased vascular surgical specialization on general surgery trainees, practicing surgeons, and the provision of vascular surgical care. *J. Am. Coll. Surg.* 208, 692–697, NaN-699. doi:10.1016/j.jamcollsurg.2008.12.029.

Kheradvar, A., Groves, E.M., Falahatpisheh, A., Mofrad, M.K., Hamed Alavi, S., Tranquillo, R., Dasi, L.P. et al., 2015. Emerging trends in heart valve engineering: Part IV. Computational modeling and experimental studies. *Ann. Biomed. Eng.* 43, 2314–2333. doi:10.1007/s10439-015-1394-4.

Linte, C.A., Camp, J.J., Holmes, D.R., Rettmann, M.E., Robb, R.A., 2013a. Toward online modeling for lesion visualization and monitoring in cardiac ablation therapy. *Med. Image Comput. Comput. Assist. Interv.* 16, 9–17.

Linte, C.A., Davenport, K.P., Cleary, K., Peters, C., Vosburgh, K.G., Navab, N., Edwards, P.J. et al., 2013b. On mixed reality environments for minimally invasive therapy guidance: Systems architecture, successes and challenges in their implementation from laboratory to clinic. *Comp. Med. Imag. Graph* 37, 83–97.

Linte, C.A., Moore, J., Wedlake, C., Peters, T.M., 2010a. Evaluation of model-enhanced ultrasound-assisted interventional guidance in a cardiac phantom. *IEEE Trans. Biomed. Eng.* 57, 2209–2218. doi:10.1109/TBME.2010.2050886.

Linte, C.A., Moore, J., Wiles, A.D., Wedlake, C., Peters, T.M., 2009. Targeting accuracy under model-to-subject misalignments in model-guided cardiac surgery. *Med. Image Comput. Comput. Assist. Interv.* 12, 361–368.

Linte, C.A., White, J., Eagleson, R., Guiraudon, G.M., Peters, T.M., 2010b. Virtual and augmented medical imaging environments: Enabling technology for minimally invasive cardiac interventional guidance. *IEEE Rev. Biomed. Eng.* 3, 25–47. doi:10.1109/RBME.2010.2082522.

Litynski, G.S., 1999. Endoscopic surgery: The history, the pioneers. *World J. Surg.* 23, 745–753.

Mack, M.J., 2006. Minimally invasive cardiac surgery. *Surg. Endosc.* 20 (Suppl 2), S488–S492. doi:10.1007/s00464-006-0110-8.

Mack, M.J., Aronoff, R.J., Acuff, T.E., Douthit, M.B., Bowman, R.T., Ryan, W.H., 1992. Present role of thoracoscopy in the diagnosis and treatment of diseases of the chest. *Ann. Thorac. Surg.* 54, 403–408–409.

Marmurek, J., Wedlake, C., Pardasani, U., Eagleson, R., Peters, T., 2006. Image-guided laser projection for port placement in minimally invasive surgery. *Stud. Health Technol. Inform.* 119, 367–372.

McLeod, A.J., Currie, M.E., Moore, J.T., Bainbridge, D., Kiaii, B.B., Chu, M.W.A., Peters, T.M., 2016. Phantom study of an ultrasound guidance system for transcatheter aortic valve implantation. *Comput. Med. Imaging Graph. Off. J. Comput. Med. Imaging Soc.* 50, 24–30. doi:10.1016/j.compmedimag.2014.12.001.

Miyazaki, S., Shah, A.J., Xhaët, O., Derval, N., Matsuo, S., Wright, M., Nault, I. et al., 2010. Remote magnetic navigation with irrigated tip catheter for ablation of paroxysmal atrial fibrillation. *Circ. Arrhythm. Electrophysiol.* 3, 585–589. doi:10.1161/CIRCEP.110.957803.

Moore, J., Wiles, A., Wedlake, C., Kiaii, B., Peters, T.M., 2010. Integration of transesophageal echocardiography with magnetic tracking technology for cardiac interventions, in: *Proceedings of the SPIE Medical Imaging 2010: Visualization, Image-Guided Procedures and Modeling*, San Diego, CA, p. 76252Y–1–10.

Moore, J.T., Chu, M.W.A., Kiaii, B., Bainbridge, D., Guiraudon, G., Wedlake, C., Currie, M., Rajchl, M., Patel, R.V., Peters, T.M., 2013. A navigation platform for guidance of beating heart transapical mitral valve repair. *IEEE Trans. Biomed. Eng.* 60, 1034–1040. doi:10.1109/TBME.2012.2222405.

Peters, T., Cleary, K. (Eds.), 2008. *Image-Guided Interventions Technology and Applications.* Springer Science+Business Media, New York.

Rausch, M.K., Bothe, W., Kvitting, J.-P.E., Swanson, J.C., Miller, D.C., Kuhl, E., 2012. Mitral valve annuloplasty. *Ann. Biomed. Eng.* 40, 750–761. doi:10.1007/s10439-011-0442-y.

Rettmann, M.E., Holmes III, D.R., Packer, D.L., Robb, R.A., 2011. Incorporating a Gaussian model at the catheter tip for improved registration of preoperative surface models. In: Wong, K.H., Holmes III, D.R. (Eds.), p. 796411. doi:10.1117/12.879242.

Rettmann, M.E., Holmes, D.R., 3rd, Cameron, B.M., Robb, R.A., 2009. An event-driven distributed processing architecture for image-guided cardiac ablation therapy. *Comput. Methods Programs Biomed.* 95, 95–104. doi:10.1016/j.cmpb.2009.01.009.

Soares, G.M., Murphy, T.P., 2005. Clinical interventional radiology: Parallels with the evolution of general surgery. *Semin. Interv. Radiol.* 22, 10–14.

Tavallaei, M.A., Lavdas, M.K., Gelman, D., Drangova, M., 2016. Magnetic resonance imaging compatible remote catheter navigation system with 3 degrees of freedom. *Int. J. Comput. Assist. Radiol. Surg.* 11, 1537–1545. doi:10.1007/s11548-015-1337-4.

Trejos, A.L., Patel, R.V., Ross, I., Kiaii, B., 2007. Optimizing port placement for robot-assisted minimally invasive cardiac surgery. *Int. J. Med. Robot. Comput. Assist. Surg. MRCAS* 3, 355–364. doi:10.1002/rcs.158.

Vasilyev, N.V., Dupont, P.E., del Nido, P.J., 2012. Robotics and imaging in congenital heart surgery. *Future Cardiol.* 8, 285–296. doi:10.2217/fca.12.20.

White, J.A., Yee, R., Yuan, X., Krahn, A., Skanes, A., Parker, M., Klein, G., Drangova, M., 2006. Delayed enhancement magnetic resonance imaging predicts response to cardiac resynchronization therapy in patients with intraventricular dyssynchrony. *J. Am. Coll. Cardiol.* 48, 1953–1960. doi:10.1016/j.jacc.2006.07.046.

Wiles, A.D., Moore, J., Linte, C.A., Wedlake, C., Ahmad, A., Peters, T.M., 2008. Object identification accuracy under ultrasound enhanced virtual reality for minimally invasive cardiac surgery. 69180E–69180E–12. doi:10.1117/12.773178.

Wiles, A.D., Thompson, D.G., Frantz, D.D., 2004. Accuracy assessment and interpretation for optical tracking systems. *Presented at the Medical Imaging 2004: Visualization, Image-Guided Procedures, and Display, International Society for Optics and Photonics*, pp. 421–433. doi:10.1117/12.536128.

Wood, B.J., Zhang, H., Durrani, A., Glossop, N., Ranjan, S., Lindisch, D., Levy, E. et al., 2005. Navigation with electromagnetic tracking for interventional radiology procedures: A feasibility study. *J. Vasc. Interv. Radiol. JVIR* 16, 493–505. doi:10.1097/01.RVI.0000148827.62296.B4.

17 3D Augmented Reality-Based Surgical Navigation and Intervention

Zhencheng Fan, Cong Ma, Xinran Zhang, and Hongen Liao

CONTENTS

17.1 INTRODUCTION

An operation is easily influenced by complex anatomical structures in the intra-operative surgical scene. To guarantee the safety and accuracy of the surgery, image-guided systems, which provide preoperative medical data, such as magnetic resonance imaging (MRI) and computed tomography (CT), have been applied widely in surgery. Spatial information of the surgical tools is also shown in the guidance interface after registration, so with the assistance of information from preoperative data and intraoperative tools, surgeons can have a better understanding of the spatial relationships between critical structures, surgical targets, and tools (Cleary and Peters 2010; Fan et al. 2017c). However, common image-guided systems mainly consist of a two-dimensional (2D) display located away from the surgical scene. Consequently, surgeons must keep switching focus and attention between the 2D display and the actual surgical scene, significantly reducing the operation's efficiency and accuracy (Zhang et al. 2016).

To solve the problems mentioned above, an augmented reality (AR) system has been utilized for surgical navigation and intervention (DiGioia et al. 1998). Surgeons can both observe the navigation information and the surgical scene without eye-hand coordination problems. The AR component includes both 2D and three-dimensional (3D) approaches. With a 2D AR system, surgeons can only observe the surgical scene with 2D cross-sectional mages using a 2D image overlay method or a 2D image projection method. Reflected images in the 2D image overlay appear in a correct position using a half-silvered mirror, and an accurate registration procedure is utilized to reflect the 2D image in the desired plane, while an accurate 2D image can be projected on the surgical scene using a projector and an image redistortion procedure. In contrast to 2D AR systems, 3D AR can provide 3D information that is important for intuitive observation and operation (Liao et al. 2004b). Surgeons can observe the surgical scene with 3D navigation information and depth information. In this case, the spatial relationships between the surgical targets, the anatomical structure, and the surgical tool can be identified easily.

Generally, a 3D AR system includes either a binocular-based 3D AR system or a 3D autostereoscopic AR system. With the assistance of supplementary glasses, a binocular 3D AR system can provide 3D images simulating binocular vision. However, observers tend to suffer from visual and physical fatigue due to the supplementary glasses. Moreover, the 3D image reconstructed from two 2D images with parallax may present inaccurate spatial information because it can be easily affected by observers, which makes it unsuitable for accurate observation and operation during surgery. To overcome the eye-hand coordination problem and provide surgeons with intuitive 3D images with accurate spatial information, the 3D autostereoscopic AR system is being used more often. One promising version of 3D autostereoscopic AR systems, an Integral Videography (IV)-based 3D AR technique, has been proposed to present intuitive "see-through" images with full parallax, continuous viewing directions, and simple implementation (Liao et al. 2000, 2004b). Surgeons can look through the half-silvered mirror to observe the reflected 3D autostereoscopic images overlaid onto the real scene. Accurate patient-image registration methods that consider the optical apparatus setup ensure that the reflected images can be superimposed in the correct position. Multiple surgeons can observe the 3D AR scene intuitively without any special tracking devices or special glasses.

17.2 3D IV AR FOR SURGERY

Compared to other modes for image-guided surgery, 3D IV AR surgery has some distinct advantages. It offers surgeons intuitive autostereoscopic image guidance, which is generated through a computer generated integral videography (CGIV) algorithm. Using the guidance of the 3D IV AR system, the invasiveness of the surgery can be reduced, and the surgical accuracy can be improved. The 3D IV AR system

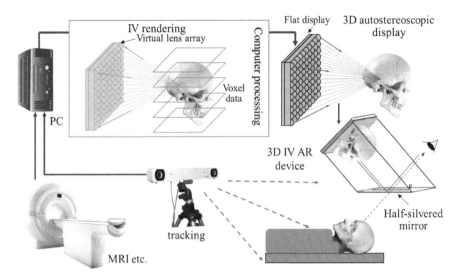

FIGURE 17.1 System configuration of 3D IV AR system. (From Liao et al. 2004b.)

includes three main parts: 3D image rendering and display, a 3D AR system and real-time tracking of targets such as patients, and surgical instruments (Figure 17.1) (Liao et al. 2014b).

17.2.1 3D Image Rendering and Display

The 3D autostereoscopic image is rendered and displayed using an IV technique. For the rendering process, light rays from the 3D image are modified by the microconvex lens array (MLA) and recorded on the elemental image array (EIA). Conventional IV employs an optical pickup method to render the EIA (Lippmann 1908). With the development of computer graphics (CG) techniques, the rendering process can be operated by simulating the light rays on the computer. The central EIA computer generation algorithms consist of the point ray-tracing rendering (PRR) algorithm (Liao et al. 2004a), real-time pickup method (Okano et al. 1997), and multiview rendering algorithm (Liao et al. 2011). The PRR algorithm, the most common CGIV rendering algorithm, includes both the surface rendering- and volume rendering-based PRR algorithms. According to actual demands, different rendering algorithms can be chosen to generate EIAs. In operation, 3D medical images can be acquired by 3D scanners, such as MRI and CT. As for the display process, a high-resolution 2D flat display, such as a liquid crystal display (LCD) is employed to display the recorded 2D EIAs. The rays from the EIA are modulated by the MLA to reconstruct the 3D image in accordance with the reversibility of the ray tracing process.

Indeed, 3D autostereoscopic images with accurate spatial information are highly sought after for surgical navigation and intervention. Using optimized parameters through quantitative calibration, an accurate 3D autostereoscopic display can be fabricated (Fan et al. 2017b). Rotational and translational calibration methods are proposed to quantitatively rectify the actual optical apparatus. Then, the principle parameters in the 3D display are evaluated through quantitative calibration of the 3D autostereoscopic display to ensure accurate 3D image rendering and display. To guarantee the real-time 3D image rendering and display, a flexible IV rendering pipeline with graphics processing unit (GPU) acceleration (Wang et al. 2013) can be utilized.

17.2.2 3D AR System

The 3D IV AR device is used to merge the displayed 3D autostereoscopic image with the patient *in situ,* via the half-silvered mirror. Surgeons can observe the 3D images reflected in the corresponding spatial position in the surgical scene when looking through the mirror.

The full set of coordinate transformations is shown in Figure 17.2 (Liao et al. 2010). The coordinates of the 3D optical tracking system are set as the reference frame. With the assistance of the optical markers mounted on the 3D IV AR device and surgical instruments, the position and orientation of the IV-based 3D autostereoscopic display device can be obtained through $_{\text{Mar}}^{\text{Tra}}T$ and $_{\text{Pat}}^{\text{Tra}}T \cdot _{\text{Img}}^{\text{Mar}}T$ can be calculated by projecting a four-point pattern onto the reflected spatial IV space by the half-silvered mirror and employing the 3D positional tracking probe to identify the four points in the registration procedure. Therefore, the transformation $_{\text{Img}}^{\text{Pat}}T$ can be obtained by the following:

$$_{\text{Img}}^{\text{Pat}}T = {}_{\text{Img}}^{\text{Mar}}T \; {}_{\text{Mar}}^{\text{Tra}}T \; {}_{\text{Tra}}^{\text{Pat}}T \tag{17.1}$$

Similarly, the IV image of the surgical instrument can be localized by the following:

$$_{\text{Img}}^{\text{Sur}}T = {}_{\text{Img}}^{\text{Mar}}T \; {}_{\text{Mar}}^{\text{Tra}}T \; {}_{\text{Tra}}^{\text{Sur}}T \tag{17.2}$$

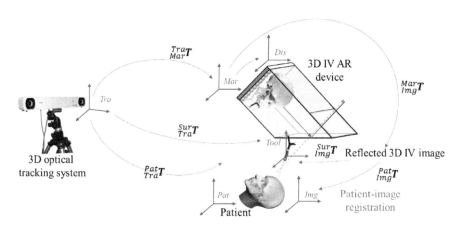

FIGURE 17.2 Coordinate transformation in 3D IV AR system. (From Liao, H. et al., *IEEE Trans. Biomed. Eng.*, 57, 1476–1486, 2010.)

17.2.3 REAL-TIME TRACKING OF TARGETS

A real-time tracking system is necessary to track the surgical instruments, the overlay device, and the patient in an IV-based 3D image overlay system. By using this tracking information, accurate 3D AR can be achieved.

Commercial clinical tracking systems may include both optical tracking systems and electromagnetic tracking systems. Spatial information relating to the targets can be acquired in real time and employed for accurate 3D AR. Moreover, the position and orientation of surgical instruments can be tracked in real time during the operation, and the 3D IV image of the instrument can be projected onto the patient according to the coordinate transformation. Therefore, surgeons can observe an accurate 3D AR image combining the patient, the 3D medical data, and the surgical instruments intuitively in real time.

17.3 ENHANCED 3D IV AR FOR MICROSURGERY

Traditional autostereoscopic IV technology is limited by the resolution and the viewing angle, which is important for the application of microsurgery. Therefore, an enhanced IV-based 3D AR system is required for effective application in microsurgery (Zhang et al. 2017).

The 3D AR system using enhanced IV display consists of four main components: (1) a high-definition IV display for displaying 3D images with high image quality, (2) a see-through microscopic device that can superimpose the displayed 3D image on the surgical scene and magnify the actual surgical scene, (3) a spatial tracking system for patient tracking and tools tracking, and (4) a workstation for image processing. The high-definition IV display comprises an LCD with high pixel density, an MLA, and a dedicated optical image enhancement module. An optical magnifier module, which is arranged between the surgical scene and observers, provides a magnified surgical scene. Therefore, based on optical reflection and the see-through microscopic device, the displayed 3D surgical guidance information can be merged onto the magnified surgical scene (Zhang et al. 2017). Observers can directly perceive a real magnified surgical scene, complemented with merged 3D surgical guidance information, as shown by Figure 17.3.

The limited spatial resolution of the conventional 3D IV display is due to the sampling effect introduced by the MLA. Therefore, optical lenses with negative focal length can be employed to increase the pixel density and spatial resolution. Dedicated optical lenses can guarantee the improvement in both resolution and viewing angle. Moreover, the resolution and the viewing angle can be flexibly adjusted by changing the optical parameters.

The optical magnifier module consists of optical lenses, which is equivalent to a positive lens. Its focal length is larger than the distance between the surgical scene and the optical center of the see-through microscopic device. To merge the displayed 3D images on the surgical scene, a patient-3D image registration method should be implemented. In contrast to conventional approaches, the scale and position changes of the image and the patient caused by the optical lenses and the half-silvered mirror need to be accounted for. Using this method, the accuracy of the proposed enhanced

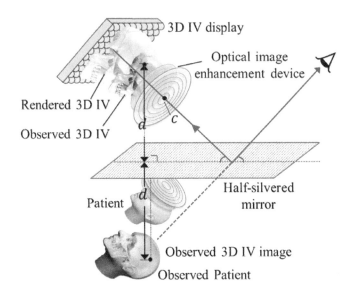

FIGURE 17.3 Configuration of enhanced IV-based 3D AR for microsurgery. (From Zhang, X. et al., *IEEE Trans. Biomed. Eng.*, 64, 1815–1825, 2017.)

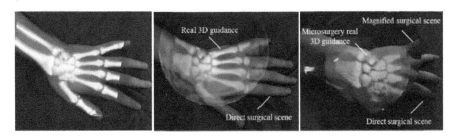

FIGURE 17.4 Real 3D see-through guidance for microsurgery. (a) Real 3D guidance superimposed on direct surgical scene; (b) Real 3D guidance with enhanced IV superimposed on direct surgical scene; (c) Real 3D guidance with enhanced IV superimposed on magnified surgical scene. (From Zhang, X. et al., *IEEE Trans. Biomed. Eng.*, 64, 1815–1825, 2017.)

IV can reach submillimeter levels and the viewing angle can be enlarged. The proposed system can provide a magnified surgical scene with high-quality 3D images, which can assist surgeons in performing accurate operations, as shown in Figure 17.4 (Zhang et al. 2017).

17.4   REGISTRATION AND SPATIAL TRACKING OF TARGETS

17.4.1   PATIENT-3D IMAGE REGISTRATION METHOD

Patient-3D image registration, which is critical for an accurate 3D AR system, consists of both marker-based and markerless registration techniques. According to external or natural anatomical features, such as landmarks and surface, a 3D image can be registered to the patient by minimizing the distance between pair-features. The Iterative Closest Point (Fitzgibbon 2003) algorithm has been widely used in this field because of its feasibility and robustness.

Marker-based registration can be easily achieved by setting and acquiring the spatial positions of the external fiducial markers, but implanted bone markers are often impractical. To resolve this problem, markerless-based registration using anatomical or surface landmarks is of great importance. Spatial positions of landmarks, or the surface in the 3D image (MRI/CT), can be calculated preoperatively. During the operation, surgeons usually use a surgical probe to confirm the spatial positions of the corresponding anatomical landmarks instead of using external markers. The spatial positions of the landmarks can be determined using a tracked surgical probe. However, during an operation, anatomical landmarks cannot be precisely identified and the time-consuming nature of the registration may cause registration error and reduce surgical efficiency (Hassfeld and Mühling 2001). Another approach to markerless registration is contour or surface matching. The contour or the surface of the target can be extracted by stereo camera (Wang et al. 2014), laser scanning (Marmulla et al. 2003), or structured light (Nicolau et al. 2011). After matching, the relationship between the patient and the 3D image coordinate systems can be calculated for accurate AR.

17.4.2 SPATIAL TRACKING OF PATIENTS AND SURGICAL TOOLS WITH DEDICATED MARKERS

During surgery, movements of the patient and surgical tools are normal and must be taken into consideration for accurate 3D AR. For example, patient motion would cause the 3D IV overlay image to be displaced from the patient. Therefore, an automatic registration method using the depth camera, which tracks the position and posture of the patient in real time would be a preferred technique for minimally invasive surgery (Figure 17.5) (Ma et al. 2016). The depth camera is used to obtain the point cloud of the patient, which contains the geometric and texture information. By employing the particle filter tracking algorithm, the position and orientation of the patient can be obtained in real time. The particle filter tracking algorithm includes three main steps. First, the position and posture of patients is predicted with random particles. Then, the weights of particles are calculated according to the evaluation formula previously constructed, which can contain both photometric and geometric information. Finally, the evaluation function is used to compare the data acquired from the depth camera with the predicted particles. Particles with large weights are resampled. Using the structural position relationship between the depth camera and the 3D IV AR device, as well as the positional information of the patient, the 3D IV image of the patient is updated to ensure that the 3D IV image is correctly fused with the patient.

With the initialization of this system, the image-patient registration is executed automatically. Then, according to the position and posture of the patient, the overlaid 3D IV image is updated. The reflected 3D IV image will fuse with the patient whether the patient moves or not.

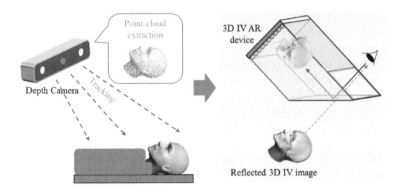

FIGURE 17.5   Fast registration process in 3D IV AR system. (From Ma, C. et al., Automatic fast-registration surgical navigation system using depth camera and integral videography 3D image overlay, *International Conference on Medical Imaging and Virtual Reality*, Springer International Publishing, Bern, Switzerland, 2016.)

Tracking surgical tools is of importance for surgical navigation and intervention. Commercial optical tracking systems use reflective balls or flat "chessboard" patterns as tracking markers. In some surgical treatments, such as cutting during an operation, detecting the tool with six degrees-of-freedom (6-DOF) is important for surgical safety. To ensure 6-DOF detection, markers are arranged in a noncollinear fashion, with the result that current surgical tools with such markers are difficult to use in a limited space due to their large spatial volume. A novel 3D spatial position measurement system using 3D image markers has been designed especially for surgical scenes with limited space (Fan et al. 2017a). The 3D image marker, which is a 2D image with encoded spatial information, has a compact size while providing spatial position measurement. The 3D image marker can be attached on the target for positioning and can be employed in a surgical tool. A novel surgical tool designed with collinear 3D image markers can generate a virtual, noncollinear set of markers (Figure 17.6) (Fan et al. 2015). Combined with the image acquisition device and the image processing method, the proposed surgical tool can be used for tracking and positioning in a limited space.

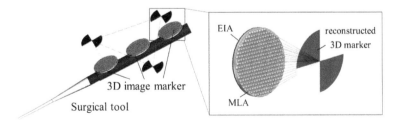

FIGURE 17.6   Novel surgical tool with three 3D image markers. (Fan, Z. et al., A spatial position measurement system using integral photography based 3D image markers, *1st Global Conference on Biomedical Engineering & 9th Asian-Pacific Conference on Medical and Biological Engineering*, Springer International Publishing, Heidelberg, Germany, pp. 150–153, 2015.)

17.5 APPLICATIONS OF 3D AR IN SURGICAL NAVIGATION AND INTERVENTION

Due to the simplicity in implementation and the ability to provide surgeons with intuitive 3D AR images, the proposed 3D AR system using IV is a promising solution in neurosurgery, oral surgery, spine surgery, and other interventions.

17.5.1 IV-Based 3D AR for Neurosurgery

Tumor extraction and therapy is especially critical in neurosurgery. To increase accuracy and safety, image-guided systems using preoperative images are becoming widespread. To provide an intuitive "see-through" scene, a 3D AR system incorporating a fast and semiautomatic tumor segmentation method was developed, especially for open MRI-guided surgery (Figure 17.7) (Liao et al. 2010).

This system consists of an IV overlay device, a 3D image scanner, a tracking device, and a workstation for image rendering and display. An IV image calibration method and a marker-based registration method was also proposed for patient-image registration in the 3D AR system, so the spatially projected 3D images can be superimposed accurately onto the patient. A fuzzy connectedness algorithm combined with 3D Slicer was used to perform intraoperative tumor segmentation. The feasibility of the proposed system was evaluated by using phantom experiments and animal experiments. Phantom experiments showed that the proposed system enables more accurate registration compared with a single-slice-based image overlay system. Animal experiments indicated that this system should be of practical use in neurosurgery and other medical fields. Moreover, surgical tools can be inserted from the required direction without changing the viewing angle, as the entire target can be observed directly and intuitively.

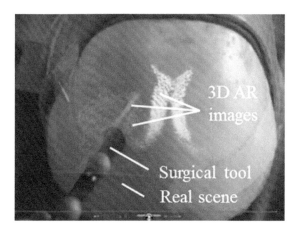

FIGURE 17.7   Observed surgical scene with superimposed 3D images in 3D AR-based neurosurgery. (From Liao, H. et al., *IEEE Trans. Biomed. Eng.*, 57, 1476–1486, 2010.)

17.5.2 IV-Based 3D AR for Oral Surgery

Oral surgery commonly consists of operations on the teeth and jaw to modify denti-tion. Basic operations in oral surgery mainly include drilling, cutting, fixation, resec-tion, and implantation. In most cases, operations are limited by the confined space and by the fact that the surgical targets may be hidden. Surgeons have to practice avoiding damaging the surrounding vital structures to guarantee surgical safety. Although computer-assisted oral surgery has been used, surgical navigation in oral surgery still suffers from the loss of 3D information and poor hand-eye coordination. Tran and Wang designed a 3D AR navigation system with automatic marker-free image registration using an IV-based 3D image overlay system and stereo tracking for oral surgery (Wang et al. 2014). The proposed system consists of a stereo cam-era for tracking patients and instruments, a real-time patient-3D image registration method, an IV-camera registration method, and an optical see-through device. The 3D AR information can guide the surgeon to observe the hidden structures as well as surgical tools intuitively. Experiments were performed to confirm the feasibility, and the overlay error of the proposed system was less than 1 mm. With the assistance of the IV-based 3D AR system, surgeons can acquire intuitive 3D information and then operate based on the 3D AR images.

17.5.3 IV-Based 3D AR for Spine Surgery

In spine surgery, pedicle screw placement can provide strong fixation to the spine, which prevents injury when the back stretches, bends, or rotates excessively. However, a screw that is improperly placed can result in neurologic and vascular complica-tions. To assist accurate placement, a navigation system is used. However, the surgi-cal target as well as surgical instruments, such as pedicle screws, may be hidden in other structures during surgery. To solve these problems, research on a 3D IV AR system complemented with ultrasound-assisted registration has been proposed for pedicle screw placement, as shown in Figure 17.8 (Ma et al. 2017). Ultrasound (US)

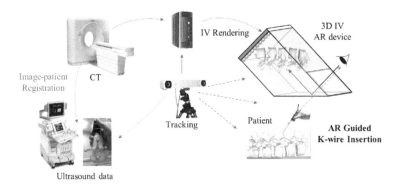

FIGURE 17.8   3D AR system for spine surgery. (From Ma, L. et al., *Int. J. Comp. Assis. Radiol. Surg.*, 12, 2205–2215, 2017.)

is used to perform registration between the preoperative medical image and patient to avoid the effect of extracting anatomical landmarks on the surface and reduce radiation exposure. The registration method is based on least-squares fitting of these two 3D point sets of anatomical landmarks from US images and preoperative images. A 3.0-mm Kirschner wire (K-wire), instead of a pedicle screw, is calibrated to acquire its orientation and tip location prior to use. An agar phantom experiment was performed to verify the feasibility of the system. Eight K-wires were successfully placed after US-assisted registration. The mean targeting and angle errors were 3.35 mm and 2.74°, respectively. Experiments demonstrate that the proposed system has acceptable targeting accuracy and repeated radiation exposure is reduced for both the patient and the surgeon.

Generally, surgical targets and tools may be hidden in other anatomical structures. As a promising solution, a 3D AR system can provide a "see-through" surgical scene with superimposed 3D images to assist surgical navigation and interventions. Moreover, combined with the microscope, the simultaneous fluoroscopy, and other therapy techniques, a 3D AR system can show a clear 3D vision of interested regions over the patient for surgical navigation and interventions.

17.6 DISCUSSION AND CONCLUSION

The described 3D AR technique solves the problem of hand-eye coordination and provides see-through 3D images with full parallax for observers, thus enabling surgeons to observe hidden anatomy directly without requiring specialized eyewear. The critical components of the 3D AR system consist of advanced 3D visualization algorithms, as well as precise patient-3D image registration and tracking methods. As a main component in the 3D AR technique, the IV-based 3D AR system, which benefits from both simplicity in implementation and the ability to provide 3D autostereoscopic AR information, has recently attracted much attention. Research on 3D visualization with high quality, flexible tracking, and novel surgical tools has been proposed to improve the performance of the IV-based 3D AR system. Moreover, we have described an enhanced 3D IV AR system, especially for microsurgery. With the benefit of intuitive visualization, 3D IV AR can be applied in neurosurgery, oral surgery, spine surgery, etc.

However, the 3D IV AR system still suffers from some problems. For instance, the spatial resolution and of the IV-based 3D display techniques, which is limited by the optical apparatus, still requires improvement (Fan et al. 2016). A high-quality 3D autostereoscopic display is required to provide clear 3D autostereoscopic images with a wide viewing angle, high resolution, and long viewing distance (Liao et al. 2004a, 2005). Although preclinical experiments have revealed its potential usage in surgery, there are some nonnegligible factors limiting further application. Structural deformation, target tracking, and patient-3D registration should be taken into consideration for accurate overlay. More experiments and evaluations must be performed for clinical efficiency and usability. However, with further improvement, we expect that 3D AR will become an integral component for image-guide surgical navigation and interventions.

REFERENCES

Cleary, K., and T. M. Peters. 2010. Image-guided interventions: Technology review and clinical applications. *Annual Review of Biomedical Engineering* 12: 119–142.

DiGioia III, A. M., B. Jaramaz, and B. D. Colgan. 1998. Computer assisted orthopaedic surgery: Image guided and robotic assistive technologies. *Clinical Orthopaedics and Related Research* 354: 8–16.

Fan, Z., G. Chen, J. Wang, and H. Liao. 2017a. Spatial position measurement system for surgical navigation using 3-D image marker-based tracking tools with compact volume. *IEEE Transactions on Biomedical Engineering* 65, no.2: 378–389.

Fan, Z., G. Chen, Y. Xia, T. Huang, and H. Liao. 2017b. Accurate 3D autostereoscopic display using optimized parameters through quantitative calibration. *Journal of the Optical Society of America A* 34, no.5: 804–812.

Fan, Z., J. Wang, and H. Liao. 2015. A spatial position measurement system using integral photography based 3D image markers. *1st Global Conference on Biomedical Engineering & 9th Asian-Pacific Conference on Medical and Biological Engineering*, Springer International Publishing, Heidelberg, Germany, pp. 150–153.

Fan, Z., S. Zhang, Y. Weng, G. Chen, and H. Liao. 2016. 3D Quantitative evaluation system for autostereoscopic display. *Journal of Display Technology* 12, no.10: 1185–1196.

Fan, Z., Y. Weng, G. Chen, and H. Liao. 2017c. 3D interactive surgical visualization system using mobile spatial information acquisition and autostereoscopic display. *Journal of Biomedical Informatics* 71: 154–164.

Fitzgibbon, A. W. 2003. Robust registration of 2D and 3D point sets. *Image and Vision Computing* 21, no.13: 1145–1153.

Hassfeld, S., and J. Mühling. 2001. Computer assisted oral and maxillofacial surgery—A review and an assessment of technology. *International Journal of Oral and Maxillofacial Surgery* 30, no.1: 2–13.

Liao, H., M. Iwahara, N. Hata, and T. Dohi. 2004a. High-quality integral videography using a multiprojector. *Optics Express* 12, no.6: 1067–1076.

Liao, H., M. Iwahara, Y. Katayama, N. Hata, and T. Dohi. 2005. Three-dimensional display with a long viewing distance by use of integral photography. *Optics Letter* 30, no.6: 613–615.

Liao, H., N. Hata, S. Nakajima, M. Iwahara, I. Sakuma, and T. Dohi. 2004b. Surgical navigation by autostereoscopic image overlay of integral videography. *IEEE Transactions on Information Technology in Biomedicine* 8, no.2: 114–121.

Liao, H., S. Nakajima, M. Iwahara, E. Kobayashi, I. Sakuma, N. Yahagi, and T. Dohi. 2000. Development of real-time 3D navigation system for intra-operative information by integral videography. *Journal of Japan Society of Computer Aided Surgery* 2, no.4: 245–252.

Liao, H., T. Dohi, and K. Nomura. 2011. Autostereoscopic 3D display with long visualization depth using referential viewing area-based integral photography. *IEEE Transactions on Visualization and Computer Graphics* 17, no.11: 1690–1701.

Liao, H., T. Inomata, I. Sakuma, and T. Dohi. 2010. 3-D augmented reality for MRI-guided surgery using integral videography autostereoscopic image overlay. *IEEE Transactions on Biomedical Engineering* 57, no.6: 1476–1486.

Lippmann, G. 1908. Epreuves reversibles donnant La Sensation Du relief. *Journal De Physique Théorique Et Appliquée* 7, no.1: 821–825.

Ma, C., G. Chen, and H. Liao. 2016. Automatic fast-registration surgical navigation system using depth camera and integral videography 3D image overlay. *International Conference on Medical Imaging and Virtual Reality*. Springer International Publishing, Bern, Switzerland, pp. 392–403.

Ma, L., Z. Zhao, F. Chen, B. Zhang, L. Fu, and H. Liao. 2017. Augmented reality surgical navigation with ultrasound-assisted registration for pedicle screw placement: A pilot study. *International Journal of Computer Assisted Radiology and Surgery* 12, no.12: 2205–2215.

Marmulla, R., S. Hassfeld, T. Lüth, and J. Mühling. 2003. Laser-scan-based navigation in cranio-maxillofacial surgery. *Journal of Cranio-Maxillofacial Surgery* 31, no.5: 267–277.

Nicolau, S., L. Soler, D. Mutter, and J. Marescaux. 2011. Augmented reality in laparoscopic surgical oncology. *Surgical Oncology* 20, no.3: 189–201.

Okano, F., H. Hoshino, J. Arai, and I. Yuyama. 1997. Real-time pickup method for a three-dimensional image based on integral photography. *Applied Optics* 36, no.7: 1598–1603.

Wang, J., H. Suenaga, X. Hoshi, L. Yang, E. Kobayashi, I. Sakuma, and H. Liao. 2014. Augmented reality navigation with automatic marker-free image registration using 3-D image overlay for dental surgery. *IEEE Transactions on Biomedical Engineering* 61, no.4: 1295–1304.

Wang, J., I. Sakuma, and H. Liao. 2013. A hybrid flexible rendering pipeline for real-time 3D medical imaging using GPU-accelerated integral videography. *International Journal of Computer Assisted Radiology and Surgery* 8: S287–S288.

Zhang, X., G. Chen, and H. Liao. 2017. High quality see-through surgical guidance system using enhanced 3D autostereoscopic augmented reality. *IEEE Transactions on Biomedical Engineering* 64, no.8: 1815–1825.

Zhang, X., Z. Fan, J. Wang, and H. Liao. 2016. 3D augmented reality based orthopaedic interventions. *Computational Radiology for Orthopaedic Interventions*. Springer International Publishing, New York, pp. 71–90.

18 Augmenting Haptic Perception in Surgical Tools

Randy Lee, Roberta L. Klatzky,
and George D. Stetten

CONTENTS

18.1 INTRODUCTION

Rendering in computer graphics refers to the process by which images (visual stimuli) are produced from two-dimensional scenes or three-dimensional (3D) models. In the context of haptics, rendering refers to the process by which tactile stimuli—for example, forces or vibrations—are presented to a user to convey information about a virtual object (Salisbury et al. 2004). High-fidelity haptic rendering therefore requires a method to sense user interaction in terms of position, velocity, or force, in multiple degrees of freedom (DoF), and subsequently to use that interaction to generate feedback forces against the user. Most commercially available haptic renderers (e.g., Geomagic Touch, Novint Falcon) are restricted to actuating in only the three translational DoF, using motors and pulleys that act on a stylus or ball. The Magnetically Levitated Haptic Device (MLHD) from Butterfly Haptics can actuate forces in all six DoF albeit over a smaller reachable volume (Berkelman and Hollis 1997, 2000).

Because haptic renderers generate forces against the user, Newton's third law requires a surface or object against which these feedback forces act in opposition. The renderers mentioned thus far are therefore called *grounded* systems: feedback forces are produced against the surface (such as a desk) on which these devices are resting or mounted. Some *ungrounded* haptic renderers exist, for example, devices mounted on one's own anatomy such that the body acts as the base against which feedback forces are produced (Solazzi et al. 2010; Maisto et al. 2017). Depending on design, ungrounded devices can also render in multiple DoF (Chinello et al. 2012; Brown et al. 2016).

It should be noted that complex haptic rendering, for example, of the interaction between a tool and a surface in a full virtual reality (VR) context, can have a high computational cost, requiring models of both the surface and tool to produce visual and tactile stimuli. The interaction between two such virtual objects may rely on calculations from the underlying physics model to render feedback forces in all six DoF. In surgical simulations, biomechanical models of tissue are complex because most tissue is heterogeneous and exhibits viscoelasticity, thus limiting the accuracy of such simulations. In augmented reality (AR), by contrast, real-world sensing provides the initial data for the force feedback. Using a sensor connected to the tool tip, AR methods can collect data on the distal interaction as it happens in real time, without requiring a complex model from which to provide the augmented force feedback. The initial computational cost is therefore much lower with AR than with VR.

The difficulty in AR haptics arises in the appropriate design and implementation of a sensing and actuation pair. Suitable sensors and actuators face challenging constraints in terms of size, weight, sensitivity, and power. AR haptics are even more difficult if multiple DOF are involved. A common solution is to render some essential subset of the available information to provide informative feedback along axes of consequence. Critical to this approach are psychophysical methods that characterize the relationship between physical stimuli and mental representations and hence indicate what kind of information should be presented to the user. This approach of presenting only the perceptible subset of the original information is used similarly to reduce bandwidth in the MP3 encoding algorithm for compressing digital audio (Musmann 2006).

In this chapter, we will discuss the need for AR haptics in surgery and the varied technologies developed thus far to augment the sense of touch. We will then present the Hand-Held Force Magnifier (HHFM), a handheld surgical robot developed by the authors, along with a series of psychophysical experiments that evaluate how such an active tool may influence the user's perception and motor control.

18.2 HAPTICS IN SURGERY

Surgery has traditionally been a "hands-on" endeavor, in which surgeons make large incisions into the body to achieve direct contact with the organs or tissues of interest in an open workspace with a clear view. However, as surgery has progressed to more indirect and displaced approaches to anatomical targets, and to smaller targets requiring visual magnification, the sense of touch is often sacrificed. In this section, we will briefly outline the corresponding need to solve this "haptic problem" by augmenting the sense of touch.

18.2.1 Minimally Invasive Surgery

In minimally invasive or laparoscopic surgery, access to an internal cavity is achieved by inserting tools, cameras, and lights through ports inserted in the body wall, called trocars. Instruments in minimally invasive surgery (MIS) are typically scissor-actuated and feature long bodies to allow for insertion and tissue manipulation. MIS approaches are associated with reduced postoperative pain and infection and shorter periods of disability compared to open surgery (Berggren et al. 1994; Jonsson and Zethraeus 2000; Boni et al. 2006).

   A significant problem associated with MIS tool design is that mechanical torques and friction forces are generated between the tool and the trocar. These extraneous forces mask the interaction forces at the distal tip, thus confounding the tactile feedback normally obtained while manipulating tissue in open surgery (van der Meijden and Schijven 2009). The long length of the tool itself further confounds the haptic feedback obtained from the interaction at the tool tip. Due to these difficulties, inaccurate control of grasping can result in tissue damage or tissue slip (Westebring-van der Putten et al. 2009a, 2009b). Vibrotactile feedback has been used in surgical training to alleviate these difficulties with some success (Westebring-van der Putten et al. 2010).

18.2.2 Microsurgery

Microsurgery refers to the set of surgical techniques that are performed beyond the limits of unassisted human eyesight (Yap and Butler 2007). As opposed to MIS, clinicians still make incisions to directly access tissues of interest, but in general they operate on relatively small structures, such as nerves, vessels, and thin membranes, and employ correspondingly smaller forces (Patkin 1977; Tsai et al. 2013). For example, Jagtap and Riviere (2004) measured average axial forces during *in vivo* microvascular puncture tasks to be as low as 75 mN. Furthermore, movements in microsurgery are performed on such a small scale that kinesthetic afferent signals are generally not differentiable (Jones 2000), and tremor becomes a significant additional component to the intended movement.

   Whereas the haptic problem in MIS is characterized by friction or other factors masking the tool-tissue interaction, the haptic problem in microsurgery derives from fundamental properties of the tissues of interest, namely that the forces are too small to perceive. A core assistive technology in such delicate procedures is the surgical microscope, which provides visual stimuli at an appropriately magnified scale, and to some extent force may be deduced by the observed movement of target tissues. However, using the surgical microscope limits the surgeon's depth of focus, thus causing structures above or below the focal plane to be blurred. Visual magnification itself can also affect operators' motor control capabilities due to the discrepancy between physical movement and observation of that movement (Vasilakos et al. 1998; Bohan et al. 2010).

18.2.3 Consequences of Perceptual Difficulties in Surgery

We believe many difficulties in MIS and microsurgery derive from inadequate perception of force informing the human sensorimotor loop. Noisy or subthreshold forces producing unreliable cutaneous sensation or movements performed over too small a scale to trigger dependable kinesthetic afferent signals may induce compensatory cognitive processes to control movement. Restoring or improving force sensing may aid the surgeon by reducing this cognitive load, leading to fewer intraoperative errors and facilitating learning for surgeons in training.

When introducing haptic augmentation, we prefer to do so *in situ*, by adding forces and torques in the same direction and location that the surgeon's hand is already expecting to feel them. In this manner, tools may be used more intuitively and thereby be integrated into existing practice more easily. Alternative approaches that provide feedback on forces through other sensory channels, i.e., via *sensory substitution*, are also possible. Auditory feedback may be used to alert the surgeon of forces beyond a certain threshold (Balicki et al. 2010), but this may not be well suited for the operating room, where ambient audio signals from medical equipment already abound. Closed-loop visual feedback systems, such as graphical displays or other force-responsive visualizations (Okamura et al. 2011), are potentially distracting and may lead to increased servo-ing when matching forces over long periods of time.

18.3 EXISTING APPROACHES TO HAPTIC FEEDBACK

A number of solutions have been developed to provide haptic feedback in telesurgery, where the tool is controlled remotely, as well as in cooperative robots, where the robot and surgeon jointly manipulate the same local tool. In the following sections, we will briefly describe some notable achievements in telesurgery (Section 18.2.1) and in cooperative robots using both grounded (Section 18.2.2) and handheld surgical systems (Section 18.2.3). For additional review, see (Hamed et al. 2012; Payne and Yang 2014; Griffin et al. 2017).

18.3.1 Pneumatic Force Feedback in Telesurgery

By far, the most widely used telerobotic system is Intuitive Surgical's *da Vinci* robot, in which a surgeon operates a bimanual master controller linked to a scaled-down slave robotic device without haptic feedback. In a project integrating haptics into the *da Vinci* (Culjat et al. 2008, 2011; King et al. 2009), piezoresistive force sensors mounted into Cadiere graspers at the end-effector of the *da Vinci* sensed the distal interaction. As with many telerobotic systems, the haptic feedback had to contend with stability problems due to data quantization and time delay effects (Diolaiti et al. 2006). Motion in the master controllers induced by the feedback actuators will typically move the end-effector, leading to unstable loops. The system avoided this problem by mounting pneumatic actuators onto the surface of the *da Vinci* grasper and deforming the operator's fingerpads to provide force feedback. Psychophysical experimentation determined the optimal arrangement of pressure actuators (King et al. 2008), and tactile feedback was found to reduce grip force in laparoscopic training tasks, especially among novice surgeons (King et al. 2009; Wottawa et al. 2013).

18.3.2 THE STEADY HAND ROBOT

In contrast to telerobotic systems, cooperative robots are based on the premise that both the human and the robot operate locally with the same tool and share its control. The Steady Hand Robot (SHR) is a cooperative robot that provides sustained force feedback during the delicate operations of retinal microsurgery, in which forces are minimally perceptible (Taylor et al. 1999; Mitchell et al. 2007; Uneri et al. 2010). Gupta and colleagues (1999) found that during retinal manipulation, 75% of all tissue interactions generate forces smaller than 7.5 mN and are perceived by the clinician only 19% of the time.

The SHR stabilizes the clinician's movement and provides force feedback through cooperative admittance control, where limits on the velocity or applied force of a surgical tool are enforced by a table-mounted robot in response to user force input. The device actuates force feedback in five DoF (three translations and two rotations). An initial prototype was successfully used to cannulate vessels in the chick chorioallantoic membrane (Fleming et al. 2008), and a subsequent version has been used to perform *in vitro* membrane peeling tasks (Balicki et al. 2010).

18.3.3 IMPERIAL COLLEGE LONDON MANIPULATORS

Imperial College London has developed a series of ungrounded, handheld surgical robots, through which stationary augmenting forces are created relative to the surgeon's own hand. The first device generates a steady feedback force through a slider to the index finger of the surgeon's hand gripping the tool (Payne et al. 2012). A piezoresistive force sensor measures the interaction force at the tool tip. Using Proportional-Integral-Derivative (PID) control, a linear motor moves the slider relative to the tool body to produce up to 2.72 N and scaling of the distal tool tip force by factors of up to 15. Subsequent approaches use optical trackers and strain gauges on the sensing side to control the user by active constraints on motion ("virtual fixtures") and feedback in the form of forces and vibrotactile stimulation (Payne et al. 2013; Payne et al. 2015). Psychophysical experiments showed that a user's absolute perceptual force threshold is reduced when using such tools, and a cadaver dissection study showed that feedback significantly reduced the time spent above a threshold of 0.3 N.

18.4 THE HAND-HELD FORCE MAGNIFIER

When designing tools that enhance sensory perception, we aim to add as little as possible to the already considerable cognitive load associated with performing a surgical procedure. Specifically, we design tools to directly amplify action-dependent forces as they would be sensed by the user—a paradigm we call *in situ* force feedback. This is opposed to using vibrotactile feedback as a force surrogate, either continuously mapped to force (Murray et al. 2003) or serving to signal when some critical force is reached. *In situ* force feedback has the benefit that force information is transmitted to the user directly as force; there is no cognitive conversion necessary, as with other approaches. Furthermore, the force feedback is superimposed on the original forces coming from the tissue interaction in the same direction and location on the tool handle so as to augment them naturally. In this section, we will describe the HHFM, which is a handheld surgical robot that provides *in situ* force feedback. We will discuss a proposed human-in-the-loop control scheme under which such a tool may be used as well as psychophysics research describing how *in situ* force feedback affects the human sensory and motor control systems.

18.4.1 Design Overview

The HHFM is a robotic surgical instrument designed to provide *in situ* force feedback (Stetten et al. 2011; Lee et al. 2013; Stetten 2015). The HHFM Model-3, depicted in Figure 18.1b, was manufactured using stereolithography and a 3D printing technology and has a total mass of 80 g. A force sensor (Motorola MPX2011DT1; 75 kPa pressure range, 1% linearity and 0.1% hysteresis) inside the handle is mechanically linked to the tool tip to measure the interaction force between the tool tip and the distal target. A voice coil actuator (Moticont LVCM-013-013-2) is rigidly connected to the handle, which is gripped by one's fingers. The voice coil magnet is mounted to a brace that fits across the palm. Therefore, instead of being grounded to the tabletop or floor, the device uses the hand as a mobile platform against which feedback

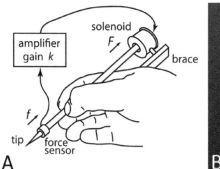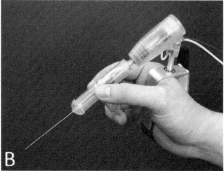

FIGURE 18.1 (a) HHFM concept; (b) HHFM model-3. (Reproduced from Stetten, G. et al., *Lect. Not. Comp. Sci.,* 6689, 90–100, 2011; Lee, R. et al., *Lect. Not. Comp. Sci.,* 7815, 77–89, 2013. With permission.)

forces are generated. By generating feedback forces between the handle and the brace, *in situ* force magnification is possible. Figure 18.1a illustrates this concept.

The HHFM operates as a first approximation under a simple control law:

$$F = k \cdot f \qquad (18.1)$$

where f is the small force of the tissue on the tool tip, measured by the internal sensor, F is the feedback force generated by the actuator, and k is the magnifier gain. The HHFM is controlled by an Analog Devices ADuC7026 microprocessor, running at 40 MHz with banks of 12-bit analog to digital and digital-to-analog converter interfaces. The microprocessor is programmed in C and operates with reliable throughput of analog inputs and outputs at 5 kHz.

In situ force feedback in the HHFM takes full advantage of the phenomenon known as distal attribution (Loomis 1992; Siegle and Warren 2010). That is, the user perceives (or "attributes") the feedback force F as originating from the distal end of the tool, where the tip contacts the tissue, rather than from the proximal end, where the voice coil is actually producing force.

18.4.2 HUMAN-IN-THE-LOOP CONTROL FRAMEWORK

A human-in-the-loop control framework comparing traditional surgery and surgery with *in situ* force feedback is illustrated in Figure 18.2 (Lee et al. 2017). In traditional surgery (Figure 18.2a), the operator's efferent (motor control) forces, F_e, are transmitted directly to the tissue, resulting in an equal and opposite force, f, the force of the tissue on the tool, that is perceived directly as the afferent force, F_a. All of these forces are functions of time.

However, with a tool that provides *in situ* force feedback (Figure 18.2b), the device actuator applies an additional feedback force, F, which not only can magnify the perception of a subthreshold distal force f to suprathreshold levels but also acts in the opposite direction of F_e by lowering the net force applied to the tissue. For this active system, note that the control framework is shown to include the gain k defined in Equation 18.1 and an electromechanical delay τ between the device measuring the distal force f and actuating F.

Thus, ignoring τ, under *in situ* force magnification the afferent force, F_a, is described by the following:

$$
\begin{aligned}
F_a &= f + F \\
&= f + k \cdot f \\
F_a &= (k + 1) \cdot f
\end{aligned}
\qquad (18.2)
$$

The net magnification is $k + 1$ or the original force plus the augmenting force. With respect to this control framework, the HHFM does not explicitly affect the motor control of the user by means of actuation. Rather, it intervenes with the user's *perception* of the distal interaction, which in turn is spontaneously leveraged by the sensorimotor system to improve motor control.

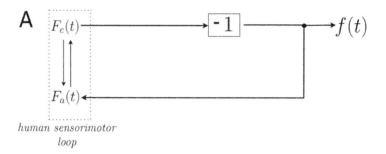

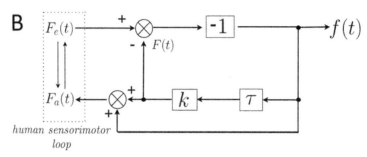

FIGURE 18.2 Human-in-the-loop control system describing (a) traditional surgery and (b) surgery with *in situ* force feedback. F_e is the efferent force, and the force produced by the user; F_a is the afferent force perceived by the user; f is the force of the tissue on the tool tip; k is the gain; and τ is the small electromechanical delay associated with HHFM control. (Reproduced from Lee, R. et al., *IEEE Trans. Hap.*, 2017. With permission.)

18.4.3 Magnification Effects on the Perceptual Pathway

The effects of *in situ* force magnification on perception were initially studied using the HHFM Model-1, a proof-of-concept prototype described in detail by Stetten and colleagues (2011). The device was controlled through analog circuitry, achieving gains as high as $k = 5.8$ before instability effects were seen.

To investigate how the HHFM affected the perceptual system, psychophysical experiments were conducted to address three fundamental questions (Stetten et al. 2011; Wu et al. 2015): (1) How does magnification affect the minimum force that can be detected? To answer, we measured users' absolute force threshold. (2) How does magnification affect the minimum difference between forces that can be discriminated? To answer, we measured users' just-noticeable-difference (JND). (3) How does magnification affect the perceived magnitude of force and mechanical stiffness? To answer, we asked users to report subjective magnitudes over a range of physical values. The perceptual experiments were performed with the HHFM Model-1 connected to a Butterfly Haptics Maglev 200, a six-DoF haptic device capable of actuating forces as high as 40 N. In all experiments, participants were tested under three conditions: HHFM-on (active magnification of actuated forces), where the HHFM gain was set to $k = 2.4$, so the overall perceptual gain as determined from Equation 18.2 was 3.4; HHFM-off, in which participants wore the HHFM but magnification was

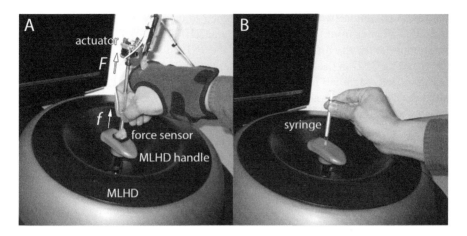

FIGURE 18.3 Experimental setup for perceptual psychophysics using the MLHD under (a) HHFM-on or HHFM-off and (b) control conditions. (Reproduced from Stetten, G. et al., *Lect. Not. Comp. Sci.,* 6689, 90–100, 2011. With permission.)

turned off; and control, where participants used a 1-mL syringe, which was identical to the handle of the HHFM Model-1, to contact the MLHD handle. Each experiment began with the tool resting on the handle, as shown in Figure 18.3.

18.4.3.1 Absolute Force Threshold

To measure the absolute force threshold (minimum detectable forces), the method of adjustment was utilized; participants used a keypad to increase or decrease the applied force until it "appeared" or "disappeared" (Jones and Tan 2013). The mean absolute threshold in the HHFM-on condition was 0.07 N, which was significantly lower than the 0.20 N threshold found in the HHFM-off condition and the 0.16 N threshold measured in the control condition without magnification, which did not differ, thus indicating no effect of wearing the device *per se*.

A measure of the perceptual gain (afferent or behavioral gain) was obtained by taking the ratio of the HHFM-off threshold to the HHFM-on threshold. It averaged 2.9, which was not significantly different from 3.4, the hypothesized gain as predicted by Equation 18.2. Hence, we verified that the perceptual pathway in our control framework (Figure 18.2b) behaves as proposed at near-threshold force levels.

18.4.3.2 JND

To measure the just noticeable difference (JND), we asked participants to compare a stimulus force against a reference force of 0.3 N. The study used an unforced adaptive procedure that targeted 75% correct detections (Kaernbach 2001). A fourth experimental condition, HHFM-off with a reference force of 1.02 N, was also tested. (This last testing condition is equivalent to the output of HHFM magnification at the 0.30 reference at an assumed perceptual magnification factor of 3.4.)

The mean JND for the 0.30 N reference force was significantly lower in the HHFM-on condition (11.04%) when compared to the HHFM-off (15.39%) and control (15.15%) conditions, which were statistically equivalent. The JND in the last

HHFM-off condition (with a 1.02 N reference force) was 9.58%, which was significantly different from the JND found in the HHFM-off condition at the 0.30 N force. Importantly, the difference between the JND in the HHFM-on condition at 0.30 N and the JND in the HHFM-off condition at 1.02 N was not significant. These data show that magnified forces are perceived by individuals as essentially equivalent to the corresponding non-magnified values and that *in situ* force magnification enhances a user's ability to detect small differences in force.

18.4.3.3 Subjective Estimation of Force and Stiffness

Force and stiffness in a medical context are valuable in identifying pathologic tissue, such as a malignant tumor or calcified tissue, or in differentiating between anatomical landmarks. We hypothesized that the ability to estimate both quantities would be aided by force magnification, but the effect on stiffness estimation may be reduced due to the additional uncertainty in estimating deformation (Wu et al. 2011). Two separate experiments measured the perceived magnitudes of force and stiffness.

The force study examined how participants subjectively experience tool tip force under magnification (Stetten et al. 2011). Each participant was presented with a randomly ordered series of force stimuli with magnitudes of 0.1, 0.2, 0.3, or 0.4 N. In the control condition, forces of 0.5, 1.0, and 1.5 N were also presented to produce similar stimuli to those in the HHFM-on condition, where distal forces were magnified by the magnification factor of 3.4. Participants were instructed to assign a numerical score to each stimulus based on its perceived intensity, with the only restriction being that subjectively stronger stimuli should be assigned higher numbers. The data were normalized by dividing each response by the participant's mean for a given condition, then multiplying by the overall mean for all participants (Stevens 1975).

Average magnitudes are presented in Figure 18.4. As expected, for the same distal stimuli, forces were judged to be subjectively more intense with the HHFM turned on (see Figure 18.4a). The average perceptual gain, obtained by taking the ratio

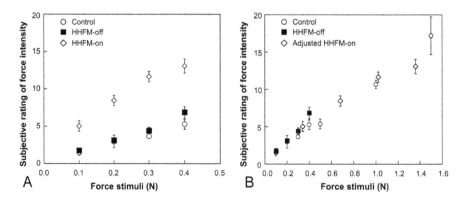

FIGURE 18.4 (a) Subjective estimation of force by stimulus strength. (b) Subjective ratings with HHFM-on condition rescaled by hypothesized perceptual gain of 3.4. Error bars represent ±1 SEM. (Reproduced from Stetten, G. et al., *Lect. Not. Comp. Sci.,* 6689, 90–100, 2011. With permission.)

of HHFM-on ratings to HHFM-off ratings, was 2.14 ± 0.18, which was somewhat lower than the expected gain of 3.4.

Multiplying the force stimuli by the hypothesized perceptual gain of 3.4 in the HHFM-on condition enables us to replot the magnitude data over the range of stimuli as they were actually perceived. This reorganization of data is shown in Figure 18.4b. Given the close overlap between the ratings obtained in the control condition and those from the rescaled HHFM-on condition, we can conclude that feedback forces generated by our device are perceived similarly to real forces of similar magnitude.

The second study of subjective magnitudes investigated how force magnification affects the perception of mechanical stiffness (Wu et al. 2015). Over a series of trials, virtual springs with stiffnesses of 20, 40, 60, and 80 N/m were rendered in the MLHD, and participants were allowed to freely interact with them. In addition, springs of stiffness 100 and 200 N/m were rendered in the control condition. Again, the only restriction placed on the numerical estimates was that subjectively stiffer springs should be assigned higher numbers. The data showed an average perceptual gain for the weakest (20 N/m) spring of 2.7, which was not statistically different from the hypothesized perceptual gain of 3.4. However, the perceptual gain declined with stiffness, setting a target for future iterations of the HHFM to expand the effective range of magnification.

18.4.4 Magnification Effects on Motor Control

The previous studies were concerned with the perceptual consequences of magnified forces. An additional experiment was conducted to assess how *in situ* force augmentation affects motor control, specifically, the generation of an isometric force (Lee et al. 2017). In modern surgery, controlling contact with a surface while applying minimal force is a critical skill, especially in applications such as electrocautery, or ablative surgery, where energy-delivering probes, rather than sharp blades, are used to dissect tissue (Neumyer and Ghalyaie 2017).

The HHFM Model-3 (see Figure 18.1) was utilized in this experiment, albeit with a somewhat shorter tip and a pronounced 90° hook with which users could connect to a small hole in the cylindrical target depicted in Figure 18.5.

Participants took part in a series of trials that required them to maintain contact while minimizing force. Three Light Emitting Diodes (LEDs) guided the participant to a maximum force, 15 g (147 mN), at which point the LEDs were extinguished. A subsequent six-second period without visual feedback was the critical part of the trial captured for analysis. Participants were instructed that, during this period, they should maintain contact with the target while applying as little force as possible. The task was tested in the push and pull directions, and under three magnification levels induced by the HHFM: $k = 0$, 2, and 4.

The data analysis focused on the last five seconds of the six-second task period to avoid perturbing effects of task onset. The analysis was further limited only to when the tool tip was actually in contact with the force sensor during that period. To detect contact, we applied a Welch's t-test to force measured during the 250 ms prior to the beginning of each trial (the control period) and that measured during each successive

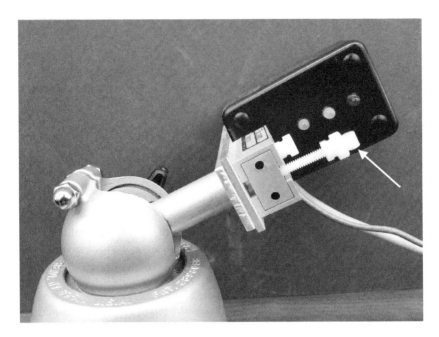

FIGURE 18.5 Apparatus for isometric force generation experiments. GS0-100 force sensor (A-Tech. Instruments) measures interaction force applied to cylindrical target (white arrow). LEDs provide visual feedback. (Reproduced from Lee, R. et al., *IEEE Trans. Hap.*, 2017. With permission.)

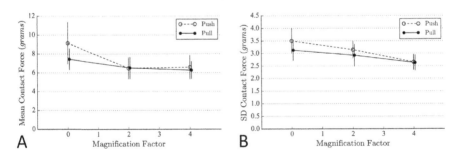

FIGURE 18.6 (a) Mean and (b) standard deviation of contact force during isometric force generation as a function of magnification factor and direction. Error bars represent ±1 SEM. (Reproduced from Lee, R. et al., *IEEE Trans. Hap.*, 2017. With permission.)

30-ms interval of the target task. Contact was signaled by a significant difference in force relative to the pretrial control. Figure 18.6 shows the means and standard deviation of the force applied during periods of contact as a function of magnification and direction. Magnification led to a decrease in both measures, independent of direction.

Power spectra on raw force data were calculated for three frequency bands: 1–4 Hz, 4–7 Hz, and 7–10 Hz. The first two bands are taken to assess voluntary control of action (Tan et al. 1994; Jones 2000) and involuntary motion in the form of tremor (Timmer et al. 1996; Safwat et al. 2009; MacLachlan et al. 2012), respectively.

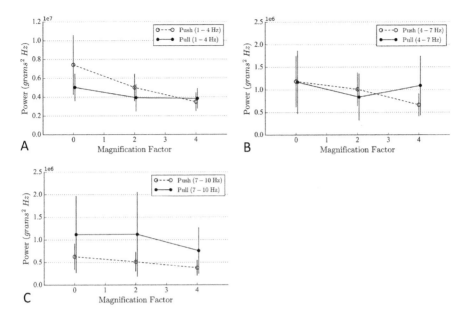

FIGURE 18.7 Power spectra of applied force in (a) 1–4 Hz, (b) 4–7 Hz, and (c) 7–10 Hz frequency bands. Error bars represent ±1 SEM. (Reproduced from Lee, R. et al., *IEEE Trans. Hap.*, 2017. With permission.)

The last band is taken to encompass the higher frequency components of tremor (Allum et al. 1978; Brown et al. 1982).

Figure 18.7 shows the power in each band as a function of magnification and direction. Although the mean power trends suggested that magnification tended to reduce power, the sole reliable effect was a significant interaction between magnification and direction in the second power band, 4–7 Hz, taken to primarily represent tremor. The effect is that power decreases with magnification for the push but not the pull direction.

As systemic effects of magnification were consistently observed across the mean, standard deviation, and power, a principal-components analysis was conducted on the *slope* of the magnification function for each of these variables, within each direction (push and pull). On the first component, nine of the ten variables showed loadings greater than 0.5, which accounted for 64.2% of the variance. The exception was the standard deviation of force in the pull direction, which loaded greater than 0.5 on a second factor. This second factor accounted for an additional 18.3% of variability and also showed greater than 0.5 loadings for the power in the first two frequency bands, exclusively for the pull direction. Note that there is a direct mathematical relationship between total power and standard deviation in a signal, as they both derive from the sums of squares of signal amplitude. The overall pattern for the second factor, then, suggests it is related to an effect of magnification on the variability in pulling. Movements of the wrist in the pull direction are known to involve more dexterity than pushing motions (Di Domizo and Keir 2010; Seo et al. 2010; Klatzky et al. 2013; Gershon et al. 2015).

18.5   DISCUSSION

Our research into the perceptual effects of *in situ* force magnification shows reductions in the absolute threshold (minimum detectable force) by a factor of $k + 1$ as predicted by Equation 18.2, as well as improved force discrimination. Subjective perception of force and stiffness also follow an approximate $k + 1$ factor increase though the effect is somewhat compressed at higher forces. Thus, the threshold and suprathreshold measures both point to effective magnification along the perceptual pathway, following the framework depicted in Figure 18.2b.

Examining motor control consequences of *in situ* force augmentation, we found that magnification minimizes and stabilizes the applied force. Preliminary data also show that tremor in the push direction may be reduced with *in situ* force feedback, due to the application of a counterforce. Magnification may also broadly stabilize pull forces. Additionally, given that these benefits were seen in naïve participants who were handling the HHFM for the first time, *in situ* force feedback seems to be readily transparent to the user, bolstering its potential usability.

Underlying our design effort is the recognition that the clinician plays a critical part in the human-machine loop when using AR tools. We respect this executive role by enforcing no external restrictions on the surgeon's behavior. Compared to other robotic tools that enforce global rules on applied force or tool velocity, we believe that an open-ended control scheme will better present a perceptually seamless and a more intuitive experience when using AR tools.

To implement this design philosophy requires extensive knowledge of how the user perceives force and the interplay between sensation and motor control such that a user's natural reactions are anticipated by our system and then corrected as necessary. This effort is worthwhile, however, because in the end, the surgeon is the ultimate judge of whether or not to incorporate a technology into their practice. The progress of medical intervention is, after all, an exercise in controlled chaos, and clinicians are reluctant to gamble away their hard-earned collective knowledge with the advent of each new technology. Perhaps a new set of surgical techniques are necessary before AR tools such as the HHFM are adopted in the surgical theater. These kinds of advances are only adopted when clinicians devote themselves to performing surgery with such tools. Therefore, it is prudent to design our tools such that their capabilities are adaptable far into the future, rather than set hard limits based on our current (and imperfect) knowledge. Psychophysical studies provide a valuable design input. Using these broad techniques, not only can we gain deeper insight into the perception of touch, but researchers and engineers can also better preserve the sensorimotor benefits due to augmentation as we move beyond the initial prototypes.

REFERENCES

Allum, J. H. J., V. Dietz, and H.-J. Freund. 1978. Neuronal mechanisms underlying physiological tremor. *Journal of Neurophysiology* 41 (3): 557–571.

Balicki, M., A. Uneri, I. Iordachita, J. Handa, P. Gehlbach, and R. Taylor. 2010. Micro-force sensing in robot assisted membrane peeling for vitreoretinal surgery. *Lecture Notes in Computer Science* 6363: 303–310. doi:10.1007/978-3-642-15711-0_38.

Berggren, U., T. Gordh, D. Grama, U. Haglund, J. Rastad, and D. Arvidsson. 1994. Laparoscopic versus open cholecystectomy: Hospitalization, sick leave, analgesia and trauma responses. *British Journal of Surgery* 81 (9): 1362–1365. doi:10.1002/bjs.1800810936.

Berkelman, P. J., and R. L. Hollis. 1997. Dynamic performance of a magnetic levitation haptic device. *Proceedings of SPIE Telemanipulation and Telepresence IV* 3206. doi:10.1117/12.295578.

Berkelman, P. J., and R. L. Hollis. 2000. Lorentz magnetic levitation for haptic interaction: Device design, function, and integration with simulated environments. *International Journal of Robotics Research* 19 (7): 644–667. doi:10.1177/027836490001900703.

Bohan, M., D. S. McConnell, A. Chaparro, and S. G. Thompson. 2010. The effects of visual magnification and physical movement scale on the manipulation of a tool with indirect vision. *Journal of Experimental Psychology: Applied* 16 (1): 33–44. doi:10.1037/a0018501.

Boni, L., A. Benevento, F. Rovera, G. Dionigi, M. D. L. Giuseppe, C. Bertoglio, and R. Dionigi. 2006. Infective complications in laparoscopic surgery. *Surgical Infections* 7 (S2): S109–S112. doi:10.1089/sur.2006.7.s2-109.

Brown, J. D., M. Ibrahim, E. D. Z. Chase, C. Pacchierotti, and K. J. Kuchenbecker. 2016. Data-driven comparison of four cutaneous displays for pinching palpation in robotic surgery. In *Proceedings of the 2016 IEEE Haptics Symposium*, edited by S. Choi, K. J. Kuchenbecker, and G. Gerling (Piscataway, NJ: IEEE), pp. 147–154. doi:10.1109/HAPTICS.2016.7463169.

Brown, T. I. H., P. M. H. Rack, and H. F. Ross. 1982. Different types of tremor in the human thumb. *Journal of Physiology* 332: 113–123.

Chinello, F., M. Malvezzi, C. Pacchierotti, and D. Prattichizzo. 2012. A three DoFs wearable tactile display for exploration and manipulation of virtual objects. In *Proceedings of the 2012 IEEE Haptics Symposium*, edited by K. MacLean and M. K. O'Malley (Piscataway, NJ: IEEE), pp. 71–76. doi:10.1109/HAPTIC.2012.6183772.

Culjat, M. O., C. King, M. L. Franco, C. E. Lewis, J. W. Bisley, E. P. Dutson, and W. S. Grundfest. 2008. A tactile feedback system for robotic surgery. In *Proceedings of the 30th Annual International Conference of the IEEE Engineering in Medicine and Biology Society* (Piscataway, NJ: IEEE), pp. 1930–1934. doi:10.1109/IEMBS.2008.4649565.

Culjat, M. O., J. W. Bisley, C.-H. King, C. Wottawa, R. E. Fan, E. P. Dutson, and W. S. Grundfest. 2011. Tactile feedback in surgical robotics. In *Surgical Robotics: Systems Applications and Visions*, edited by J. Rosen, B. Hannaford, and R. M. Satava (Boston, MA: Springer), pp. 449–468. doi:10.1007/978-1-4419-1126-1_19.

Di Domizio, J., and P. J. Keir. 2010. Forearm posture and grip effects during push and pull tasks. *Ergonomics* 53 (3): 336–343.

Diolaiti, N., G. Niemeyer, F. Barbagli, and J. K. Salisbury. 2006. Stability of haptic rendering: Discretization, quantization, time delay, and coulomb effects. *IEEE Transactions on Robotics* 22 (2): 256–268.

Fleming, I., M. Balicki, J. Koo, I. Iordachita, B. Mitchell, J. Handa, G. Hager, and R. Taylor. 2008. Cooperative robot assistant for retinal microsurgery. *Lecture Notes in Computer Science* 5242: 543–550. doi:10.1007/978-3-540-85990-1_65.

Gershon, P., R. L. Klatzky, and R. Lee. 2015. Handedness in a virtual haptic environment: Assessments from kinematic behavior and modeling. *Acta Psychologica* 155: 37–42. doi:10.1016/j.actpsy.2014.11.014.

Griffin, J. A., W. Zhu, and C. S. Nam. 2017. The role of haptic feedback in robotic-assisted retinal microsurgery systems: A systematic review. *IEEE Transactions on Haptics* 10 (1): 94–105. doi:10.1109/TOH.2016.2598341.

Gupta, P. K., P. S. Jensen, and E. de Juan Jr. 1999. Surgical forces and tactile perception during retinal microsurgery. *Lecture Notes in Computer Science* 1679: 1218–1225. doi:10.1007/10704282_132.

Hamed, A., S. C. Tang, H. Ren, A. Squires, C. Payne, K. Masamune, G. Tang, J. Mohammadpour, and Z. T. H. Tse. 2012. Advances in haptics, tactile sensing, and manipulation for minimally invasive surgery, noninvasive surgery, and diagnosis. *Journal of Robotics.* doi:10.1155/2012/412816.

Jagtap, A. D., and C. N. Riviere. 2004. Applied force during vitreoretinal microsurgery with handheld instruments. In *Proceedings of the 26th International Conference of the IEEE Engineering in Medicine and Biology Society* (Piscataway, NJ: IEEE, 2004), pp. 2771–2773. doi:10.1109/IEMBS.2004.1403792.

Jones, L. A. 2000. Kinesthetic sensing. In *Human and Machine Haptics*, edited by M. R. Cutkosky, R. D. Howe, K. Salisbury, and M. A. Srinivasan (Cambridge, MA: MIT Press).

Jones, L. A., and H. Z. Tan. 2013. Application of psychophysical techniques to haptic research. *IEEE Transactions on Haptics* 6 (3): 268–284. doi:10.1109/TOH.2012.74.

Jonsson, B., and N. Zethraeus. 2000. Costs and benefits of laparoscopic surgery—A review of the literature. *European Journal of Surgery* 166 (S585): 48–56.

Kaernbach, C. 2001. Adaptive threshold estimation with unforced-choice tasks. *Perception and Psychophysics* 63 (8): 1377–1388. doi:10.3758/BF03194549.

King, C.-H., M. O. Culjat, M. L. Franco, C. E. Lewis, E. P. Dutson, W. S. Grundfest, and J. W. Bisley. 2009. Tactile feedback induces reduced grasping force in robot-assisted surgery. *IEEE Transactions on Haptics* 2 (2): 103–110. doi:10.1109/ToH.2009.4.

King, C.-H., M. O. Culjat, M. L. Franco, J. W. Bisley, E. Dutson, and W. S. Grundfest. 2008. Optimization of a pneumatic balloon tactile display for robot-assisted surgery based on human perception. *IEEE Transactions on Biomedical Engineering* 55 (11): 2593–2600. doi:10.1109/TBME.2008.2001137.

Klatzky, R. L., P. Gershon, V. Shivaprabhu, R. Lee, B. Wu, G. Stetten, and R. H. Swendsen. 2013. A model of motor performance during surface penetration: From physics to voluntary control. *Experimental Brain Research* 230 (2): 251–260. doi:10.1007/s00221-013-3648-4.

Lee, R., B. Wu, R. L. Klatzky, V. Shivaprabhu, J. Galeotti, S. Horvath, M. Siegel, J. S. Schuman, R. Hollis, and G. Stetten. 2013. Hand-held force magnifier for surgical instruments: Evolution toward a clinical device. *Lecture Notes in Computer Science* 7815: 77–89. doi:10.1007/978-3-642-38085-3_9.

Lee, R., R. L. Klatzky, and G. D. Stetten. 2017. *In-situ* force augmentation improves surface contact and force control. *IEEE Transactions on Haptics.* doi:10.1109/TOH.2017.2696949.

Loomis, J. M. 1992. Distal attribution and presence. *Presence: Teleoperators and Virtual Environments* 1 (1): 113–119. doi:10.1162/pres.1992.1.1.113.

MacLachlan, R. A., B. C. Becker, J. Cuevas Tabares, G. W. Podnar, L. A. Lobes Jr., and C. N. Riviere. 2012. Micron: An actively stabilized handheld tool for microsurgery. *IEEE Transactions on Robotics* 28 (1): 195–212.

Maisto, M., C. Pacchierotti, F. Chinello, G. Salvietti, A. De Luca, D. Prattichizzo. 2017. Evaluation of wearable haptic systems for the fingers in augmented reality applications. *IEEE Transactions on Haptics.* doi:10.1109/TOH.2017.2691328.

Mitchell, B., J. Koo, I. Iordachita, P. Kazanzides, A. Kapoor, J. Handa, G. Hager, and R. Taylor. 2007. Development and application of a new steady-hand manipulator for retinal surgery. In *Proceedings of the 2007 IEEE International Conference on Robotics and Automation* (Piscataway, NJ: IEEE), pp. 623–629. doi:10.1109/ROBOT.2007.363056.

Murray, A. M., R. L. Klatzky, and P. K. Khosla. 2003. Psychophysical characterization and testbed validation of a wearable vibrotactile glove for telemanipulation. *Presence* 12 (2): 156–182. doi:10.1162/105474603321640923.

Musmann, H. G. 2006. Genesis of the MP3 audio coding standard. *IEEE Transactions on Consumer Electronics* 52 (3): 1043–1049. doi:10.1109/TCE.2006.1706505.

Neumyer, L., and N. Ghalyaie. 2017. Principles of preoperative and operative surgery. In *Sabiston Textbook of Surgery: The Biological Basis of Modern Surgical Practice,*

20th ed., edited by C. M. Townsend, R. D. Beauchamp, B. M. Evers, and K. L. Mattox (Philadelphia, PA: Elsevier), pp. 201–240.

Okamura, A. M., L. N. Verner, T. Yamamoto, J. C. Gwilliam, and P. G. Griffiths. 2011. Force feedback and sensory substitution for robot-assisted surgery. In *Surgical Robotics: Systems Applications and Visions*, edited by J. Rosen, B. Hannaford, and R. M. Satava (Boston, MA: Springer), pp. 419–448. doi:10.1007/978-1-4419-1126-1_18.

Patkin, M. 1977. Ergonomics applied to the practice of microsurgery. *Australian and New Zealand Journal of Surgery* 47 (3): 320–329. doi:10.1111/j.1445-2197.1977. tb04297.x.

Payne C. J., H. J. Marcus, and G.-Z. Yang. 2015. A smart haptic hand-held device for neurosurgical microdissection. *Annals of Biomedical Engineering* 43 (9): 2185–2195. doi:10.1007/s10439-015-1258-y.

Payne, C. J., and G.-Z. Yang. 2014. Hand-held medical robots. *Annals of Biomedical Engineering* 42 (8): 1594–1605. doi:10.1007/s10439-014-1042-4.

Payne, C. J., K.-W. Kwok, and G.-Z. Yang. 2013. An ungrounded hand-held surgical device incorporating active constraints with force-feedback. In *Proceedings of the 2013 IEEE/ RSK International Conference on Intelligent Robots and Systems*, edited by N. Amato (Piscataway, NJ: IEEE), pp. 2559–2565. doi:10.1109/IROS.2013.6696717.

Payne, C. J., W. T. Latt, and G.-Z. Yang. 2012. A new hand-held force amplifying device for micromanipulation. In *Proceedings of the 2012 IEEE International Conference on Robotics and Automation* (Piscataway, NJ: IEEE), pp. 1583–1588. doi:10.1109/ ICRA.2012.6225306.

Safwat, B., E. L. M. Su, R. Gassert, C. L. Teo, and E. Burdet. 2009. The role of posture, magnification, and grip force on microscopic accuracy. *Annals of Biomedical Engineering* 37 (5): 997–1006. doi:10.1007/s10439-009-9664-7.

Salisbury, K., F. Conti, and F. Barbagli. 2004. Haptic rendering: Introductory concepts. *IEEE Computer Graphics and Applications* 24 (2): 24–32. doi:10.1109/MCG.2004.1274058.

Seo, N. J., T. J. Armstrong, and J. G. Young. 2010. Effects of handle orientation, gloves, handle friction and elbow posture on maximum horizontal pull and push forces. *Ergonomics* 53 (1): 92–101.

Siegle, J. H., and W. H. Warren. 2010. Distal attribution and distance perception in sensory substitution. *Perception* 39 (2): 208–223. doi:10.1068/p6366.

Solazzi, M., A. Frisoli, and M. Bergamasco. 2010. Design of a novel finger haptic interface for contact and orientation display. In *Proceedings of the 2010 IEEE Haptics Symposium* (Piscataway, NJ: IEEE), pp. 129–132. doi:10.1109/HAPTIC.2010.5444667.

Stetten, G. 2015. Portable haptic force magnifier. U.S. Patent no. 8,981,914, filed September 27, 2011, awarded March 17, 2015.

Stetten, G., B. Wu, R. L. Klatzky, J. Galeotti, M. Siegel, R. Lee, F. Mah, A. Eller, J. Schuman, and R. Hollis. 2011. Hand-held force magnifier for surgical instruments. *Lecture Notes in Computer Science* 6689: 90–100. doi:10.1007/978-3-642-21504-9_9.

Stevens, S. S. 1975. *Psychophysics: Introduction to its Perceptual, Neural, and Social Prospects* (New York: John Wiley).

Tan, H. Z., M. A. Srinivasan, B. Eberman, and B. Cheng. 1994. Human factors for the design of force-reflecting haptic interfaces. In *Dynamic Systems and Control*, vol. 55–61, edited by C. J. Radcliffe (New York: ASME).

Taylor, R., P. Jensen, L. Whitcomb, A. Barnes, R. Kumar, D. Stoianovici, P. Gupta, Z. Wang, E. de Juan, and L. Kavoussi. 1999. A steady-hand robotic system for microsurgical augmentation. *International Journal of Robotics Research* 18 (12): 1201–1210. doi:10.1177/02783649922067807.

Timmer, J., M. Lauk, and G. Deuschl. 1996. Quantitative analysis of tremor time series. *Electroencephalography and Clinical Neurophysiology* 101: 461–468. doi:10.1016/0924-980X(96)94658-5.

Tsai, T.-M., J. M. Breyer, and J. B. Panattoni. 2013. History of microsurgery: Curiosities from the sixties and seventies. *Microsurgery* 33 (2): 85–89. doi:10.1002/micr.22066.

Uneri, A., M. A. Balicki, J. Handa, P. Gehlbach, R. H. Taylor, and I. Iordachita. 2010. New steady-hand eye robot with micro-force sensing for vitreoretinal surgery. In *Proceedings of the 3rd IEEE RAS and EMBS International Conference on Biomedical Robotics and Biomechatronics* (Piscataway, NJ: IEEE), pp. 814–819. doi:10.1109/BIOROB.2010.5625991.

van der Meijden, O. A. J., and M. P. Schijven. 2009. The value of haptic feedback in conventional and robot-assisted minimal invasive surgery and virtual reality training: A current review. *Surgical Endoscopy* 23 (6): 1180–1190. doi:10.1007/s00464-008-0298-x.

Vasilakos, K., L. Glass, and A. Beuter. 1998. Interaction of tremor and magnification in a motor performance task with visual feedback. *Journal of Motor Behavior* 30 (2): 158–168. doi:10.1080/00222899809601333.

Westebring-van der Putten, E. P., J. J. van den Dobbelsteen, R. H. M. Goossens, J. J. Jakimowicz, and J. Dankelman. 2009a. Force feedback requirements for efficient laparoscopic grasp control. *Ergonomics* 52 (9): 1055–1066. doi:10.1080/00140130902912803.

Westebring-van der Putten, E. P., J. J. van den Dobbelsteen, R. H. M. Goossens, J. J. Jakimowicz, and J. Dankelman. 2009b. Effect of laparoscopic grasper force transmission ratio on grasp control. *Surgical Endoscopy* 23 (4): 818–824. doi:10.1007/s00464-008-0107-6.

Westebring-van der Putten, E. P., J. J. van den Dobbelsteen, R. H. M. Goossens, J. J. Jakimowicz, and J. Dankelman. 2010. The effect of augmented feedback on grasp force in laparoscopic grasp control. *IEEE Transactions on Haptics* 3 (4): 280–291. doi:10.1109/ToH.2010.23.

Wottawa, C. R., J. R. Cohen, R. E. Fan, J. W. Bisley, M. O. Culjat, W. S. Grundfest, and E. P. Dutson. 2013. The role of tactile feedback in grip force during laparoscopic training tasks. *Surgical Endoscopy* 72: 1111–1118. doi:10.1007/s00464-012-2612-x.

Wu, B., R. Klatzky, R. Lee, V. Shivaprabhu, J. Galeotti, M. Siegel, J. S. Schuman, R. Hollis, and G. Stetten. 2015. Psychophysical evaluation of haptic perception under augmentation by a handheld device. *Human Factors* 57 (3): 523–537. doi:10.1177/0018720814551414.

Wu, B., R. L. Klatzky, and R. L. Hollis. 2011. Force, torque, and stiffness: Interactions in perceptual discrimination. *IEEE Transactions on Haptics* 4 (3): 221–228. doi:10.1109/TOH.2011.3.

Yap, L. H., and C. E. Butler. 2007. Principles of microsurgery. In *Grabb and Smith's Plastic Surgery*, 6th ed., edited by C. H. Thorne (Philadelphia, PA: Lippincott Williams & Wilkins), pp. 66–72.

Index

Note: Page numbers in *italic* and **bold** refer to figures and tables respectively.

Printed and bound by CPI Group (UK) Ltd, Croydon, CR0 4YY

24/10/2024

01778304-0005